Oxford Case Histories

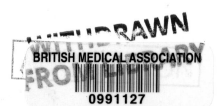

Oxford Case Histories

Series Editors

Sarah Pendlebury and Peter Rothwell

Published:

Neurological Case Histories (Sarah Pendlebury, Philip Anslow, and
Peter Rothwell)

Oxford Case Histories in Cardiology (Rajkumar Rajendram, Javed Ehtisham,
and Colin Forfar)

Oxford Case Histories in Gastroenterology and Hepatology (Alissa Walsh,
Otto Buchel, Jane Collier, and Simon Travis)

Forthcoming:

Oxford Case Histories in Nephrology (Chris Pugh, Chris O'Callaghan,
Aron Chakera, Richard Cornall, and David Mole)

Oxford Case Histories in Respiratory Medicine (John Stradling, Andrew
Stanton, Anabell Nickol, Helen Davies, and Najib Rahman)

Oxford Case Histories in Rheumatology (Joel David, Anne Miller, Anushka
Soni, and Lyn Williamson)

Oxford Case Histories in Stroke and TIA (Sarah Pendlebury, Ursula Schulz,
Aneil Malhotra, and Peter Rothwell)

Oxford Case Histories in Cardiology

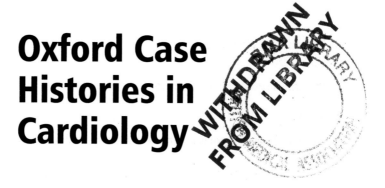

Dr Rajkumar Rajendram

Specialist Registrar
General Medicine and Intensive Care
John Radcliffe Hospital
Oxford, UK

Dr Javed Ehtisham

Cardiology Specialist Registrar
John Radcliffe Hospital
Oxford, UK

Professor Colin Forfar

Consultant Cardiologist and Senior Lecturer in Medicine
John Radcliffe Hospital and Oxford University
Oxford, UK

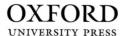

OXFORD
UNIVERSITY PRESS

OXFORD

UNIVERSITY PRESS

Great Clarendon Street, Oxford OX2 6DP

Oxford University Press is a department of the University of Oxford.
It furthers the University's objective of excellence in research, scholarship,
and education by publishing worldwide in

Oxford New York

Auckland Cape Town Dar es Salaam Hong Kong Karachi
Kuala Lumpur Madrid Melbourne Mexico City Nairobi
New Delhi Shanghai Taipei Toronto

With offices in

Argentina Austria Brazil Chile Czech Republic France Greece
Guatemala Hungary Italy Japan Poland Portugal Singapore
South Korea Switzerland Thailand Turkey Ukraine Vietnam

Oxford is a registered trade mark of Oxford University Press
in the UK and in certain other countries

Published in the United States
by Oxford University Press Inc., New York

British Library Cataloguing in Publication Data
Data available

Library of Congress Cataloging in Publication Data
Data available

Typeset in Minion by Glyph International Bangalore, India
Printed in Great Britain
on acid-free paper by
Ashford Colour Press Ltd., Gosport, Hampshire

ISBN 978–0–19–955678–6

10 9 8 7 6 5 4 3 2 1

Oxford University Press makes no representation, express or implied, that the drug
dosages in this book are correct. Readers must therefore always check the product
information and clinical procedures with the most up-to-date published product
information and data sheets provided by the manufacturers and the most recent codes of
conduct and safety regulations. The authors and the publishers do not accept responsibility
or legal liability for any errors in the text or for the misuse or misapplication of material in
this work. Except where otherwise stated, drug dosages and recommendations are for the
non-pregnant adult who is not breastfeeding.

Preface

Post-graduate medicine is evolving. The core curriculum developed for all medical specialties is a competence-based document dictating the knowledge, skills and attitudes which a trainee should obtain before a certificate of completion of training (CCT) can be awarded. Mandatory knowledge and performance-based assessments are being conducted in order to ensure these standards are met. Although 'student-centred learning' is encouraged in order to develop mastery of the core curriculum, there are few books available to direct higher trainees preparing for these examinations.

We firmly believe that the use of clinical material is one of the best methods of learning and teaching medicine. This is just as true for experienced consultants as for first year clinical medical students. However, although many collections of cases are available for medical students and as preparation for the MRCP(UK), there are few that challenge the experienced clinician or trainee specialist. It is for this reason that the cases are not only challenging, but also, we hope, entertaining and informative.

The general medical council is now issuing licences to practice and re-validation will soon be a requirement. We envisage that use of advanced clinical texts such as this could be included in a portfolio of continuing medical education that could be used to support a process of specialist re-validation.

The book consists of 50 case presentations each describing the clinical history and progress of a patient. Each case includes a set of questions to which we have given detailed evidence-based answers. Where evidence is unclear and clinical judgement is required we have expressed our opinion.

The selection of cases covers the breadth of cardiology including acute emergencies requiring rapid diagnosis and treatment and chronic diseases which require thoughtful management.

The major topics of the cardiology core curriculum are covered but it is not the aim of this book to give the answers to all cardiological questions. Rather the Socratic method of questions and answers is intended to guide towards deeper thought about clinical issues.

The questions and answers format also ensures that this book will be suitable for those preparing for specialist examinations in acute medicine and cardiology. However, perhaps more importantly, this book bridges the gap between the acute physician and the cardiologist through the discussion of cases from their initial acute presentation to the on-take team through to the management initiated by cardiologists in a tertiary centre.

We would like to thank the many colleagues who contributed cases and illustrations and made helpful comments on the manuscript, in particular Dr Jim Newton for providing several echocardiographic images. We also thank our families for their support whilst we worked late evenings, early mornings, and weekends!

Contents

Abbreviations

2D	2-dimensional	aVR	Augmented vector right
AAA	Abdominal aortic aneurysm	AVR	Aortic valve replacement
A-a pO2	Arterial–alveolar oxygen	AVID	Antiarrhythmas vs implantable defibrillators trial
ABG	Arterial blood gas		
ACC/AHA	American College of Cardiology/American Heart Association	aVL	Augmented vector left
		AVN	Atrioventricular node
		BMW	Balanced middle weight
ACE	Angiotensin-converting enzyme	BP	Blood pressure
		BPEG	British Pacing and Electrophysiology Group
ACS	Acute coronary syndrome		
ADP	Adenosine diphosphate	bpm	Beats per minute
AF	Atrial fibrillation	BSA	Body surface area
AIDS	Acquired immuno deficiency syndrome	CABG	Coronary artery bypass graft
AL	Amyloid light chain	CAD	Coronary artery disease
ALCAPA	Anomalous left coronary artery arising from the pulmonary artery	CASH	The Cardiac Arrest Study Hamburg
		CCB	Calcium channel blockade
ALP	Alkaline phosphatase	CCU	Coronary care unit
ALT	Alkaline transaminase	CEA	Carcinoembryonic antigen
AP	Anterior–posterior	CFA	Common femoral artery
APTT	Activated partial thromboplastin times	CHB	Complete heart block
		CI	Confidence interval
ARB	Angiotensin receptor blocker	CIDS	Canadian Implantable Defibrillator Study
ARDS	Acute respiratory distress syndrome		
		CIN	Contrast-induced nephropathy
ARF	Acute renal failure	CK	Creatine kinase
ARVC	Arrhythmogenic right ventricular cardiomyopathy	CKD	Chronic kidney disease
		CK-MB	Creatine Kinase-muscle and bone isoform
ARVD	Arrhythmogenic right ventricular dysplasia		
		CLOSURE 1	A prospective, multicenter, randomized controlled trial to assess the safety and efficacy of the STARFlex® septal closure device against medical therapy after a stroke and/or transient ischemic attack due to presumed paradoxical emboslism through a patent foramen ovale.
AS	Aortic stenosis		
ASD	Atrial septal defect		
AST	Aspartate transaminase		
AT	Anaerobic threshold		
ATN	Acute tubular necrosis		
ATP	Adenosine triphosphatase		
AV	Aortic valve		
aVF	Augmented vector foot		

CMRI	Cardiovascular magnetic resonance imaging
CMT	Circus movement tachycardia
CMR	Cardiac magnetic resonance
CNS	Central nervous system
CO	Cardiac output
COPD	Chronic obstructive pulmonary disease
COPE	COlchicine for acute PEricarditis
CPAP	Continuous positive airways pressure
CPEX	Cardiopulmonary exercise
CPVT	Catecholaminergic polymorphic ventricular tachycardia
CRP	C-reactive protein
CPR	Cardiopulmonary resuscitation
CRT	Cardiac resynchronization therapy
CSF	Cerebrospinal fluid
CT	Computerise tomography
CTEPH	Chronic thromboembolic pulmonary hypertension
cTnI	Cardiac troponin I
cTnT	Cardiac troponin T
CTPA	Computed tomographic pulmonary angiography
CURE	Clopidogrel in Unstable Angina to precent Recurrent Events
CVA	Cerebrovascular accident
CXR	Chest X-ray
DBP	Diastolic blood pressure
DC	Direct current
DCM	Dilated cardiomyopathy
DDDR	Dual-chamber rate-responsive
DIC	Disseminated intravascular coagulopathy
DIGAMI	Diabetes Mellitus, insulin Glucose infusion in Acute myocardial infarction
DVLA	Driver and Vehicle Licensing Agency
DVT	Deep vein thrombosis
ECG	Electrocardiograph

ED	Emergency department
EDD	Estimated delivery date
EEG	Electroencephalography
EF	Ejection fraction
eGFR	Estimated glomerular filtration rate
ELISA	Enzyme-linked immuno sorbent assays
ELISPOT	Enzyme-linked immunospot
EMD	Electromechanical dissociation
ENT	Ear, nose, and throat
ESC	European Society of Cardiology
ESD	End systolic diameter
ESR	Erythrocyte sedimentation rate
ET	Endotracheal
ETT	Exercise tolerance test
EuroSCORE	European System for Cardiac Operative Risk Evaluation
FBN-1	Fibrillin-1 gene
FFP	Fresh frozen plasma
GCS	Glasgow coma score
GFR	Glomerular filtration rate
GGT	Gamma-glutamyl transferase
GI	Gastrointestinal
GISSI	Gruppo Italiano per l0 studio della Streptochinasi nell' infarto miocardico (Itallian Group for the study of the survival of myocardial infraction)
GP	General practitioner
GTN	Glyceryl trinitrate
GUSTO	Global utilization of streptokinase and tissue plasminogen activator for occluded coronary arteries
HACEK	Group of slow growing gram negative organisms
Hb	Haemoglobin
HCM	Hypertrophic cardiomyopathy
HDL	High density lipoproten
H&E	Haematoxylin and eosin
HERG	Human Ether-à-go-ge Related Gene
HGV	Heavy goods vehicle

HIV	Human immunodeficiency virus	LVOT	Left ventricular outflow tract
HR	Heart rate	MAP	Mean arterial pressure
IABP	Intra-aortic balloon pump	MCV	Mean cell volume
IAS	Interatrial septum	MDR	Multidrug-resistant
ICD	Implantable cardioverter defibrillator	MDRD	Modification of diet in renal disease study
IFN	Interferon	MET	Metabolic equivalent of task
IgG	Immunoglobulin G	MFS-2	Marfan's syndrome type 2
IgM	Immunoglobulin M	MI	Myocardial infarction
IHD	Ischaemic heart disease	MR	Mitral regurgitation
INR	International normalised ratio	MRI	Magnetic resonance imaging
IPAH	Idiopathic PAH	MV	Mitral valve
IPPV	Intermittent positive pressure ventilation	MVR	Mechanical mitral valve replacement
ITU	Intensive care unit	NAC	N-acetylcysteine
iv	Intravenous	NASPE	North American Society of Pacing and Electrophysiology
IVC	Inferior vena cava		
IVS	Interventricular septum	NKDA	No known drug allergies
IVUS	Intravascular ultrasound	NICE	National Institute for Health and Clinical Excellence
JVP	Jugular venous pressure		
KCNH2	Gene encoding potassium channel	NR	Normal ranage
		NSAIDS	Non-steroidal anti-inflammatory drugs
KDOQI	Kidney Disease Outcomes & Quality Initiative	NSTE-ACS	Non-ST elevation acute coronary syndrome
LA	Left atrium	NSTEMI	Non-ST elevation myocardial infarction
LAD	Left anterior descending		
LAO	Left-anterior-oblique	NSVT	Non-sustained ventricular tachycardia
LBBB	Left bundle branch block		
LDH	Lactate dehydrogenase	NYHA	New York Heart Association
LDL	Low density lipoprotein	OASIS	Organization to assess strategies in ischemic syndromes
LM	Left main coronary artery		
LMWH	Low-molecular-weight heparin		
LQTS	Long QT syndrome	od	Once daily
LR	Likelihood ratio	OGD	Oesophagogastroduodensocopy
LV	Left ventricular	OM1	First obtuse marginal
LVAD	Left ventricular assist devices	OR	Odds ratio
LVEDP	Left ventircular end diastotic pressure	PA	Posteroanterior
		PA	Pulmonary artery
LVEF	Left ventricular ejection fraction	PAC	Preoperative assessment clinic
		PAH	Pulmonary artery hypertension
LVF	Left ventricular ejection fraction	PAP	Pulmonary artery pressure
		PAR	Pulmonary arterial resistance
LVH	Left ventricular hypertrophy	PCI	Percutaneous coronary intervention

PCM	Peripartum cardiomyopathy	RV	Right ventricular
PCR	Polymerase chain reaction	RVH	
PE	Pulmonary embolism	RVOT	Right ventricular outflow tract
PEEP	Positive end expiratory pressure	RVSP	Right ventricular systolic pressure
PFO	Patent foramen ovale	SAM	Systolic anterior motion
PH	Pulmonary hypertension	SAP	Serum amyloid P-component
PLE	Protein-losing enteropathy	SBP	Spontaneous bacterial peritonitis
PLV	Posterior left ventricular		
po	Per os (oral)	SCD	Sudden cardiac death
POISE	Perioperative Ischemic Evaluation	SCD-HeFT	Sudden cardiac death in heart failure trial
PRKAR1a	Cyclic adenosine monophosphate-dependent protein kinase A	SEC	Spontaneous echo contrast
		SHOCK	SHould we emergently revascularize Occluded Coronaries for cardiogenic shock
PPM	Permanent pacemaker		
PR	Pulmonary regurgitation		
PS	Pressure support	SLE	Systemic lupus erythematosus
PVL	Paravalvular leak	SPECT	Single photon emission computed tomography
PVR	Pulmonary vascular resistance		
PVT	Prosthetic valve thrombosis	SpO2	Oxygen saturation
PW	Pulsed wave	STEMI	ST elevation myocardial infarction
qds	Four times a day		
RA	Right atrium	SVC	Superior vena cava
RALES	Randomized aldactone evaluation study	SVR	Systemic vascular resistance
		SVT	Supraventricular tachyarrhythmia
RAO	Right-anterior-oblique		
RAP	Right atrial pressure	TB	Tuberculosis
RBBB	Right bundle branch block	TCPC	Total cavopulmonary connection
RBC	Red blood cell		
RCA	Right coronary artery	TGF	Transforming growth factor
RCRI	Revised cardiac risk index	THR	Total hip replacement
RCT	Randomized controlled trials	TIA	Transient ischaemic attack
RESPECT	Randomized evaluation of recurrent stroke comparing PFO closure to established current standard of care	TIMI	Thrombolysis in myocardial infarction
		TOE	Transoesophageal echocardiography
		TOF	Tetralogy of Fallot
RIFLE	Risk, injury, failure, loss, endstage renal disease (ESRD)	TR	Tricuspid regurgitation
		TT	Thrombin time
RLN	Recurrent laryngeal nerve	TTE	Trans-thoracic echocardiogram?
RR	Respiratory rate		
RRT	Renal replacement therapy	UA	Unstable angina
rtPA	Recombinant tissue plasminogen activator	UFH	Unfractionated heparin
		VA	Ventriculoatrial

VF	Ventricular fibrillation	VTE	Venous thrombo-embolism
VLDL	Very low density lipoprotein	VVI	Single-chamber ventricular demand
VP	Ventriculo-peritoneal		
V/Q	Ventilation/perfusion	WBC	White blood cell
VSD	Venticular septal defect	WCC	White cell count
VT	Ventricular tachycardia	WPW	Wolff–Parkinson–White

Case 1

A 79-year-old man with type II diabetes mellitus, New York Heart Association (NYHA) class II–III heart failure, and a permanent pacemaker (PPM) presented to the emergency department (ED) with a 3-week history of increasing shortness of breath. His exercise tolerance had reduced and he also reported orthopnoea and paroxysmal nocturnal dyspnoea. He denied chest pain, palpitations, or loss of consciousness. The PPM had been implanted for complete heart block 7 years prior to this presentation.

Examination revealed a regular tachycardia (120 beats per minute (bpm)), blood pressure (BP) 102/68 mmHg and a jugular venous pressure (JVP) that was visible at his ear lobes sitting upright. On auscultation, a pansystolic murmur was audible and coarse crackles consistent with pulmonary oedema were present in the mid and lower zones bilaterally.

The admission electrocardiograph (ECG) is shown in Fig. 1.1. The cardiology registrar was asked to review the patient. Immediately after initiation of the appropriate treatment the heart rate slowed and the patient's breathlessness began to improve. The ECG was then repeated (Fig. 1.2). Echocardiography demonstrated moderate to severe impairment of left ventricular (LV) function and an estimated left ventricular ejection fraction (LVEF) of 30%.

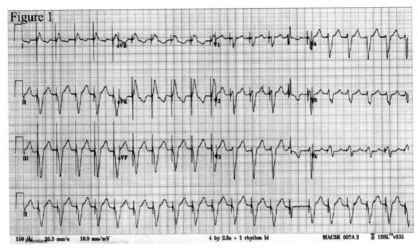

Fig. 1.1 ECG on admission.

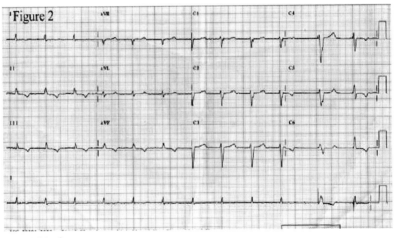

Fig. 1.2 ECG after treatment.

Questions

1. Report the admission ECG shown in Fig. 1.1.
2. Report the repeat ECG shown in Fig. 1.2.
3. If the patient did not know the type of pacemaker that was implanted or the manufacturer how could this information be obtained?
4. What was the cardiology registrar asked to do? What intervention was made?
5. What is the effect of placing a magnet over a PPM? Is the response different with an implantable cardioverter defibrillator (ICD)?
6. How should the patient's current arrhythmia be treated?
7. What are the chances of improvement in cardiac function?

Answers

1) **Report the admission ECG shown in Fig. 1.1.**

   Figure 1.1 shows a broad complex tachycardia at a rate of 120 bpm with left axis deviation. The pacing potential before each QRS complex suggests that this is a paced tachycardia. The left bundle branch block (LBBB) pattern demonstrates that the patient is being paced from the right ventricle. Atrial pacing potentials are not seen. The fast ventricular response suggests an atrial wire is present with inappropriate sensing and ventricular response.

   There is a narrow complex fusion beat at the 14th paced complex on the rhythm strip. This is conducted along the normal activation pathway. However, it is followed by an inverted T wave. T-wave changes can be classified as primary or secondary. Primary T-wave changes are caused by changes in the shape of the action potential and may be due to ischaemia or electrolyte abnormalities. Secondary T-wave changes are caused by alterations of the activation sequence such as during ventricular pacing, intermittent LBBB, ventricular tachycardia, ventricular extrasystoles, and ventricular pre-excitation. These secondary changes can persist after the normal supraventricular activation pattern resumes. The mechanism underlying this T-wave 'memory' is not yet understood.

2) **Report the repeat ECG shown in Fig. 1.2.**

   The ECG in Fig. 1.2 was recorded after the pacemaker was checked. It demonstrates atrial fibrillation (AF) with a ventricular response rate of 72 bpm. Ventricular pacing is initiated when the rate slows at end of the rhythm strip. The period of pacing is followed by a fusion beat with normal conduction. The QRS axis is normal. There is infero-lateral T-wave inversion. Although this could represent myocardial ischaemia, persisting T-wave memory is more likely as his pacemaker has recently been active.

3) **If the patient did not know the type of pacemaker that was implanted or the manufacturer how could this information be obtained?**

   Most patients will carry a card with information about their pacemaker. However, if this is not available, the patient's general practitioner (GP) or cardiologist should be contacted as soon as possible. Examination of the surface ECG may reveal pacing potentials and bundle branch block [usually LBBB morphology if the pacing lead is located within the right ventricular (RV)] if the patient is paced. However, this information may not be available if the patient is not pacemaker dependent. A chest X-ray can reveal the type of pacemaker (single or dual chamber, biventricular, ICD) and the manufacturer (logo visible by X-ray).

   A pacemaker can be interrogated by the programmer provided by the manufacturer of that pacemaker. Most departments will have programmers for the most commonly used makes (Medtronic, St Jude, Boston Scientific, and Biotronik). If the manufacturer is not known, interrogation can be attempted with the programmers from each manufacturer until the correct one is found. The pacemaker programmer performs several functions. It can assess battery status, modify pacing settings, and access diagnostic information stored in the pacemaker (e.g. heart rate trends and tachyarrhythmia recordings).

4) **What was the cardiology registrar asked to do? What intervention was made?**

A pacemaker should not pace at a rate of 120 bpm in a patient at rest. As malfunction was suspected, a cardiology registrar was asked to review the patient and interrogate the pacemaker. Interrogation revealed that it was a functioning dual-chamber device, with leads in the right atrium and ventricle, programmed to an atrio-ventricular synchronising dual-chamber rate-responsive (DDDR) mode (see Table 1.1 for the naming conventions of pacing modes). The electrocardiograms obtained from these endocardial leads demonstrated that the underlying rhythm was AF. The AF sensed by the atrial lead was triggering the pacemaker, which was pacing the ventricle at 120 bpm, the set upper rate limit.

The pacemaker should have automatically switched to a single-chamber ventricular demand (VVI) mode when the patient developed AF. However, the mode-switching algorithm was disabled. When this algorithm was enabled the pacemaker automatically switched to VVIR pacing and ignored the atrial lead inputs. This slowed the heart rate. The previous pacemaker check had found paced sinus rhythm only and so the initial programming error was not spotted.

Classification of cardiac pacemakers

The North American Society of Pacing and Electrophysiology (NASPE) and the British Pacing and Electrophysiology Group (BPEG) have published a joint pacemaker code (Table 1.1). The code was initially published in 1983 and was last revised in 2002. It describes the five-letter code for operation of implantable pacemakers and defibrillators.

The first two positions of this code indicate the chambers paced and sensed. The third position indicates the programmed response to a sensed event, which can be either to inhibit further pacing or to trigger it. Of the most frequently used modes, VVI is the simplest form, utilizing a single lead (V- -) that is able to sense ventricular activity (- V -) and inhibit pacing if it is present (- - I) or pace at a set rate.

DDD offers maintenance of atrial and ventricular synchrony with two leads (A - - + V - - = D - -) by allowing the atrial lead to sense intrinsic activity, inhibiting atrial pacing (I) and triggering ventricular pacing (- - I + - - T = - - D) in the absence of sensed ventricular activity. Rate responsiveness is achieved by ventricular tracking of atrial activity. The fourth position, rate modulation, increases the patient's heart rate in response to patient exercise and is useful in dual-chamber mode when sinus node dysfunction is present and with single-chamber ventricular pacing. A number of parameters (such as QT interval, movement, blood temperature, chest wall impedence, and pressure) are used to detect patient exercise. As the exercise wanes, the sensor indicated rate returns to the programmed lower rate. The fifth position describes multisite pacing functionality—ventricular multisite pacing is a treatment for heart failure in the presence of dysynchonous LV contraction.

Dual-chamber pacing is desirable to optimize atrio-ventricular synchrony. However, ventricular tracking of rapid atrial rates can occur during supraventricular tachyarrhythmias (SVT) if standard dual-chamber pacing modes are used. In the early 1990s, the introduction of mode-switching algorithms allowed automatic switching from DDD to VVI, preventing inappropriate tracking of the atrial response. This case emphasizes the importance of enabling automatic mode switching at implantation to ensure safe functioning, especially in patients with known paroxysmal AF or SVT.

Table 1.1 NASPE/BPEG Revised in 2002 Pacemaker Code

Position I	**Position II**	**Position III**	**Position IV**	**Position V**
Chamber paced	Chamber sensed	Response to sensed event	Programmability, rate modulation	Multisite pacing
O	O	O		O
A	A	I		A
V	V	T	O	V
D	D	D	R	D
(A & V)	(A & V)	(T & I)		(A & V)

O, none; A, atrium; I, inhibited; V, ventricle; T, triggered; D, dual; R, rate modulation.

5) **What is the effect of placing a magnet over a pacemaker? Is the response different with an ICD?**

Placing a magnet over the pacemaker pulse generator closes an internal magnet-sensitive 'reed switch' but this was never intended for the management of pacemaker emergencies. The response to switch closure varies between pacemaker manufacturers, models, and programmed settings (magnet mode). Sensing is usually inhibited and the PPM is often set to pace in an asynchronous (non-sensing of native electrical activity), fixed rate ('magnet rate'), overdrive mode in either a single- or dual-chamber configuration (VOO/DOO; see Table 1.1).

Importantly, this reprogramming response is not universal and is usually only temporary (i.e. whilst the magnet is *in situ*). Most models have unique asynchronous rates set for the 'beginning of life', an 'elective replacement indicator', and the 'end of life'. Hence, magnet placement can determine whether the battery needs replacement. However, application of a magnet to a pacemaker with depleted batteries may result in pacing output instability and could even stop pacing output. Some possible responses to placement of a magnet and the corresponding magnet modes are listed in Table 1.2. Manufacturers can provide information on the magnet modes of each model of pacemaker.

The response of ICDs differs from that of pacemakers. Some ICDs are temporarily programmed to monitor-only mode (will not deliver a shock even if programmed criteria are met) whilst the magnet remains *in situ*. Other ICDs will remain in monitor-only mode permanently if activation of the reed switch is sustained for >25 seconds. This response depends on the magnet mode program of the device.

Table 1.2 Pacemaker responses to magnet placement and magnet modes

i.	**Asynchronous high-rate pacing (rate varies by model)**	a. Sustained
		b. Brief (10–100 beats) burst then return to standard program
ii.	**No apparent rhythm or rate change**	a. No magnet sensor (no reed switch)
		b. Magnet mode disabled
		c. ECG storage mode enabled
		d. Program rate pacing in already paced patient
		e. Inappropriate monitor settings (pace filter on)
iii.	**Continuous or transient loss of pacing**	Diagnostic threshold test mode

6) **How should the patient's current arrhythmia be treated?**

If AF has persisted for over 48 hours, management must take into consideration the risk of thromboembolism. If the onset cannot be determined, patients should be managed as if the AF has been present for over 48 hours. This is discussed further in Case 44.

7) **What are the chances of improvement in cardiac function?**

Tachycardia can induce changes in ventricular structure and function if persistent and prolonged. Fortunately these changes may be reversed with rate or rhythm control. The mechanisms responsible are unclear. However, once heart failure develops, adrenergic stimulation could enhance the ventricular response, resulting in a vicious cycle with further reduction of cardiac output and amplification of cardiac failure. Improvement in LV function generally begins within days to weeks after termination of the tachycardia and may continue over months.

In this case there was immediate symptomatic improvement, with further resolution over the next few months. An echo performed 3 months after presentation demonstrated only mild impairment in LV function (EF 45%).

Further reading

Guidelines for cardiac pacing and cardiac resynchronization therapy (2007). The Task Force for Cardiac Pacing and Cardiac Resynchronization Therapy of the European Society of Cardiology. *Eur Heart J*; **28**: 2256–2295.

ACC/AHA/HRS (2008). Guidelines for Device-Based Therapy of Cardiac Rhythm Abnormalities: A Report of the American College of Cardiology/American Heart Association Task Force on Practice Guidelines. *Circulation*; **117**: 350–408.

Kaszala K, Huizar JF, Ellenbogen KA (2008). Contemporary pacemakers: what the primary care physician needs to know. *Mayo Clin Proc*; **83**: 1170–1186.

Trohman RG, Kim MH, Pinski SL (2004). Cardiac pacing: the state of the art. *Lancet*; **364**: 1701–1719.

Rajappan, K (2009). Education in Heart: Permanent pacemaker implantation technique. *Heart*; Part I **95**: 259–264; Part II **95**: 334–342.

Case 2

A 45-year-old male presented with shortness of breath and fast palpitations that developed suddenly 1 hour prior to presentation. The admission ECG is shown in Fig. 2.1. Intravenous adenosine was administered whilst a rhythm strip was recorded from lead V2 (Fig. 2.2).

Questions

1. What is the differential diagnosis of a broad complex tachycardia?
2. Report the findings in ECG Fig. 2.1.
3. What are the contraindications to administration of adenosine?
4. Which drugs interact with adenosine?
5. How should adenosine be administered for the diagnosis or treatment of an SVT?
6. What is the effect of adenosine on this arrhythmia? What is the mechanism of this action?
7. What drugs should be avoided in this condition?
8. How should the patient be managed acutely?
9. What is the long-term management?

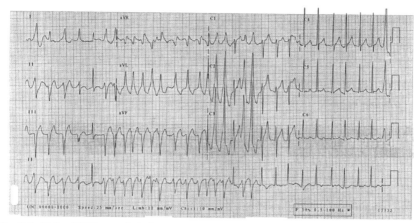

Fig. 2.1 12 lead ECG on admission.

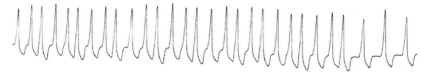

Fig. 2.2 10-second rhythm strip recorded from lead V2 after administration of adenosine.

Answers

1) **What is the differential diagnosis of a broad complex tachycardia?**

   Causes of broad complex QRS tachycardia may be of ventricular or supraventricular origin and may be regular or irregular. See Cases 33–35, Table 2.1, and further discussion below for further discussion of broad complex tachycardia.

Table 2.1 Causes of regular and irregular broad complex tachycardias

Supraventricular
Regular
SVT, AF, and AV nodal re-entry tachycardia with pre-existing or functional bundle branch block
[1]Orthodromic CMT with pre-existing or functional bundle branch block
Antidromic CMT with anterograde conduction via an accessory pathway and retrograde conduction via AV node
SVT with conduction though an accessory pathway
Irregular
AF with bundle branch block with aberrant conduction (pre-existing or functional)
AF with pre-excitation
Ventricular
Regular
Monomorphic ventricular tachycardia
[2]Fascicular tachycardia
Right ventricular outflow tract tachycardia
Paced ventricular rhythm
Irregular
Polymorphic ventricular tachycardia

[1] CMTs are described in more detail below.
[2] Fascicular tachycardia is an uncommon arrhythmia that originates around of the fascicles of the left bundle branch (usually posterior) and propagates partly via Purkinje fibres. It is often misdiagnosed as an SVT as the QRS complexes are relatively narrow (0.11–0.14 seconds). The QRS complexes have an RBBB pattern with left axis deviation if it originates from the posterior fascicle but right axis deviation if the anterior fascicle is the origin. Fascicular tachycardias are rare and generally do not respond to lignocaine but can be terminated by intravenous verapamil.

2) **Report the findings in ECG Fig. 2.1**

   Fig. 2.1 shows a tachyarrhythmia. During the last 4 seconds of the rhythm strip there is an irregularly irregular narrow complex tachycardia AF at a rate of approximately 150 bpm. During this arrhythmia the QRS axis is probably normal. The QRS complex of the single narrow complex capture beat in leads I and II is predominantly positive. This part of the ECG demonstrates AF, which is conducted via the atrioventricular node (AVN) to the ventricles.

During the first 6 seconds of the ECG, the rhythm is obviously different. An irregularly irregular broad complex tachycardia predominates. The rate varies from 150 to 280 bpm. The QRS complexes are broad and the initial upstroke is slurred and slow rising (delta wave). During this rhythm the QRS axis is deviated to the left and there is right bundle branch block (RSR pattern V1). These findings demonstrate that conduction is antegrade via a left-sided accessory pathway.

This ECG demonstrates AF in a patient with Wolff–Parkinson–White (WPW) syndrome. Conduction of the atrial arrhythmia to the ventricles is intermittently occurring via a left-sided accessory pathway likely posteroseptal. This diagnosis is supported by the broad complex tachycardia with unusual and changing QRS complex morphology in a young patient. The irregularly irregular QRS complexes in this case distinguish AF from circus movement tachycardia (CMTs) in WPW. In the context of WPW syndrome if there is any doubt about the regularity of the rhythm, treat for AF with direct current (DC) cardioversion.

Arrhythmias in Wolff–Parkinson–White syndrome

The incidence of WPW is approximately 1/1000 population. However, a minority experience sustained tachyarrhythmias, therefore asymptomatic individuals who are incidentally found to have WPW on routine ECG do not require further investigation unless involved in high-risk activities such as rock climbing or for vocational reasons such as commercial flying.

Although several arrhythmias can occur in patients with WPW, the most common are CMTs. Circus movement tachycardias are triggered either by a premature atrial ectopic beat occurring during the refractory period of the accessory pathway or by a ventricular ectopic conducting retrogradely to the atrium through the accessory pathway. Both can trigger CMT through completion of the circuit via the accessory pathway or AVN, respectively.

This results in a regular narrow complex CMT, usually limited by the refractory period of the AVN. Regular narrow complex CMTs are difficult to differentiate from paroxysmal supraventricular tachycardia (PSVT) due to AV nodal re-entry because the delta wave is lost.

Antidromic CMT can be triggered by antegrade transmission of an ectopic via the accessory pathway. Antidromic CMT are regular, broad complex tachycardias that are potentially faster than orthodromic CMT because of the relatively short refractory period of most accessory pathways. Antidromic CMT are much less common than orthodromic CMT but retain the delta wave within the broad QRS complex.

Differential diagnoses include ventricular tachycardia (VT) and supraventricular tachycardia (SVT) with aberrant conduction. However, all regular broad-complex tachycardias should be treated as VT until proven otherwise. Most regular broad-complex CMT associated with WPW syndrome can be treated with adenosine cardio-vert to sinus rhythm.

AF is common in patients with WPW with an incidence of up to 40%. AF is the most serious arrhythmia in WPW as it can deteriorate into ventricular fibrillation (VF).

The relatively long refractory period of the AVN protects normal hearts from excessively high ventricular rates. However, accessory pathways often have short anterograde refractory periods, allowing much faster ventricular rates. Furthermore, sympathetic discharge secondary to hypotension may shorten the refractory period further and increase the ventricular rate.

AF conducted through an accessory pathway (pre-excited AF; Fig. 2.1) appears as an unusual, irregular, broad-complex tachycardia on ECG. Pre-excited AF should be considered in young patients with broad-complex tachycardias that exhibit unusual or changing QRS complex morphologies.

3) **What are the contraindications to administration of adenosine?**

The contraindications to adenosine include:

- sinus bradycardia, sinus node disease, second or third degree atrioventricular block, unless the patient has a functioning PPM
- cardiac transplant
- risk of bronchospasm (asthma)—caution is required in patients with chronic obstructive pulmonary disease (COPD)
- previous adverse reaction to adenosine
- patient refusal

Adenosine may be administered in a patient with WPW with a regular SVT with caution. Most regular wide-complex CMT in patients with WPW syndrome can be converted to sinus rhythm by adenosine. However, preparation should be made for immediate DC cardioversion should the patient's cardiovascular status degenerate. Adenosine should not be administered to a patient with WPW with AF (see answer 6).

4) **What drugs interact with adenosine?**

Methylxanthines (theophylline and caffeine) are competitive adenosine receptor antagonists. Consider increasing the dose of adenosine in patients on theophylline.

Adenosine is broken down by adenosine deaminase, present in red blood cells and vessel walls. Dipyridamole inhibits adenosine deaminase. This allows adenosine to accumulate in the circulation and potentiates the vasodilatation. The dose of adenosine should be reduced in patients taking dipyridamole.

5) **How should adenosine be administered for the diagnosis or treatment of a SVT?**

When given for the diagnosis or treatment of an SVT 6 mg adenosine should be given as a fast intravenous bolus. As the half-life of adenosine is very short, the cannula used for administration should be sited as close to the heart as possible (e.g. antecubital fossa or external jugular vein). The adenosine bolus should be immediately followed by a flush of 0.9% saline. If there is no effect (i.e. transient AV block does not occur), 12 mg adenosine can be given 2 minutes later. If this has no effect, 18 mg can be administered 2 minutes later.

6) **What is the effect of adenosine on this arrhythmia? What is the mechanism of this action?**

After administration of adenosine the AF was conducted only through the accessory pathway, as demonstrated by the rhythm strip in Fig. 2.2. Figure 2.2 shows an irregularly irregular broad complex tachycardia (AF conducted via an accessory pathway). The first 26 complexes on the rhythm strip are transmitted at rates up to 250 bpm. The patient felt lightheaded and nauseated, and his BP fell to 90/40. Fortunately, the half-life of adenosine is less than 10 seconds so the effect was short-lived. Figure 2.2 shows that the heart rate slows significantly for the remaining three complexes. Adenosine blocks AV nodal conduction and shortens the cycle length of AF, allowing increased rates of conduction through an accessory pathway.

7) **What drugs should be avoided in this condition?**

Digoxin and dihydropyridine calcium channel blockers are contraindicated in patients with WPW syndrome and AF caused by anterograde conduction through the accessory pathway. These agents promote anterograde conduction through the accessory pathway. This can increase the ventricular rate and promote degeneration into VF.

8) **How should the patient be managed acutely?**

The aim of treatment of the common, non-pre-excited AF is to increase the refractory period of the atrioventricular node to limit conduction of irregular atrial activity to the ventricles. This is discussed in Case 44. The management of pre-excited AF is very different. To slow the ventricular rate, conduction via the accessory pathway must be reduced. The anterograde refractory period of the accessory pathway must be increased relative to that of the AV node.

Type I (disopyramide, procainamide, flecainide, propafenone) or type III (amiodarone) antiarrhythmic agents may be used. However, amiodarone should be administered slowly (over 1–4 hours). If the patient is compromised haemodynamically then electrical cardioversion is required.

The management of fast AF should take into consideration the cardiovascular status of the patient and the risk of thromboembolism. In this case, the onset of AF was clearly defined and less than 48 hours prior to presentation so the risk of thromboembolism is low. The patient was haemodynamically stable and so intravenous flecainde 50 mg was administered. The patient subsequently cardioverted to sinus rhythm. The ECG after administration of flecainide is shown in Fig. 2.3. This demonstrates sinus rhythm at a rate of 84 bpm. The most striking abnormalities are the short pr interval (0.12 seconds) and the delta waves visible in all QRS complexes. These findings demonstrate the presence of an accessory pathway. The RSR pattern in V1 suggests that the accessory pathway is left sided.

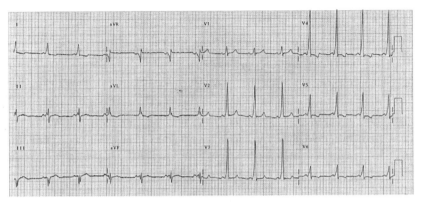

Fig. 2.3 ECG recorded after administration of flecainide.

9) What is the long-term management?

In the long term, prevention of recurrent arrhythmias may require a combination of agents. Amiodarone and bisoprolol are commonly used. Radiofrequency ablation of the accessory pathway is indicated for most patients with WPW, especially if they are intolerant of medication or have frequent, disabling arrhythmias. Ablation is curative and no further drug treatment is required. This was undertaken successfully in this patient a few days after presentation.

Further reading

Fengler BT, Brady WJ, Plautz CU (2007). Atrial fibrillation in the Wolff–Parkinson–White syndrome: ECG recognition and treatment in the ED. *Am J Emerg Med*; **25**: 576–583.

Case 3

A 74-year-old man was admitted for elective stenting of a left common femoral artery (CFA) stenosis under general anaesthesia. Comorbidities included treated hypertension, hyperlipidaemia, and type II diabetes mellitus.

He had suffered an ischaemic cerebrovascular accident (CVA) 4 years before and had been diagnosed with benign prostatic hypertrophy and renal impairment 2 years ago. Renal tract ultrasound and magnetic resonance imaging (MRI) showed normal-sized kidneys with mild–moderate bilateral renal artery stenoses and a calcified distal aorta. He was followed up by the renal physicians regularly and was assessed to currently have Kidney Disease Outcomes & Quality Initiative (KDOQI) Stage 2 chronic kidney disease (CKD) with a creatinine of 115 μmol/L.

Current medications consisted of aspirin, clopidogrel, bisoprolol, simvastatin, metformin, insulin, losartan, and doxazosin. On the advice of the vascular surgical team, clopidogrel had been stopped 10 days prior to admission and metformin was stopped 2 days prior to admission.

The left CFA stenosis was stented using a combined open and endovascular approach. There were no complications during this procedure, but 3 days later he sustained a non-ST elevation myocardial infarction (NSTEMI). Intravenous unfractionated heparin was started and coronary angiography with follow-on percutaneous coronary intervention (PCI) was performed 2 days later (see report; Fig. 3.1).

The next day the patient's urine output was less than 200 mL in 24 hours (creatinine 230 μmol/L). Losartan and metformin were stopped. Urine dipstick testing revealed blood + and protein ++, but urine microscopy excluded red cell casts. Urine sodium was 90 mmol/L. Immunological investigations were negative. Despite supportive therapy the renal function continued to deteriorate. On the 7th postoperative day the patient was anuric (creatinine 550 μmol/L). Throughout the postoperative period, cardiovascular and abdominal examinations were unremarkable and peripheral pulses remained intact.

CARDIAC CATHETERISATION REPORT

...Access was gained via right femoral artery with a 7 French gauge sheath...

...Coronary angiography revealed an 80–90% stenosis in a diffusely diseased intermediate vessel and a 90% stenosis in the first diagonal branch...

...Follow on double vessel percutaneous coronary intervention (PCI) to the intermediate and diagonal vessels was performed with drug eluting stent implantation and an excellent final result...

...Contrast agent used: 250ml Omnipaque™ 350...

Fig. 3.1 Coronary angiogram and PCI procedure report.

Questions

1. What are the KDOQI stages of CKD? What is stage 2?
2. How is renal function assessed in CKD?
3. How is acute renal failure diagnosed? What are the RIFLE criteria?
4. What is the differential diagnosis for his renal failure and which is the most likely diagnosis?
5. What are the risk factors for contrast-induced nephropathy (CIN)?
6. What is the pathogenesis of CIN and how can it be prevented?

Answers

1) **What are the KDOQI stages of CKD? What is stage 2?**

The five KDOQI stages of CKD are based on glomerular filtration rate (GFR), which can be either measured or estimated (eGFR; see answer to question 2). The definitions of each stage are outlined in Table 3.1. Note that stage 2 CKD is often over-diagnosed if based on eGFR rather than measured values. When renal function is near normal, eGFR calculations provide falsely low values for GFR.

Table 3.1 The KDOQI stages of chronic kidney disease. The diagnosis of CKD requires two estimates of GFR ≥90 days apart

Stage	GFR (mL/min/1.73 m^2)	Definition
1	>90	Renal disease with normal renal function
2	60–89	Renal disease with mildly impaired renal function
3 A/B	45–59/30–44	Moderately impaired renal function
4	15–29	Severely impaired renal function
5	<15 or on dialysis	End-stage renal failure

2) **How is renal function assessed in CKD?**

In CKD estimates of GFR, which are standardized to body surface area, are more representative of renal function than serum creatinine measurements or urine output. Glomerular filtration rate can be estimated from equations that take into account several variables (e.g. age, gender, race, and size) in addition to the serum creatinine. The Cockcroft–Gault and the modification of diet in renal disease study (MDRD) equations (see Equations 1 and 2) are the most useful in adults. Because these equations were originally validated in young and middle-aged individuals there can be discordance between these estimates and the actual measured GFR in the elderly. Specifically, the MDRD equation tends to overestimate and the Cockcroft–Gault equation to underestimate kidney function in subjects aged over 65 years. In addition, the use of urine collections to measure creatinine clearance is often inaccurate as collections are usually incomplete. In the present case, the baseline eGFR was 61 mL/min/1.73 m^2 using the MDRD equation.

Equation 1: MDRD study equation for eGFR

♂ $\quad$ eGFR (mL/min/1.73 m^2) $=186 \times ($creatinine$\times 0.0113) - 1.154 \times (age) - 0.203$

♀ $\quad$ eGFR (mL/min/1.73 m^2) $= 186 \times ($creatinine$\times 0.0113) - 1.154 \times (age) - 0.203 \times 0.74$

Equation 2: The Cockcroft–Gault equation for eGFR

$$\text{eGFR} = \frac{(140 - \text{age}) \times \text{mass(in kilograms)} \times [0.85 \text{ if female}]}{72 \times \text{serum creatinine (in mg/dL)}}$$

3) **How is acute renal failure diagnosed? What are the RIFLE criteria?**

Acute renal failure (ARF) is diagnosed after a rapid and significant rise in serum creatinine that is usually associated with a fall in urine output. In order to make the diagnosis, previous measurements of serum creatinine are useful for comparison, particularly in patients with CKD, where the baseline creatinine is already raised. The RIFLE criteria are validated for the diagnosis of ARF and are outlined in Table 3.2.

Table 3.2 The RIFLE criteria for diagnosis of acute renal failure

RIFLE criteria	Definition
Risk	Increased serum creatinine (a single reading >1.5 × baseline) or urine output <0.5 mL/kg for 6 hours
Injury	Increased creatinine (a single reading >2 × baseline) or urine output <0.5 mL/kg for 12 hours
Failure	Increased creatinine (a single reading >3 × baseline) or serum creatinine >355 μmol/L (with a rise of >44) or urine output <0.3 mL/kg for 24 hours
Loss	Persistent ARF or need for renal replacement therapy (RRT) for over 4 weeks
End-stage	Complete loss of renal function (need for RRT) for over 3 months

4) **What is the differential diagnosis for his renal failure and which is most likely?**

Acute renal failure is usually secondary to a combination of pre-renal, renal, or obstructive post-renal insults. In this case, hypovolaemia, postoperative bleeding, or aortic dissection should be considered but are unlikely if the patient has been haemodynamically stable and all the peripheral pulses are normal. Rhabdomyolysis can occur after prolonged operations and serum creatine kinase (CK) should be checked. Obstruction should be excluded by renal tract ultrasound. Doppler ultrasound of the renal vessels can be used to detect thromboembolic or renovascular disease. All potentially nephrotoxic drugs should be discontinued. A urinary catheter should be inserted to monitor urine output and guide fluid management.

In this case, abdominal examination excluded urinary retention. A renal tract ultrasound excluded hydronephrosis, and confirmed that the bladder was empty but otherwise showed similar findings to those performed prior to this presentation. Urine sodium (90 mmol/L) suggested that acute tubular necrosis (ATN) was more likely than a pre-renal cause of renal failure. A urinary catheter was inserted to guide fluid management.

Cholesterol embolization syndrome due to atheromatous plaque disruption can complicate endovascular procedures. This can be difficult to diagnose as it typically manifests 1–4 weeks after the intervention. However, this delay in onset of renal impairment and the usual subsequent progressive deterioration in renal function can help to distinguish cholesterol embolism from contrast nephropathy. Other diagnostic clues include a skin rash, raised erythrocyte sedimentation rate, hypocomplementaemia, and modest proteinuria with or without haematuria. The diagnosis can be confirmed by biopsy of skin, muscle, kidney, or any other involved organs.

Intravenous contrast (250 mL Omnipaque™ 350) was administered during the coronary angiography (Fig. 3.1) and the stenting of the CFA stenosis (40 mL Omnipaque™ 350). Intravenous contrast is nephrotoxic. However, CIN is a diagnosis of exclusion. Although angiotensin receptor blockade and reduction in renal perfusion post myocardial infarction may have contributed, CIN is the most likely cause of ARF in this case.

Contrast-induced nephropathy is a serious and potentially life-threatening non-coronary complication of cardiac catheterization. Classically, the renal dysfunction peaks at around day 3 and has reached baseline in most by day 10. Only a minority of patients have persisting renal impairment, although the requirement for haemofiltration or dialysis in the acute phase is a poor prognostic sign.

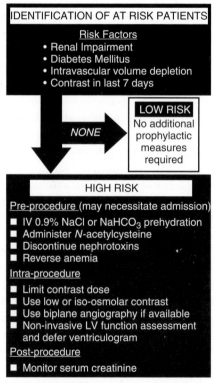

Fig. 3.2 Risk stratification and prophylaxis of CIN in patients undergoing coronary angiography. Renal impairment for risk stratification is defined as an eGFR <60 mL/min and >30 mL/min. In those with eGFR <30 mL/min liaison with the nephrology team prior to cardiac catheterization is advisable.

5) **What are the risk factors for CIN?**

Contrast-induced nephropathy has been defined as an increase in serum creatinine (>25% or >44 µmol/L) within 48 hours of contrast administration. The most important risk factors for CIN are listed in Fig. 3.2. Significantly, postoperative anaemia may also have contributed in this case, as a low haematocrit predisposes to CIN.

In patients with advanced CKD the incidence of CIN is over 50%. The risk factors are additive. In patients with mild–moderate renal impairment, the incidence of CIN is 5–10%. However, if the patient also has diabetes mellitus the incidence increases to 10–40%. The incidence in patients with no risk factors is negligible. Simple risk assessment scoring tools are available (see Further reading section below).

6) **What is the pathogenesis of CIN and how can it be prevented?**

Contrast-induced nephropathy is thought to be due to a combination of a contrast-induced reduction or redistribution of renal blood flow and direct renal tubular injury mediated by free radicals. It affects 3% of patients after percutaneous coronary intervention, leading to a 20% increase in in-hospital mortality and a 30% increase in mortality at 5 years. However, it may be prevented if high-risk patients are identified and prophylactic treatments are administered. Pre-procedural volume expansion, pretreatment with N-acetylcysteine (NAC), and reducing the use of high osmolar contrast agents can improve outcomes.

Evidence for the prevention of CIN by volume expansion with intravenous isotonic saline is based on animal models and clinical trials. The addition of forced diuresis does not improve outcomes, nor does oral hydration alone. The use of intravenous isotonic sodium bicarbonate may confer additional benefit by increasing renal medullary pH or minimizing tubular damage induced by reactive oxygen species.

N-acetylcysteine is used as prophylaxis against CIN based on its antioxidant properties. Pretreatment with oral or intravenous NAC (600 mg twice daily for 2 days) and volume expansion results in a relative risk reduction of 56%.

Ionic and non-ionic contrast media differ in their osmolality. The conventional ionic contrast agents have significantly higher osmolality (1500 mOsm/kg) than the non-ionic compounds (600–800 mOsm/kg), which are still hyperosmolar to plasma (280–300 mOsm/kg). Low osmolar (nonionic) contrast agents (e.g. Omnipaque) are less nephrotoxic in patients with renal impairment and diabetes mellitus. Newer multimeric iso-osmolar (290 mOsm/kg) radiocontrast agents (Visipaque) are available. Although there is no additional benefit over low osmolar agents in low-risk patients, there may be advantages in CKD.

Risk assessment for CIN and use of proven preventative measures should be considered for all patients who undergo coronary angiography (Fig. 3.2). If CIN develops, management is generally supportive.

In this case, the patient was referred to intensive care when he became anuric. He was started on haemofiltration. The patient remained anuric for 3 days.

Urine output resumed on the 10th postoperative day. Haemofiltration was discontinued and the patient was discharged from the intensive care unit back to the cardiology ward. The creatinine gradually improved and was 130 μmol/L on discharge home 5 days later. The clopidogrel, metformin, and losartan were restarted.

Further reading

Mehran R, Aymong ED, Nikolsky E, Lasic Z, Iakovou I, Fahy M, Mintz GS, Lansky AJ, Moses JW, Stone GW, Leon MB, Dangas G. (2004). A simple risk score for prediction of contrast-induced nephropathy after percutaneous coronary intervention: development and initial validation. *J Am Coll Cardiol*; **44**: 1393–1399.

McCullough PA (2008). Contrast-induced acute kidney injury. *J Am Coll Cardiol*; **51**: 1419–1428.

Tepel M, Aspelin P, Lameire N (2006). Contrast-induced nephropathy: A clinical and evidence-based approach. *Circulation*; **113**: 1799–1806.

Case 4

A 39-year-old south Asian man presented to the ED with a 3-week history of chest pain. This burning, central, lower chest pain was not clearly associated with exertion. It did not radiate and there were no associated symptoms. He smoked 20 cigarettes per day. There was no past medical history but his father had died of a heart attack at the age of 41 and there was a family history of diabetes. He had presented twice in the preceding 3 weeks. On both previous occasions ECG and cardiac enzymes were reported to be normal. On the second occasion gastro-oesophageal reflux was diagnosed and he was prescribed Ranitidine 150 mg bd.

On examination he was anxious but pain free. His pulse was regular at 75 bpm, with a BP of 145/80 mmHg, O_2 saturations of 98% breathing room air, and respiratory rate 14 breaths/min. Cardiovascular examination was unremarkable. The chest pain was not reproducible with manual pressure. His admission ECG is shown in Fig. 4.1 and his admission and 12-hour cardiac troponin I (cTnI) measurements were normal. A cardiology opinion was sought.

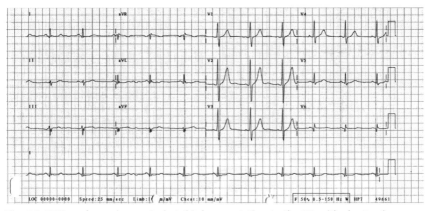

Fig. 4.1 ECG performed on arrival at third presentation to the ED with chest pain.

Questions

1. Discuss the differential diagnosis for this presentation.
2. Describe typical angina.
3. Report the ECG in Fig. 4.1.
4. What is the differential diagnosis for the ECG findings? What is the most likely diagnosis in this case?
5. What is the most correct next management step?

Answers

1) **Discuss the differential diagnosis for this presentation.**

In the present case, it initially appears that the patient's presentation is not consistent with any cause of chest pain. The broad differential diagnosis of chest pain must be considered whenever a patient is assessed (see Case 36). This is particularly important if the presentation is atypical. Significant complications can occur if a patient is labelled with an incorrect diagnosis and this is not challenged when the patient is reviewed.

In one study of patients presenting to an ED with chest pain only, the most common eventual diagnoses were non-cardiac (55%), acute coronary syndrome (ACS; 17%), and stable angina (6%), whilst 21% had other cardiac diagnoses (e.g. pulmonary embolism and acute aortic dissection). However, in one in five cases eventually diagnosed to have an ACS, the patient was initially discharged from the ED with another diagnosis. Misdiagnosis and inappropriate discharge are most common in women younger than 55 years old, non-caucasians, and those with normal ECGs. Consequently, these patients have a significantly higher risk of mortality.

In most cases, cardiac chest pain is a manifestation of the ischaemia which has occurred as a result of a discrepancy between myocardial oxygen supply and demand. It is mainly due to atherosclerotic plaque rupture with coronary occlusion or narrowing with distal thrombotic embolization. Less commonly, it can be associated with coronary artery spasm, either in normal arteries or near atherosclerotic plaques, coronary dissection, coronary emboli, congenital coronary anomalies, and myocardial bridging (a segment of an epicardial coronary artery with an intra-myocardial course and arterial constriction can occur when the overlying muscle shortens in systole).

Rarely, other disease processes involving the ostia of the coronary arteries (e.g. aortic dissection, connective tissue disorders, and syphilitic aortitis) can acutely impair coronary flow. Non-flow-limiting coronary disease may become clinically apparent if oxygen supply falls for other reasons (e.g. anaemia) or demand rises (e.g. sepsis and thyrotoxicosis). Non-coronary causes of reduced perfusion pressure (e.g. aortic stenosis, aortic regurgitation) or increased oxygen demand (e.g. hypertrophic cardiomyopathy) can precipitate myocardial ischaemia, which can be exacerbated with increases in heart rate that reduce diastolic perfusion time.

2) **Describe typical angina.**

Typical angina is the chest pain commonly associated with myocardial ischaemia. It is described as a heavy chest pressure or squeezing sensation that often radiates to the shoulders (usually left), neck/jaw, and/or arms, and often builds in intensity over several minutes after exercise or psychological stress (Table 4.1). Any deviation from this description makes the chest pain 'atypical' and reduces the probability that it represents acute myocardial injury or ischaemia. However, infero-posterior wall myocardial ischaemia can mimic an acute abdomen (nausea, vomiting, and upper abdomen pain) or trigger vagal reflexes, causing dizziness, syncope, bradycardia, and hypotension.

Pleuritic pain, constant or fleeting pain, abdominal pain primarily in the middle or lower zones, pain which can be easily localized at the tip of one finger, particularly over the apex of the heart, or pain reproduced with movement or palpation of the chest wall or arms is generally regarded as atypical of cardiac ischaemia.

However, atypical presentations of ACS are not uncommon, particularly in younger (25–40 years) and older (>75 years) patients, diabetics, and women. Myocardial ischaemia can cause pain predominantly at rest, epigastric pain, mimicking recent onset indigestion, stabbing chest pain, chest pain with some pleuritic features, or increasing dyspnoea. In the Multicenter Chest Pain Study, acute myocardial ischaemia was diagnosed in 22% of patients presenting to EDs with sharp or stabbing chest pain, in 13% of those with chest pain that had some pleuritic features, and in 7% of those whose chest pain was fully reproduced by palpation.

Table 4.1 Typical angina: markers of impending infarction

Prolonged symptoms (≥20 minutes)
Retrosternal discomfort
Radiation to arms (usually left), back, neck, or lower jaw
Pain is pressing, heavy, or tight band
Breathing or posture does not influence pain severity

3) **Report the ECG in Fig. 4.1.**

The admission ECG is not normal. It demonstrates sinus rhythm at a rate of 66 bpm with left axis deviation. There are dominant R waves in all the right precordial leads, including V1 and low voltage R waves inferiorly and laterally. The T waves anteriorly are upright and lateral T waves are biphasic. There is a suspicion of a Q wave in V6.

4) **What is the differential diagnosis for the ECG findings? What is the most likely diagnosis in this case?**

The diagnosis for this patient was missed at the medicine–cardiology interface when the ECG was reported incorrectly. When reporting a 12 lead ECG, the assessment of the QRS complex should include a specific review of lead V1, in which the S wave should dominate. A dominant R wave in V1 may be abnormal; causes are listed in Tables 4.2 and 4.3. In this case, the mode of presentation, with a 3-week history of symptoms that may represent coronary ischaemia, suggests that the ECG findings are due to a completed posterior myocardial infarction (MI). Acute posterior infarction presents with anterior ST depression that involves V1–3 and is a mirror of ST elevation (see Fig. 4.2). If untreated, full thickness infarction occurs in this territory, with posterior Q waves that appear instead as dominant R waves on the anterior recording leads. The chest pain he is experiencing is likely to be due to post-infarct angina (normal troponin).

Table 4.2 Common causes of a tall R waves in the right precordial leads (R/S ratio >1 in lead V1)

Right ventricular hypertrophy (the most common cause)	*Distinguishing right ventricular hypertrophy (RVH) from posterior MI* RVH: 1. Obligatory repolarization abnormality producing a down-sloping ST segment and an inverted T wave in V1 2. Usually right-axis deviation Posterior MI: 1. Upright T wave in V1 2. Left-axis deviation due to associated inferior infarction	
Posterior myocardial infarction		See Figs 4.1 and 4.2
Right bundle branch block	The QRS duration is prolonged and typical waveforms are present	
WPW syndrome	1. Left-sided accessory pathway locations produce prominent R waves with an R/S ratio >1 in V1 2. Delta wave may be present	
Incorrect ECG electrode placement	1. Reversal of right precordial electrodes may result in labelling of lead V1 as V3 2. Assess the P waves 3. The net area of the P wave in V1 is always the most negative of the precordial P waves (V1–6)	

Table 4.3 Rare causes of dominant R wave in V1

Normal variant	◆ Early precordial QRS transition ◆ Diagnosed on clinical grounds
Duchenne/Becker muscular dystrophy	
Chronic constrictive pericarditis	
Dextrocardia	◆ Standard electrode placement gives appearance of lead reversal ◆ Standard lead V1 may really be lead V2 ◆ The alerting sign is in lead I. The QRS is negative, with an inverted P wave and T wave ◆ Repeat the ECG with right-sided chest leads and reversal of limb leads

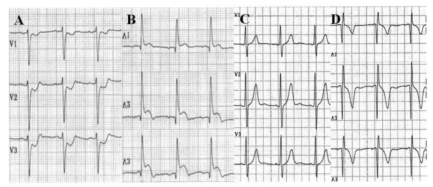

Fig. 4.2 The evolution of a posterior infarction. The 12 lead ECG in the acute phase demonstrates anterior ST depression (A), which is in fact posterior ST elevation seen from the other side of the heart and can be seen if the leads are inverted (B) or if posterior leads (V7–9) are recorded. If full thickness posterior infarction occurs then anterior R waves develop with upright T waves (C) reflecting posterior Q waves and inverted T waves when the trace is inverted (D).

5) **What is the most correct next management step?**

The diagnosis should be confirmed with a coronary angiogram. In this patient this demonstrated moderate diffuse atheroma in the left anterior descending and circumflex coronary arteries with a critical proximal stenosis in a dominant right coronary artery (RCA).

After confirming viability in this territory by stress echocardiography, angioplasty and stenting of the proximal RCA stenosis were performed. After this a large posterior left ventricular (PLV) branch was clearly visible, consistent with the posterior, inferior, and lateral ECG signs (Fig. 4.3).

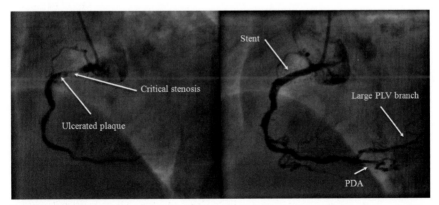

Fig. 4.3 Coronary angiogram. Right oblique view of right coronary artery demonstrating severe proximal stenosis with plaque ulceration (A). After stenting an extensive distal territory is clearly visualized with a large PLV branch now apparent (B).

The patient made a good recovery after angioplasty and stopped smoking. He was discharged on aspirin, clopidogrel, simvastatin ramipril, and bisoprolol for outpatient review.

Further reading

Pope JH, Aufderheide TP, Ruthazer R, Woolard RH, Feldman JA, Beshansky JR, Griffith JL, Selker HP. (2000). Missed diagnoses of acute cardiac ischemia in the emergency department. *N Engl J Med*; **342**: 1163–1170.

Task Force for Diagnosis and Treatment of Non-ST-Segment Elevation Acute Coronary Syndromes of European Society of Cardiology, Bassand JP, Hamm CW, Ardissino D, Boersma E, Budaj A, Fernández-Avilés F *et al.* (2008). Non-ST-segment elevation acute coronary syndromes. *Eur Heart J*; **28**: 1598–1660.

Geleijnse ML, Elhendy A, Kasprzak JD, Rambaldi R, van Domburg RT, Cornel JH, Klootwijk AP, Fioretti PM, Roelandt JR, Simoons ML. (2000) Safety and prognostic value of early dobutamine–atropine stress echocardiography in patients with spontaneous chest pain and a non-diagnostic electrocardiogram. *Eur Heart J*; **21**: 397–406.

Rouan GW, Lee TH, Cook EF, Brand DA, Weisberg MC, Goldman L (1989). Clinical characteristics and outcome of acute myocardial infarction in patients with initially normal or nonspecific electrocardiograms (a report from the Multicenter Chest Pain Study). *Am J Cardiol*; **64**: 1087–1092.

Canto JG, Fincher C, Kiefe CI, Allison JJ, Li Q, Funkhouser E, Centor RM, Selker HP, Weissman NW. (2002). Atypical presentations among Medicare beneficiaries with unstable angina pectoris. *Am J Cardiol*; **90**: 248–253.

Case 5

A 35-year-old body-builder was referred to the rapid access chest pain clinic. He gave a 6-month history of occasional exertional chest tightness on the days after weight training. However, he was asymptomatic whilst weight training three times a week. He thought these pains were muscular and so stopped training, but as his symptoms failed to settle, he sought his GP's advice. He had smoked 10 cigarettes a day for 20 years, admitted to smoking marijuana but denied any other drug use (including anabolic steroids). There was no relevant family history. The fasting blood glucose was 4.3 mmol/L, with a total cholesterol of 7.7 mmol/L and triglycerides of 1.9 mmol/L. Cardiovascular examination was unremarkable and his BP was 130/90 mmHg.

An exercise tolerance test (ETT) was performed but had to be stopped at 7 minutes when the patient developed chest tightness and was unable to continue; the ECG recorded at this time point did not show any significant ST changes. The patient's symptoms persisted into the recovery phase of the test and some ECG data recorded during this period are shown in Fig. 5.1.

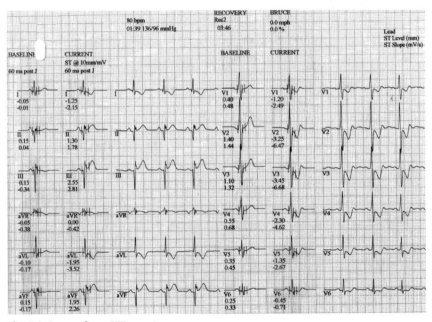

Fig. 5.1 Extract from ETT report.

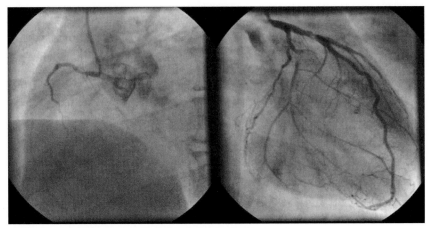

Fig. 5.2 Coronary angiogram. Selected views of right and left coronary arteries.

Questions

1. Report the exercise tolerance test ECG data shown in Fig. 5.1.
2. Explain the symptoms he has and why he remains asymptomatic whilst weight training.
3. What are his modifiable risk factors?
4. What is the differential diagnosis for this patient's chest pain and ETT findings?
5. Report the angiograms in Fig. 5.2.

Answers

1) **Report the results shown in Fig. 5.1.**

   The figure shows a summary page from the ETT recorded at 3 minutes 46 seconds into the recovery phase. The ECG tracings show infero-lateral down-sloping ST-segment depression of more than 0.1 mV, which persisted for more than 0.06–0.08 seconds after the J-point. This fulfils the criteria for a positive test. In about 15% of patients, the diagnostic ST-segment changes only appear during the recovery phase following exercise. As the patient had complained of chest tightness, the test was terminated prematurely at 7 minutes but his symptoms were slow to resolve during recovery, therefore this ETT was strongly positive and diagnostic of myocardial ischaemia.

2) **Explain the symptoms he has and why he remains asymptomatic whilst weight training.**

   The exercise test confirms that the patient has myocardial ischaemia and that the chest pain is likely to be angina. Angina occurs if there is a mismatch between oxygen supply to and demand in the myocardium. Oxygen demand increases with increasing heart rate and so for stable angina symptoms to occur a threshold rate must be exceeded.

   This case highlights the difference in myocardial oxygen demand between isometric burst anaerobic exercise and prolonged aerobic exercise (usually associated with sustained heart rate increases). This patient only developed symptoms during the prolonged aerobic exercise of walking when his heart rate exceeded his angina threshold.

3) **What are his modifiable risk factors?**

   Nine modifiable risk factors have been identified as targets for primary and secondary prevention (Table 5.1). Taken together these factors account for more than 90% of the risk of ischaemic heart disease. They are consistent across geographic regions and ethnic groups.

   The modifiable risk factors present in this case are smoking and hyperlipidaemia. Lipid-lowering (low density lipoprotein (LDL) and very low density lipoprotein (VLDL)) strategies for primary and secondary prevention are well established. Statins have revolutionized treatment and significantly reduce the risk of adverse cardiovascular events. The high density lipoprotein (HDL) cholesterol is protective and reduced levels confer increased risk. However, it is uncertain whether increasing HDL cholesterol lowers cardiovascular risk for an individual.

   In this case, the abnormal lipid profile could also be secondary to illicit use of anabolic steroids and growth hormone, which have both been linked to premature coronary artery disease. When confronted, the patient admitted to having used both agents when preparing for competitions around a year ago.

   Although not present in this case, hypertension is strongly associated with atherosclerotic vascular disease, contributing to over half the total cerebrovascular and

IHD burden. Numerous randomized trials confirm the efficacy of BP reduction in primary and secondary prevention of cardiovascular disease. In general, the increasing prevalence of obesity has lead to the metabolic syndrome and type 2 diabetes mellitus becoming more common. The risk of cardiovascular death is increased six-fold in patients with type 2 diabetes with the number needed to treat to prevent one cardiovascular event over 8 years being estimated at 5. Of note, anabolic steroids and growth hormone can cause hypertension and excessive protein supplementation (e.g. creatine) is associated with renal failure.

Table 5.1 Modifiable risk factors for cardiovascular disease. Data for the odds ratio of each taken from the INTERHEART study

Identified modifiable risk factors for cardiovascular disease	Attributable risk–odds ratio
Abnormal lipids (e.g. ApoB/ApoA1 ratio)	4.1
Diabetes	3.5
Smoking	3.0
Psychosocial	2.7
Hypertension	2.6
Abdominal obesity	2.3
Consumption of fruits and vegetables	0.7 (protective)
Alcohol	0.6 (protective)
Physical activity	0.6 (protective)

4) **What is the differential diagnosis for this patient's chest pain and ETT findings?**

Although atherosclerosis is the most common cause of myocardial ischaemia, non-atheromatous causes should be considered, especially in young patients (Table 5.2). Cocaine is the second most commonly used illicit drug after marijuana and should be considered in the differential in such cases, since 40% of patients presenting to the ED after using cocaine report chest discomfort. The patient denied cocaine abuse on direct questioning but although it could have precipitated the acute chest pain, these effects are short lived and would not explain the positive ETT. Cocaine inhibits reuptake of norepinephrine and dopamine at pre-synaptic adrenergic terminals. The resulting build up of catecholamines produces a powerful sympathomimetic effect, causing tachycardia, vasoconstriction, hypertension, increased myocardial contractility, and oxygen demand. These effects are potentiated by the consumption of alcohol or cigarettes. Those with pre-existing coronary artery disease are at greatest risk. Cocaine-associated MI usually occurs soon after ingestion. Cocaine can also cause aortic dissection.

5) **Report the angiograms in Fig. 5.2.**

The coronary angiograms (Fig. 5.2) demonstrate a non-dominant, severely dis-eased RCA, a dominant circumflex coronary artery with an occluded large first obtuse marginal (OM1) that filled via collaterals, and a tight proximal left anterior descending (LAD) artery stenosis (Fig. 5.3). The present case required surgical revascularization with arterial grafts to the LAD and OM1 territories. He made a good postoperative recovery and resumed light training after 4 months.

Table 5.2 Causes of myocardial ischaemia to be considered after exclusion of atherosclerosis

Mechanism of myocardial ischaemia		
1. *Coronary artery luminal narrowing*	a) Arteritis	i. Granulomatous (e.g. Takayasu disease)
		ii. Polyarteritis nodosa
		iii. Mucocutaneous lymph node (Kawasaki) syndrome
		iv. Systemic lupus erythematosus
		v. Rheumatoid arthritis
		vi. Ankylosing spondylitis
	b) Mural or intimal changes	i. Mucopolysaccharidoses (e.g. Hurler disease)
		ii. Homocysteinuria
		iii. Fabry disease
		iv. Amyloidosis
		v. Juvenile intimal sclerosis—an idiopathic arterial calcification of infancy
		vi. Intimal hyperplasia associated with contraceptive steroids or with the postpartum period
		vii. Pseudoxanthoma elasticum
		viii. Coronary fibrosis caused by radiation therapy
	c) Other	i. Coronary arteries spasm—*Prinzmetal angina* with normal coronary arteries, cocaine abuse
		ii. Aortic dissection/coronary artery dissection
2. *Congenital coronary artery anomalies*	a) Aberrant anatomical origin (e.g. left coronary artery from anterior (right) sinus of Valsalva)	
	b) Coronary arteriovenous fistulas	
	c) Coronary artery aneurysms	
3. *Myocardial oxygen demand–supply disproportion*	a) Aortic stenosis (congenital and acquired)	
	b) Aortic insufficiency	
	c) Carbon monoxide poisoning	
	d) Thyrotoxicosis	
	e) Prolonged hypotension	
	f) Anaemia	

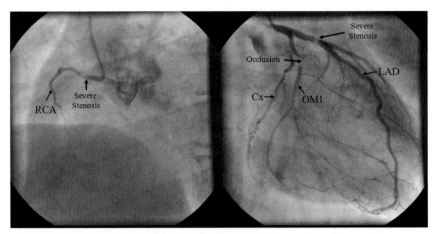

Fig. 5.3 Coronary angiogram demonstrating severe coronary artery disease. The coronary angiograms demonstrate a non-dominant, severely diseased RCA, a dominant circumflex coronary artery with an occluded large OM1 that filled via collaterals, and a tight proximal LAD artery stenosis.

Further reading

INTERHEART Study Investigators Yusuf S, Hawken S, Ounpuu S, Dans T, Avezum A, Lanas F *et al.* (2004). Effect of potentially modifiable risk factors associated with myocardial infarction in 52 countries (the INTERHEART study): case–control study. *Lancet*; **364**: 937–952.

The Task Force on the Management of Stable Angina Pectoris of the European Society of Cardiology Fox K, Garcia MA, Ardissino D, Buszman P, Camici PG, Crea F, Daly C, De Backer G, Hjemdahl P, Lopez-Sendon J, Marco J, Motais J, Pepper J, Sechtem U, Simoons M, Thygesen K, Priori SG, Blanc JJ, Budaj A, Camm J, Dean V, Deckers J, Dickstein K, Lekakis J, Mc Gregor K, Metra M, Morais J, Osterspey A, Tamargo J, Zamorano JL. (2006). Guidelines on the management of stable angina pectoris. *Eur Heart J*; **27**: 1341–1381.

Fletcher GF, Balady GJ, Amsterdam EA, Chaitman B, Eckel R, Fleg J, Froelicher VF, Leon AS, Piña IL, Rodney R, Simons-Morton D, Williams MA, Bazzarre T. (2001). Exercise standards for testing and training: a statement for healthcare professionals from the American Heart Association. *Circulation*;**104**: 1694–1740.

Mirza A. (2003). Myocardial infarction resulting from nonatherosclerotic coronary artery diseases. *Am J Emerg Med*; **21**: 578–584.

Case 6

A 31-year-old visiting Chinese post-doctoral student was found collapsed in his room by his landlady. He had been unwell with flu-like symptoms for the previous 2 days. He was conscious but drowsy and was clutching his chest complaining of pain. She called for help and a paramedic ambulance crew were on the scene 10 minutes later.

They found him still in pain, drowsy, and peripherally shut down, with a Glasgow coma score (GCS) of 14/15, BP of 90/70 mmHg, a regular tachycardia of 115 bpm, a respiratory rate of 30 per minute and saturation of 100% on high-flow oxygen.

The paramedics performed a 12 lead ECG (Fig. 6.1) and gave him loading doses of aspirin and clopidogrel. An intravenous cannula was sited and bolus thrombolytic was administered. Intravenous opiates were required for ongoing pain, and he remained tachypnoeic, hypotensive, and tachycardic. Intravenous fluids were started and he was rapidly transferred to the nearest ED.

On arrival in hospital the emergency team performed another ECG (Fig. 6.2) as he was still in pain. Blood was drawn for routine tests and a blood gas was sent. The chest X-ray was normal.

The team considered re-thrombolysis but wanted a cardiology opinion before proceeding. While the cardiology registrar was on his way the blood results in Table 6.1 were obtained and the emergency team gave an intravenous bolus of a medication and started an infusion based on these results.

When the cardiology registrar arrived, the patient was less drowsy and further history was forthcoming: he had diabetes and hypertension and smoked 20 cigarettes per day. His regular medications were insulin and ramipril.

The cardiology registrar requested another 12 lead ECG (Fig. 6.3). As this was being performed he noticed three small blisters with an erythematous base below the left axilla.

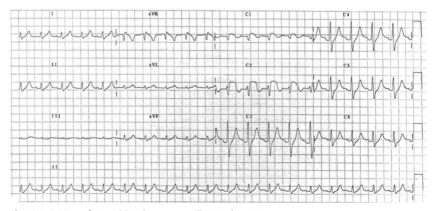

Fig. 6.1 ECG performed by the paramedics at the scene.

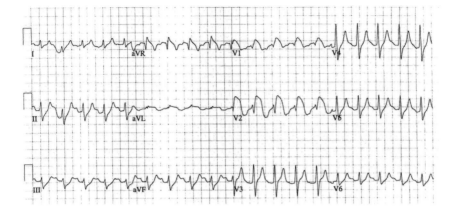

Fig. 6.2 ECG on arrival in the ED.

Table 6.1 Results of arterial blood gas analysis

Arterial blood gas		Biochemistry		Haematology	
pH	7.29	Na	136 mmol/L	Hb	14.2 g/dL
PaCO$_2$	3.4 kPa	K	Haemolysed		
PaO$_2$	35.2 kPa	Glucose	18.9		
HCO$_3^-$	12 mmol/L				
BE	−16 mmol/L				

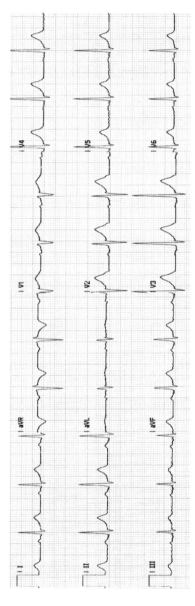

Fig. 6.3 ECG performed by cardiology registrar.

Questions

1. What is the differential diagnosis of the ECG abnormalities shown in Fig. 6.1?

2. What investigation should the paramedics have performed before initiating treatment?

3. What diagnosis had the paramedics made? Do you agree with their management?

4. What treatment do you expect the ED team gave before the cardiology registrar arrived?

5. Report the ECG performed by the cardiology registrar in Fig. 6.3.

6. What are the correct diagnoses and management?

7. What may have caused the chest pain in this case? How would you confirm this?

Answers

1) **What is the differential diagnosis of the ECG abnormalities shown in Fig. 6.1?**

The ECG recorded by the paramedics at the scene shown in Fig. 6.1 demonstrates sinus tachycardia at a rate of 120 bpm. There is ST segment elevation in V1 (2 mm) and V2 (4 mm), with T-wave inversion. There are tall T waves in the rest of the precordial leads. The axis is normal and there is no QRS duration prolongation. The PR interval is at the upper limit of normal.

These findings are consistent with an anterior ST elevation MI. However, ST segment changes do not always represent ischaemia or the ECG pattern of myocardial injury. Other causes of ST segment elevation are listed in Table 6.2.

Table 6.2 Most frequent causes of ST segment elevation other than coronary artery disease

Normal variants	Chest abnormalities
	Early repolarization
	High vagal tone
Racial variants	
Athletes	ST segment elevation can occur with or without negative T waves (need to exclude hypertrophic cardiomyopathy)
Pericarditis	Acute pericarditis (early stages)
	Myopericarditis
Pulmonary embolism	
Hyperkalaemia	Tall peaked T waves are more common than ST segment elevation
Hypothermia	
Brugada's syndrome	
Arrhythmogenic right ventricular cardiomyopathy	
Dissecting aortic aneurysm	
Left pneumothorax	
Coronary artery spasm	Cocaine abuse

After complete coronary occlusion, the ECG pattern of subendocardial ischaemia appears first (increase in T-wave amplitude due to delay in repolarization), followed by sub-epicardial ischaemia (flattened or negative T waves are observed). With increasing degrees of ischaemia the pattern of injury starts to appear (ST-segment elevation). The onset of necrosis is characterized by the development of a Q-wave pattern.

Several other conditions can also affect T-wave morphology. The most frequent causes of a hyperacute T waves are summarized in Table 6.3, and those of negative

Table 6.3 Causes of a hyperacute T wave besides IHD

Normal variants: vagotonia, athletes, elderly
Alcoholism
Moderate LV hypertrophy in heart diseases with diastolic overload
Stroke
Hyperkalaemia
Advanced AV block (tall and peaked T wave in the narrow QRS complex escape rhythm)

or flattened T waves in Table 6.4. Note that normal T waves are usually in the same direction as the QRS complex except in the right precordial leads (V1, V2). Normal T waves are always upright in leads I, II, and V3–6, and are always inverted in lead aVR.

Pathological Q waves are defined as being either 25% or more of the height of the succeeding R wave; and/or ≥0.04 seconds in width (1 small square) and ≥2 mm in depth. Q waves fitting this definition may still not be pathological in lead III if there are no accompanying pathological Q waves in aVF and II. Q waves present in lead III alone often disappear on deep inspiration. Although the specificity of pathological Q waves for diagnosing MI is high, similar Q waves can be seen in other conditions (Table 6.5). The pattern of ischaemia or injury accompanying a pathological Q wave is supportive of the Q wave being secondary to IHD. However, in 5–25% of Q-wave infarctions (with the highest incidence in inferior wall infarction) the Q wave disappears with time, hence the poor sensitivity of Q waves in old MI.

Table 6.4 Causes of negative or flattened T waves besides ischaemic heart disease

Normal variants	◆ Children
	◆ Black race
	◆ Hyperventilation
	◆ Females
Pericarditis	
Cor pulmonale and pulmonary embolism	
Myocarditis and cardiomyopathies	
Alcoholism	
Stroke	
Myxoedema	
Athletes	
Medications	◆ Amiodarone
	◆ Thioridizine

(Continued)

Table 6.4 (continued) Causes of negative or flattened T waves besides ischaemic heart disease

Hypokalaemia	
Post-tachycardia	
Left ventricular hypertrophy	
Left bundle branch block	
Post-intermittent depolarization abnormalities ('electrical memory')	◆ Pacemakers ◆ WPW syndrome ◆ LBBB

Table 6.5 Pathological Q wave not secondary to myocardial infarction

Acute pattern	a. Acute myocarditis	
	b. Pulmonary embolism	
	c. Cardiotoxic chemical agents	
Chronic pattern	a. Recording artefact	
	b. Normal variants	◆ aVL in the vertical heart ◆ III in the dextro-rotated and horizontal heart
	c. Qs in V1	◆ Septal fibrosis ◆ Emphysema
	d. Right ventricular hypertrophy (chronic cor pulmonale)	
	e. Left ventricular hypertrophy	
	f. Hypertrophic cardiomyopathy	
	g. Dilated cardiomyopathy	
	h. Infiltrative processes	◆ Amyloidosis ◆ Sarcoidosis ◆ Cardiac tumours ◆ Chronic myocarditis
	i. WPW syndrome	
	j. Dextrocardia	

2) **What investigation should the paramedics have performed before initiating treatment?**

   In patients presenting with reduced conscious states blood glucose estimation is mandatory. Bedside testing for ketones is also possible and may have helped in the diagnosis of this patient.

3) **What diagnosis had the paramedics made? Do you agree with their management?**

The paramedics made a diagnosis of anterior myocardial infarction based on the history of chest pain and the initial ECG findings. Pre-hospital thrombolysis is recommended by the treatment algorithms used by the paramedics. However, given the overall clinical picture, MI does not explain all the clinical features of this case and so delaying thrombolysis until full assessment in hospital may have been preferable.

4) **What treatment do you expect the ED team gave before the cardiology registrar arrived?**

The blood gas analysis showed a metabolic acidosis with a raised glucose level. This suggests the alternative diagnosis of diabetic ketoacidosis. Although the sample was haemolysed, the ECG changes seen in this context should suggest a possible non-ischaemic cause for the ST elevation, with the most likely being hyperkalaemia. Indeed, the blood gas was repeated and the potassium was raised at 5.8 mmol/L. In addition, high levels of ketones were present on blood and urine analysis at the bedside.

Management of hyperkalaemia: urgent treatment is required if:

A. serum potassium ≥7 mmol/L

B. hyperkalaemia (>5.5 mmol/L) accompanied by ECG changes or symptoms.

Hyperkalaemia should be managed by:

I   Cardioprotective measures:

  ◆ Calcium reduces cardiac membrane excitability.

  ◆ Calcium gluconate or calcium chloride given i.v.; if hyperkalaemic ECG changes present (Table 6.6).

  ◆ Onset of cardioprotection is immediate but duration of action is only a few minutes, so serum potassium must be reduced rapidly.

  ◆ Be aware that hypercalcaemia potentiates the myocardial toxicity of digoxin and intravenous calcium should be administered slowly in digitalized patients.

II Prevention of further accumulation of K$^+$:

  ◆ Drugs which cause hyperkalaemia should be stopped immediately [e.g. angiotensin-converting enzyme (ACE) inhibitors, angiotensin receptor blockers, potassium-sparing diuretics (e.g. spironolactone, amiloride), non-steroidal anti-inflammatory drugs (NSAIDS) and potassium-containing laxatives (e.g. Movicol®, Klean-Prep®, and Fybogel®)].

  ◆ Consider stopping beta-blockers and digoxin as they prevent intracellular buffering of potassium and reduce the effectiveness of insulin and beta-2 agonists.

III Redistribution into cells:

- ◆ If patients are hypovolaemic fluid resuscitation will improve acid base status and hyperkalaemia.
- ◆ Intracellular uptake of potassium can be increased by insulin:
  - binds specific membrane receptors and stimulates the sodium–potassium adenosine triphosphatase (ATP) pump
  - although uraemia can attenuate the hypoglycaemic response to insulin it does not affect the hypokalaemic action
  - the onset of the hypokalaemic effect is within 15 minutes, lasts for around 60 minutes and reduces plasma potassium 0.65–1.0 mmol/L.
- ◆ Salbutamol indirectly activates the Na^+K^+ ATP pump increasing intracellular K^+ uptake:
  - reduces plasma potassium 0.8–1.5 mmol/L within around 30 minutes
  - if IHD is present or suspected the tachycardia produced by salbutamol is undesirable.

IV Elimination of K^+ from the body:

- ◆ Other strategies to reduce plasma potassium are to encourage renal loss or prevent further gastrointestinal (GI) absorption.
- ◆ Loop diuretics such as furosemide produce a direct kaliuresis and promote renal loss of potassium both acutely and in the long term.
- ◆ Polystyrene sulfonate (e.g. calcium resonium) is a binding resin that binds K within the intestine and can help in the medium term to prevent recurrent episodes of hyperkalaemia by reducing intestinal absorption and increasing removal from the body by defecation.
- ◆ The definitive and most effective treatment for hyperkalaemia is haemodialysis or haemofiltration. It is indicated in patients who are anuric or if hyperkalaemia is resistant to medical treatment. Rapid reduction in potassium by as much as 1.2–1.5 mmol/L is possible in the first hour.

Table 6.6 ECG changes associated with hyperkalaemia

Approximate level of hyperkalaemia (mmol/L)	Associated ECG changes
6–7	Tall T waves >5 mm
	Small broad P waves
	Absent P waves
	ST elevation
7–8	Wide QRS complex
8–9	Sinusoidal QRST
	Atrio-ventricular dissociation
>9	Ventricular tachycardia/fibrillation

5) **Report the ECG performed by the cardiology registrar in Fig. 6.3.**

The ECG performed after the arrival of the cardiology registrar demonstrates that the ST segment elevation seen in Figs 6.1 and 6.2 has resolved. However, the tall and tented T waves in the anterior leads persist. This may signify that although the hyperkalaemia has been reduced, further treatment is required.

6) **What are the correct diagnoses and management?**

The correct diagnosis is diabetic ketoacidosis with hyperkalaemia and dehydration. Further questioning revealed that the patient had had influenzal symptoms and his supply of insulin had run out.

The effects of the hyperkalaemia were countered by rehydration with intravenous 0.9% saline and treatment with a bolus of insulin and 50% dextrose. The hyperkalaemia and ECG abnormalities resolved completely with these measures. Urinary ketones were 4+. The patient was fluid resuscitated and an insulin infusion was started. Subsequent troponin levels were normal.

It is important to be aware of differential diagnoses that can masquerade as ACS. Inadequate assessment can result in a cascade of potentially harmful management decisions. The authors' practice is to perform venous blood gas and electrolyte analysis prior to administration of antiplatelet agents, anticoagulation, or thrombolysis. In this way acidosis, anaemia, hyperglycaemia, and electrolyte abnormalities can often be excluded within 2 minutes.

7) **What may have caused the chest pain in this case? How would you confirm this?**

In this case, the chest pain was probably due to reactivation of varicella zoster virus, causing shingles, which would explain the vesicles below the left axilla found on examination. The diagnosis of shingles is usually clinical based on a prodromal history of characteristic neuropathic pain and the subsequent appearance of a characteristic dermatomal vesicular rash. If the diagnosis is uncertain, culture of vesicle fluid, electron microscopy, and immunofluorescence of vesicle fluid or detection of viral DNA in vesicle fluid using polymerase chain reaction (PCR) may be used to confirm the presence of the *Varicella zoster virus*.

The diagnosis of acute anterior myocardial infarction was clearly in doubt from the beginning. Transthoracic echocardiography (TTE) can facilitate the early assessment of such patients. The interruption of coronary flow initially causes ventricular diastolic dysfunction and then systolic dysfunction with regional wall motion abnormalities; the chest pain and ECG abnormalities associated with ischaemia develop subsequently. The regional wall motion abnormalities correspond closely to the affected coronary artery territories.

Echocardiography has a diagnostic sensitivity of approximately 90–95%, and a high negative predictive value (approximately 95%), but the positive predictive value is low and more variable. This may partly relate to interpretation difficulties in the presence of previous myocardial infarction and aggressive interpretation of minor abnormalities by physicians anxious to avoid false negatives.

Further reading

Wang K, Asinger RW, Marriott HJ (2003). ST-segment elevation in conditions other than acute myocardial infarction. *N Engl J Med*; **349**: 2128–2135.

American Heart Association Electrocardiography and Arrhythmias Committee, Council on Clinical Cardiology; American College of Cardiology Foundation; Heart Rhythm Society, Wagner GS, Macfarlane P, Wellens H, Josephson M, Gorgels A, Mirvis DM *et al.* (2009). AHA/ACCF/HRS recommendations for the standardization and interpretation of the electrocardiogram: part VI: acute ischemia/infarction: a scientific statement from the American Heart Association Electrocardiography and Arrhythmias Committee, Council on Clinical Cardiology; the American College of Cardiology Foundation; and the Heart Rhythm Society. *J Am Coll Cardiol*; **53**: 1003–1011.

Khanna A, White WB (2009). The management of hyperkalemia in patients with cardiovascular disease. *Am J Med*; **122**: 215–221.

Case 7

A 50-year-old man with hypertension and a recent history of crescendo chest pains on exertion called for an ambulance when he developed severe crushing central chest pain at rest. The pain radiated into his jaw and down both arms.

The paramedics found him to be in pain, sweaty, clammy, and peripherally shut down. They gave sublingual glyceryl trinitrate (GTN), but this did not relieve the symptoms. Because the pain had now been present for over 1 hour, a clinical diagnosis of MI was made.

A loading dose of aspirin and clopidogrel was given. An ECG recorded at the scene (Fig. 7.1) was transmitted to the coronary care unit (CCU) at the heart attack centre. The ECG was reviewed by a member of the primary angioplasty team, who advised urgent transfer to the ED rather than triggering direct transfer to the catheter laboratory.

On arrival at the ED another ECG was recorded (Fig. 7.2). Examination found a regular pulse of 80 bpm, a BP of 110/70 mmHg that was equal in both arms, O_2 saturations of 98% on air and a respiratory rate of 20 breaths per minute. There were no signs of heart failure and auscultation of the heart and lungs was normal. There was no calf swelling. There was no mediastinal widening on chest X-ray. He was reviewed by the cardiology registrar on call, who recorded an ECG from leads positioned posteriorly (Fig. 7.3).

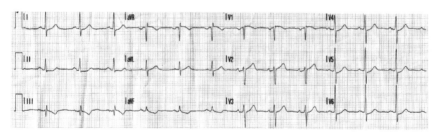

Fig. 7.1 ECG recorded at the scene by paramedics.

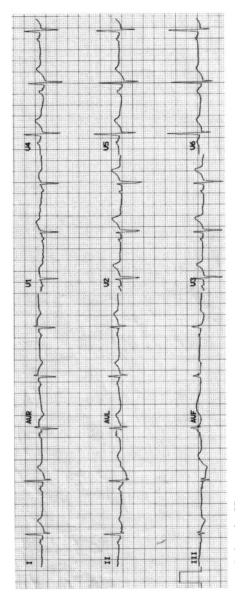

Fig. 7.2 ECG on arrival at the ED.

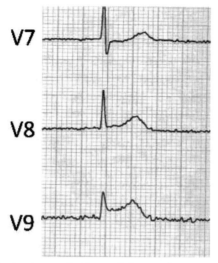

Fig. 7.3 Three posterior leads recorded by cardiology registrar.

Questions

1. Report the ECG in Fig. 7.1. Was the decision to divert the patient correct?
2. Report the ECG in Fig. 7.2.
3. How are the ECG tracings in Fig. 7.3 obtained and what do they show?
4. What bedside test could be performed to support the ECG findings?
5. How should the patient be managed?
6. What was the cause of the initial ECG discrepancy?

Answers

1) **Report the ECG in Fig. 7.1. Was the decision to divert the patient correct?**

   The ECG performed at the scene (Fig. 7.1) shows sinus rhythm at a rate of 78 bpm, with a normal axis and PR/QRS duration. There is 1-mm ST segment depression in leads II and augmented vector foot (aVF), and possibly lead III. There are no formal criteria met for an ECG diagnosis of an ST elevation MI. Although localized, isolated inferior ST segment depression is sometimes associated with epicardial coronary artery occlusion, and has been reported in the context of antero-lateral papillary muscle infarction, it usually indicates regional subendocardial ischaemia. Hence, the decision to divert the patient to the ED was reasonable.

   It is important to note that, in contrast, widespread (≥6 leads) isolated ST segment depression (≥1 mm) is highly specific for coronary occlusion and transmural infarction (96.5%), suggesting left main stem involvement. In addition, localized, isolated ST depression in V2–3 can be due to circumflex artery occlusion and posterior wall transmural infarction. Finally, any ST depression can be associated with non-occlusive coronary events with partial thickness infarction and is a high-risk marker in NSTEMI (see Case 37 for discussion of risk stratification).

2) **Report the ECG in Fig. 7.2.**

   The ECG recorded on admission to the ED in Fig. 7.2 demonstrates sinus rhythm at a rate of 65 bpm, with a normal axis and PR/QRS duration. There is minor (<1 mm) ST depression in III and aVF with T-wave inversion. There are no pathological Q waves. The differential diagnosis includes the spectrum of acute coronary syndromes (ACSs) and possibly other acute diagnoses such as aortic dissection but the subtle changes in V1 between the first (Fig. 7.1) and second (Fig. 7.2) traces, where the T wave is now upright, suggest a posterior wall coronary event.

3) **How are the ECG tracings in Fig. 7.3 obtained and what do they show?**

   The posterior leads (V7–9) are recorded from three electrodes lateral to V6. V7 is recorded from an electrode placed in the posterior axillary line in the 6th intercostal space. V9 is recorded from an electrode placed beneath the tip of the scapula in the 6th intercostal space. The V8 electrode is placed midway between the V7 and V9 electrodes. These leads record the potentials over the far lateral aspect of the LV. Figure 7.3 demonstrates increasing ST elevation from V7 to V9 (>2 mm). The most likely diagnosis is a posterior wall MI.

4) **What bedside test could be performed to support the ECG findings?**

   Transthoracic echocardiography can be used to detect regional wall motion abnormalities. In this case, TTE demonstrated a large akinetic but unthinned posterio-lateral wall suggestive of an acute transmural MI in the circumflex territory.

5) **How should the patient be managed?**

   The patient was treated with loading doses of aspirin and clopidogrel; a bolus of intravenous heparin was given. He was then consented and transferred to the

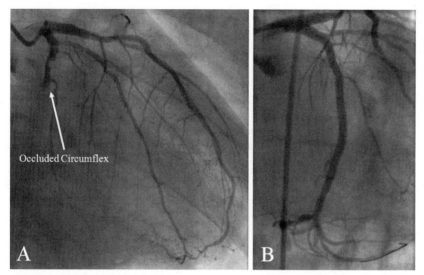

Fig. 7.4 Emergency angiogram. The right anterior oblique (RAO) view shows an occlusion of the proximal circumflex coronary artery (A). This was successfully reopened and the vessel stented (B). STEMI is due to acute intracoronary thrombotic occlusion. Treatment strategies have developed to provide rapid, complete, and lasting restoration of coronary blood flow.

catheter laboratory for emergency angiography. This demonstrated an occluded circumflex coronary artery (Fig. 7.4). The artery was reopened and stented, the patient's symptoms resolved and the ECG returned to normal. Peak cardiac troponin I was 15 ng/mL.

Fibrinolytics

The landmark trials of fibrinolytic therapy were conducted in the mid 1980s (GISSI-1 and ISIS-2) and demonstrated a 23% reduction in 30-day mortality in patients randomized to streptokinase (9.8% vs 12.4% events; odds ratio (OR) 0.77; 95% confidence interval (CI) 0.72–0.83). These results were confirmed in nine further trials, but fibrinolysis was also associated with a small but significant excess risk of intracranial haemorrhage (0.4% vs 0.1% events). Accelerated or front-loaded alteplase reduced mortality by a further 15% compared to streptokinase (GUSTO-1: 6.3% vs 7.3% events; OR 0.85; 95% CI 0.78–0.94) but the risk of intracranial haemorrhage was slightly higher (0.7% vs 0.5% events). Pre-hospital fibrinolysis reduced mortality by 18% at 30 days when compared with in-hospital treatment.

Bolus fibrinoytics, although more suitable for pre-hospital use, have no additional benefit over accelerated alteplase on 30-day mortality. However, in one trial patients treated with one particular bolus agent, tenecteplase (ASSENT-2), had a lower rate of intracerebral haemorrhage (26.4% vs 29.0%) and need for blood transfusion (4.3% vs 5.5%).

Although fibrinolytics promote epicardial vessel patency, tissue perfusion is not always restored. The fibrin-rich components of the thrombus may be lysed, but platelet-rich areas are not, and these thrombus fragments promote distal micro-embolization and microvascular obstruction.

Adjunctive antiplatelet agents

Aspirin is associated with a 23% risk reduction in 35-day mortality (ISIS-2 9.4% vs 11.8% events; OR 0.77; 95% CI 0.70–0.85) and enhances the effect of fibrinolysis in ST elevation myocardial infarction (STEMI). Although more aggressive strategies with GP-IIb/IIIa inhibitors (GUSTO-5 and ASSENT-3 trials: abciximab) reduce re-infarction rate, mortality is not affected as the incidence of major bleeding complications is increased, particularly in the elderly (4.6% vs 2.4% events; OR 2.1; 95% CI 1.7–2.4).

Adjunctive heparin

Paradoxically, thrombin released after fibrinolysis of the thrombus induces a proco-agulant state, and so addition of low molecular weight heparin (LMWH; ASSENT-3 trial: enoxaparin) improved 30-day mortality and reduced re-infarction without significantly increasing the risk of bleeding complications. Direct thrombin inhibitors (e.g. bivalirudin) have similar benefits to LMWH but the incidence of bleeding complications is reduced.

Failed thrombolysis

Fibrinolysis does not restore coronary arterial patency in 20–45% of cases, and there is an associated 5–10% early and 30% late re-occlusion rate. Mechanical reperfusion by primary angioplasty is more likely to be successful and is associated with a signifi-cantly lower incidence of re-infarction, stroke, and intracranial haemorrhage (30% reduction in 30-day mortality compared with fibrinolysis).

In centres where angioplasty is not readily available, the issue of how failed throm-bolysis should be managed remains. The choice is between repeating thrombolysis and mechanical reperfusion strategies. Rescue PCI for STEMI allows mechanical reper-fusion after failed fibrinolysis. Epicardial blood flow may be restored whilst the myocar-dium is still viable. This improves long-term clinical outcomes (open-artery hypothesis). The REACT trial is the largest trial of rescue PCI. This nationwide trial compared rescue PCI with repeated fibrinolysis and conservative care in 427 patients. Percutaneous coronary intervention was performed for thrombolysis in myocardial infarction (TIMI) flow <3 in the presence of a coronary artery stenosis >50%. The primary endpoint was composite all-cause mortality, recurrent infarction, stroke, and heart failure at 6 months. This occurred in 15.3, 31, and 29.8% of patients, respectively ($P < 0.01$), with lower rates in the rescue PCI group being driven by a lower re-infarction rate.

Early reperfusion

The concept of the golden hour and the exponential loss of benefit with time are well established for fibrinolysis. The data for primary angioplasty are less clear. It may be that the loss of efficacy with time is less dramatic than with fibrinolytics, and equivalent results may be achievable even if primary angioplasty is delayed for up to 90 minutes. This may be due to the more effective restoration of vessel patency, less re-occlusion, and improved residual LV function without the potentially detrimental effects that thrombolysis may have on acutely infracted myocardium. Infrastructure and logistical challenges must be overcome to prevent delays in delivery of primary angioplasty, which is now the gold standard treatment for coronary occlusion with evidence for mortality reduction (compared to thrombolysis) up to 12 hours after ST elevation MI.

6) **What was the cause of the initial ECG abnormalities?**

This case demonstrates transmural infarction in the circumflex artery territory presenting with isolated inferior ST segment depression. The ECG changes seen in the standard leads are reciprocal, mirroring the ST segment elevation that was only visible when posterior leads (V7–V9) were recorded.

Further reading

Dabrowska B, Walczak E, Prejs R, Zdzienicki M. (1996). Acute infarction of the left ventricular papillary muscle: electrocardiographic pattern and recognition of its location. *Clin Cardiol*; **19**: 404–407.

Menown IB, Mackenzie G, Adjey AA. (2000). Optimizing the initial 12-lead electrocardiographic diagnosis of acute myocardial infarction. *Eur Heart J*; **21**: 275–283.

O'Keefe JH Jr, Sayed-Taha K, Gibson W, Christian TF, Bateman TM, Gibbons RJ. (1995). Do patients with left circumflex coronary artery-related acute myocardial infarction without ST-segment elevation benefit from reperfusion therapy? *Am J Cardiol*; **75**: 718–720.

Keeley EC, Boura JA, Grines CL. (2003) Primary angioplasty versus intravenous thrombolytic therapy for acute myocardial infarction: a quantitative review of 23 randomised trials. *Lancet*; **361**: 13–20.

The Task Force on the Management of ST-Segment Elevation Acute Myocardial Infarction of the European Society of Cardiology, Van de Werf F, Bax J, Betriu A *et al.* (2008). Management of acute myocardial infarction in patients presenting with persistent ST-segment elevation. *Eur Heart J*; **29**: 2909–2945.

Case 8

A 40-year-old heavy goods vehicle (HGV) driver was referred to the cardiology clinic for a Driver and Vehicle Licensing Agency (DVLA) assessment of fitness to drive Group 2 vehicles (public transport vehicles) because of a 6-month history of epigastric ache that was sometimes associated with exertion, particularly after eating. He had thought his symptoms were indigestion but went to see his GP when antacids failed to work. His risk factors for coronary disease were smoking, a total cholesterol of 6.4 mmol/L and a strong family history of IHD. He was not taking any medication and physical examination was unremarkable with a resting BP of 135/70 mmHg.

Resting ECG was normal and he completed 9 minutes of the full Bruce protocol ETT. His heart rate reached 162 bpm (90% of his age-predicted maximum heart rate). No symptoms or ECG changes occurred during the test or recovery period. The patient was reassured that he could continue driving his Group 2 HGV and was commenced on a proton pump inhibitor. He was given smoking cessation and dietary advice.

Whilst driving the next day, he developed his usual chest pain. In view of the advice he had received, he attempted to ignore these symptoms. However, he eventually presented to the ED 8 hours later as his symptoms had continued. An ECG revealed ST segment elevation in leads V2–V4 and thrombolysis with recombinant tissue plasminogen activator (rtPA) was given.

The ECG changes had normalized by 90 minutes. Peak troponin I was 0.5 ng/mL and creatinine kinase was 110 iu/dL, and an echocardiogram demonstrated preserved systolic function with no regional wall motion abnormalities. However, subsequent coronary angiography demonstrated a critical stenosis of the LAD artery that was treated with a 3.5 × 28 mm drug-eluting coronary stent.

Questions

1. What are the current UK DVLA guidelines for the assessment of Group 2 licence holders with suspected IHD?

2. What is the sensitivity and specificity of exercise treadmill testing?

3. What alternative non-invasive modalities exist and how do they compare?

4. What is the role of angiography in the DVLA guidelines for the investigation of chest pain?

Answers

1) **What are the current UK DVLA guidelines for the assessment of Group 2 licence holders with suspected IHD?**

   Group 2 vehicles include large lorries (category C) and buses (category D). The DVLA medical standards for Group 2 drivers are higher than those for Group 1 (motor cars and motor cycles) because of the size and weight of the vehicles involved and the length of time spent at the wheel.

   When Group 2 drivers present with chest pain careful and thorough assessment is required. Exercise testing should be performed on a treadmill or bicycle. To retain their Group 2 licence drivers must complete three stages of the standard Bruce protocol or equivalent safely. There should be no signs of cardiovascular dysfunction or ST segment shift indicative of myocardial ischaemia (usually >2 mm horizontal or down-sloping) during exercise or the recovery period.

   Those who cannot exercise will require a gated myocardial perfusion scan, stress echo study, and/or specialist cardiological opinion.

   Anti-anginal medication (nitrates, beta-blockers, calcium channel blockers, nicorandil, ivabradine, and ranolazine) should be stopped 48 hours prior to the exercise test. However, any of these drugs prescribed purely for control of hypertension or an arrhythmia may be continued.

2) **What is the sensitivity and specificity of exercise treadmill testing?**

   Treadmill ETT during 12 lead ECG monitoring is a useful test to assess myocardial ischaemia in the majority of patients with suspected stable angina. However, in order to obtain maximal diagnostic information it should be conducted using a validated protocol with clear definitions of abnormal ECG changes (European Society of Cardiology(ESC)) guidelines: rectilinear or down-sloping ST-segment depression ≥0.1 mV (1 mm), persisting for at least 0.06–0.08 seconds after the J-point, in one or more ECG leads).

   It is important to continue to monitor the ECG during the recovery period after exercise (until heart rate <100 bpm). In about 15% of patients, diagnostic ST-segment changes may be limited to the recovery period only (see Case 5). The diagnostic and prognostic significance of recovery-limited ST changes is similar to that of ischaemic ST changes which develop during exercise. Other significant abnormalities that may occur during the recovery period include a delayed fall in heart rate at 1 minute (<12–18 bpm), delayed fall in systolic BP and frequent ventricular ectopics.

   Some meta-analyses have reported an average sensitivity and specificity of 68% and 75%, respectively, whereas others have suggested that the sensitivity may be lower (about 45%). Of note, if the threshold for a positive test is increased to ≥0.2 mV (2 mm), as suggested by the DVLA, then an increased specificity can be achieved, albeit at the expense of a decreased sensitivity (higher probability of a false-negative result). The sensitivity of exercise-induced ST-segment depression increases up to 90% if it is accompanied by typical angina pain.

Early ST depression, extensive lead involvement, and slow normalization after exercise are all suggestive of multi-vessel IHD. However, non-obstructive lesions or well-collateralized occlusions may not cause pathological ST depression on an ETT. The gold standard for diagnosing coronary artery disease (CAD) is the coronary angiogram. However, coronary spasm and microvascular dysfunction and significance may not be revealed by angiographic assessment of epicardial coronary anatomy. These limitations must be kept in mind when interpreting anatomical data in an individual.

The ETT has limited value in patients with basal ECG abnormalities, including LBBB, paced rhythm, or WPW syndrome, which precludes a correct interpretation of ST-segment changes. False-positive results are also more frequent in patients with resting ST-segment/T-wave abnormalities because of LV hypertrophy, electrolyte imbalance, or drug effects (e.g. digitalis).

An important issue with ETT is the diagnosis of obstructive IHD in women, in whom ST-segment depression has been found to have lower specificity (i.e. it is more often a false-positive result) than in men. However, when pre-test probability is accurately determined and patients with normal ECG at rest are selected, ETT probably has similar reliability in women and men.

Using the pre-test probability of CAD based on the age of the patient and the type of symptoms they present with (Table 8.1), a judgement on the likelihood of CAD after an ETT can be made (post-test probability). If we assume a sensitivity of 68% and a specificity of 77% for ETT (Table 8.2), then the likelihood of CAD after a positive ETT (positive likelihood ratio (+LR) = sensitivity/(1 – specificity)) is 3 and the negative likelihood ratio is 0.4 (–LR = (1 – sensitvity)/specificity). Hence, in this case, where the pre-test probability of CAD is 46% (~1:1), a positive ETT will increase this to a post-test probability of ~75% (3:1) and a negative test would reduce the likelihood of CAD to ~28% (0.4:1).

Table 8.1 Probability of important coronary disease among people with chest pain depending on age and symptoms

Age	Non-anginal chest pain		Atypical chest pain		Typical chest pain	
	Men (%)	Women (%)	Men (%)	Women (%)	Men (%)	Women (%)
30–39	5	1	22	4	70	26
40–49	14	3	46	13	87	55
50–59	21	8	59	32	92	79
60–69	28	19	67	54	94	91

3) **What alternative non-invasive modalities exist and how do they compare?**

Information about the functional status of the myocardium and the presence of ischaemia can be obtained non-invasively by several methods. Their sensitivity and specificity for detecting coronary disease differ (Table 8.2).

Myocardial perfusion scintigraphy is able to assess myocardial perfusion given that regions of myocardial ischaemia have reduced isotope uptake at peak exercise on a treadmill or bicycle that is reversible at rest. The perfusion tracers used include Thallium-201 and Technetium-99m labelled sestamibi or tetrofosmin. Whilst exercise myocardial scintigraphy is as specific as an ECG-guided ETT for cardiac ischaemia, scintigraphy is more sensitive (up to 91%). Scintigraphy is expensive and time-consuming and so is not a cost-effective alternative to ETT. However, scintigraphy is indicated if the resting ECG renders ETT uninterpretable (see above) or the results of ECG-guided ETT are inconclusive, or for detection of the location and extent of myocardial ischaemia. In those unable to exercise conventionally, pharmacological stress is an alternative and produces similar diagnostic accuracy to exercise. Dobutamine, a sympathetic agonist, simulates physical exercise by increasing myocardial oxygen consumption. Dipyridamole and adenosine are arteriolar vasodilators that work by revealing areas where the vasodilator response is attenuated by atherosclerosis and causing a coronary steal syndrome where blood is diverted away from these areas. In general, exercise is to be preferred when possible as this most closely reproduces the exercise levels associated with real-life activities.

Stress echocardiography is a well-established test for detecting myocardial ischaemia. It provides an anatomical and functional assessment of the heart through the detection of stress-induced reversible regional LV wall motion abnormalities. It is also widely available and is without radiation exposure. However, it can be limited by poor image quality (15% of patients) and image acquisition, and interpretation is considerably operator dependent. Ischaemia may be harder to detect when basal LV wall motion abnormalities exist. Pharmacological stress is used more frequently than exercise in echocardiography and the sensitivity of exercise and dobutamine stress echocardiography for the diagnosis of obstructive CAD is similar, with dipyridamole stress echocardiography being lower and specificity being similar.

Table 8.2 Sensitivities and specificities of non-invasive investigations for CAD for the assessment of chest pain patients with stable symptoms

Investigation	Sensitivity (%)	Specificity (%)
ECG-guided ETT – threshold ST depression = ≥1.0mV (1mm)	68	77
Treadmill stress echocardiography	97	64
Bicycle stress echocardiography	91	77
Dobutamine stress echocardiography	93	62
Exercise single photon emission computed tomography (SPECT) imaging	89	75
Vasodilator stress (adenosine or dipyridamole) SPECT imaging	87	73

4) **What is the role of angiography in the DVLA guidelines for the investigation of chest pain?**

For DVLA licensing purposes the functional effect of coronary disease is considered more significant than coronary artery anatomy. Stress tests are the relevant investigations for licensing purposes. It is the normal requirement that the standard of one or other of these must be met. Angiography is therefore not required for relicensing purposes. However, if the results of functional tests and recent coronary angiography conflict, relicensing will not normally be considered unless there are no flow-limiting coronary artery stenoses and the LV ejection fraction is at least 40%.

Further reading

Drivers Medical Group, DVLA. Cardiovascular disorders. In *At a Glance Guide to the Current Medical Standards of Fitness to Drive – A Guide for Medical Practitioners* Aug 2010. http://www.dvla.gov.uk/medical/ataglance.aspx, pp 19–27.

Fox K, Garcia MA, Ardissino D, Buszman P, Camici PG, Crea F, Daly C, De Backer G, Hjemdahl P, Lopez-Sendon J, Marco J, Morais J, Pepper J, Sechtem U, Simoons M, Thygesen K, Priori SG, Blanc JJ, Budaj A, Camm J, Dean V, Deckers J, Dickstein K, Lekakis J, McGregor K, Metra M, Morais J, Osterspey A, Tamargo J, Zamorano JL; Task Force on the Management of Stable Angina Pectoris of the European Society of Cardiology; ESC Committee for Practice Guidelines (CPG) (2006). Guidelines on the management of stable angina pectoris: executive summary; The Task Force on the Management of Stable Angina Pectoris of the European Society of Cardiology. (2006). *Eur Heart J*; **27**: 1341–1381.

Jelinek M, Barraclough K. (2009) Chest pain. *BMJ*; **339**: 1083–1085.

Case 9

A 75-year-old retired male librarian presented with an 8-hour history of dull central chest pain radiating to his jaw, sweating, and palpitations. The pain was not positional or pleuritic, and did not improve with sublingual nitrates. He had sustained several NSTEMIs over the past 2 years, the last of which was only 2 weeks prior to this presentation. He denied exertional chest pains in the intervening period but was short of breath on moderate exertion (NYHA II). He was not diabetic, and he had a total cholesterol of 4.4 mmol/L and triglycerides of 1 mmol/L. His brother had recently died of an MI (aged 66 years). It was difficult to elicit any further history as he was deaf. However, he had brought a copy of the discharge summary from the admission 2 weeks previously (Fig. 9.1).

Examination revealed a BP of 170/95 mmHg that was equal in both arms, a regular pulse of 70 bpm, O_2 saturations of 98% on air, and respiratory rate 18 per minute. Heart sounds and peripheral pulses were normal. There was no evidence of cardiac failure. The pain was not reproducible with sternal pressure. Figure 9.2 shows the admission ECG. Blood tests on admission revealed a raised cTnI at 84 ng/mL (normal range <0.4 ng/mL), a serum creatinine of 130 μmol/L, a C-reactive protein (CRP) of 1 mg/dL, a haemoglobin (Hb) of 12 g/dL, and a D-dimer of 75 μg/L. The chest X-ray was unremarkable. There were no regional wall motion abnormalities or structural abnormalities on transthoracic echocardiography (TTE).

Discharge Summary

Reason for admission: NSTEMI	Allergies: NKDA
Past medical history	Medication on discharge
Several NSTEMIs over the past 2 years	aspirin 75mg od
Paroxysmal AF	clopidogrel 75mg od
Hypertension	amiloride 5mg od
Deaf	Co-tenidone (atenolol & chlorthalidone) 50/12.5 T od,
Renal impairment (creatinine 125µmol/L)	fluvastatin 20mg nocte
	omeprazole 20mg od

Relevant Background History

The patient was initially admitted to his local district general hospital (DGH) with palpitations and chest pain 2 years ago. He was diagnosed with AF and although there was no Troponin rise (cardiac Troponin I; cTnI < 0.01 ng/ml) he was transferred to the regional centre for coronary angiography which was normal. He was subsequently readmitted to the DGH with similar symptoms on several occasions, but because cTnI results were negative, no further cardiac investigations were performed.

A year later, after initially presenting to the DGH, he was again transferred to the regional centre with identical symptoms. The cTnI was raised (10.2 ng/ml) and angiography demonstrated moderate atheromatous disease in the LAD with no flow limitation. A diagnosis of NSTEMI was made and he was managed medically. He was readmitted 2 weeks later with another NSTEMI (cTnI 16.8 ng/ml). Coronary angiography with intravascular ultrasound excluded flow limiting disease. Provocation testing failed to elicit vasospasm. One month later, on his 3rd admission to the regional centre with a NSTEMI, cTnI was 29 ng/ml. Cardiac MRI demonstrated a structurally normal heart. There was no perfusion defect on stress imaging. He was discharged with medical management.

Current Admission

On this admission to the regional centre (3 months after his last admission) his symptoms of chest pain and palpitations at rest were identical to those on previous admissions. Sinus rhythm was documented on telemetry throughout one episode of chest pain, sweats and palpitations. Although the cTnI was raised (39 ng/ml) his symptoms settled quickly and he was discharged after 24 hours of cardiac monitoring with cardiology outpatient follow-up. His medications were not changed. Cardiac MRI was performed as an outpatient. This was normal.

Results of investigations

cTnI 39 ng/ml (normal range < 0.4 ng/ml; >1 ng/ml diagnostic of MI)

ECG (during chest pain) sinus rhythm (rate 75 bpm), no acute ST segment or T wave changes

Chest x-ray was normal

Cardiac MRI was normal.

Follow-up

Cardiology outpatient follow-up appointment in 6 weeks

Fig. 9.1 Discharge summary from previous admission.

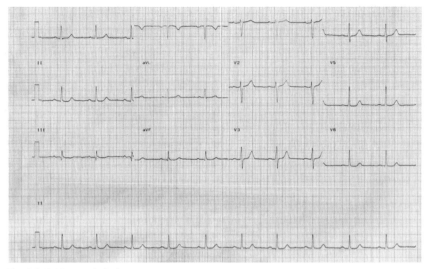

Fig. 9.2 ECG on admission.

Questions

1. Report the ECG.
2. Has this patient had an MI?
3. How is the assay for serum troponin levels performed in the laboratory?
4. Are the absolute values of cTnI results from the DGH and the regional centre comparable?
5. How do serum troponin levels change with time after an event that causes troponin release?
6. What can cause a rise in serum troponin? Which causes are relevant in this case?
7. What is the most likely cause of the raised troponin and how can this be confirmed?
8. How would you manage further admissions with chest pain?

Answers

1) **Report the ECG.**

   The resting ECG shows sinus rhythm at a rate of 60 bpm. The QRS axis is normal. There are no ST or T-wave abnormalities. The trace is within normal limits.

2) **Has this patient had an MI?**

   The patient's symptoms and the raised cTnI appear to support the diagnosis of NSTEMI. However, despite apparently having several NSTEMIs the patient's resting ECG, stress test, TTE, and cardiac magnetic resonance imaging (MRI) were all normal. It is unlikely that the patient has an ACS.

3) **How is the assay for serum troponin levels performed in the laboratory?**

   Enzyme-linked immuno sorbent assays (ELISA) for cTnI often employ two-site (sandwich) or competitive reactions that use two antibodies specific for two different cTnI epitopes. The first (capture) antibody binds cTnI in the sample. The second (label) is added after a wash phase and binds the captured cTnI. This provides a signal that can be used to quantify the cTnI concentration.

4) **Are the absolute values of cTnI results from the DGH and the regional centre comparable?**

   The cTnI results from different laboratories may not be comparable. Immunoassays for cTnI are available from several manufacturers and are not standardized. Some variability results from the antibodies used by different manufacturers, which target different cTnI epitopes. Proteolysis of cTnI produces several peptides. Some epitopes remain unchanged while others are lost or altered. The detected levels of cTnI vary between assays by factors of up to 100. However, only one assay for cTnT is available from Roche, so results from different laboratories are comparable.

   When using cTnI refer to the reference range from the laboratory that performed the assay.

5) **How do serum troponin levels change with time after an event that causes troponin release?**

   Cardiac troponins (cTnI and cTnT) are not usually detectable in the serum but are released into the circulation after cardiac strain or myocyte necrosis. Serum levels of cTn usually rise within 4–6 hours, peak at 12–24 hours, and remain elevated for 6–10 days (unless another event occurs). Troponin is cleared from the plasma by the reticulo-endothelial system or renally excreted.

   Results of a troponin immunoassay that suggest persistently high levels of serum troponin imply that either a high level of analyte (i.e. troponin) actually is present or there is analytical interference with the assay.

6) **What can cause a rise in serum troponin? Which causes are relevant in this case?**

Causes of a rise in serum troponin

Troponin consists of three single chain polypeptides which regulate muscle contraction: troponin C (binds Ca^{2+}), troponin I (binds actin-inhibiting actin–myosin interaction), and troponin T (binds tropomyosin and facilitates contraction). Cardiac muscle contains specific cTnI and cTnT isoforms. Most cTn is bound, but a small amount is free in the cytosol. The initial rise of cTn after myocyte damage is thought to be release of the unbound cytosolic cTn. This is followed by more prolonged appearance of troponin from damage to the myofilament structures.

In some conditions (e.g. unstable angina), membrane permeability is only transiently affected and cTn elevations return to baseline within a few hours. Factors released in sepsis and the inflammatory response could cause myocardial depression, degrade free cTn and increase cell membrane permeability, allowing systemic release of CTA without permanent myocyte necrosis.

Vasospasm (Prinzmetal angina), confirmed by provocation testing, is associated with troponin release in a quarter of patients. Similarly, excessive sympathetic activity induced by acute stroke or subarachnoid haemorrhage can induce coronary vasospasm and increase cTn in up to a quarter.

Demand ischaemia may also occur in the absence of CAD if myocardial oxygen demand exceeds supply. Myocardial oxygen demand increases with tachycardia, which may be caused by severe sepsis, septic shock (fall in systemic vascular resistance), hypotension or hypovolaemia, and tachyarrhythmias (e.g. AF). Oxygen supply is also reduced by tachycardia, which shortens diastole and the time available for myocardial perfusion. LV hypertrophy could cause occult subendocardial ischaemia due to the increased oxygen demand from increased muscle mass and decreased flow reserve due to remodelled coronary micro-circulation.

Trauma can damage myocytes directly. Serum cTn assays can be used to detect cardiac contusions or exclude significant myocardial injury following blunt chest trauma. Similarly, defibrillation or cardioversion from external pads or implantable cardioverter defibrillators (ICD) can release cTn.

Infiltrative disorders that cause extracellular deposits, such as amyloidosis, can compress and damage myocytes. Cardiac inflammation due to, for example, acute pericarditis, myocarditis, or the immune response after heart transplant can damage myocytes. In heart transplants, a chronically elevated troponin is a marker of poor prognosis.

The excessive wall tension occurring in ventricular volume or pressure loading has been associated with myofibrillary damage and troponin release even in the absence of myocardial ischaemia. In congestive cardiac failure there is a close correlation between troponin and B-type natriuretic peptide, a marker of right and left ventricular wall strain.

The release of cTn in ultra-endurance athletes may also be due to prolonged LV strain and sympathetic activation. cTn levels are increased in a third of cases with acute right-heart strain after pulmonary embolism and predicts increased mortality. Chronic right-heart strain due to pulmonary hypertension is associated with chronic cTn release in 10% and a significantly worse survival.

Troponins are cleared from the circulation by the reticulo-endothelial system or fragmented into molecules small enough to be renally excreted. The fragments of troponin containing the antibody binding sites will bind in the same way as the complete troponin molecule. Hence, chronic renal insufficiency is associated with a persistently elevated cardiac troponin level and for those with end-stage renal disease a higher troponin threshold for the diagnosis of coronary syndromes is required. In addition to the impaired excretion of cTn, renal failure is associated with clinically silent myocardial necrosis and increased LV mass, which may also contribute to the higher levels of cTn in these patients.

Many conditions can increase serum troponin (Table 9.1). The diagnostic and prognostic value of cTn is well established in those with a high pre-test probability of thrombotic CAD. However, if used to screen low-probability cases the positive predictive value is reduced. Thus, while a negative cTn can exclude ACS, a positive cTn is less useful as it not always specific.

Formulation of a differential diagnosis in this case

Occam's razor is 'plurality must not be posited without necessity', that is, several diagnoses should not be sought in place of one unifying diagnosis. Occam's razor suggests that a unifying diagnosis for the cause of the chest pain and the raised troponin should be sought, in which case the answer would be myocardial ischaemia. Although paroxysmal arrhythmias (e.g. AF or VT) can cause chest pain and increase cTnI (not usually to this degree), this was excluded on telemetry during the previous admission. Coronary artery vasospasm could also explain this presentation. However, an ECG recorded during an episode of chest pain was normal and vasospasm could not be provoked.

In contrast to Occam's razor, Hickam's dictum states that '*the patient can have as many diagnoses as they please*'. This suggests that a unifying diagnosis should not always be sought, especially where other diagnoses are more likely. However, in this patient alternative causes of raised troponin, including renal impairment (this could not cause the serum troponin levels seen in this case), chronic inflammation, thrombo-embolic disease, hypotension, shock, or sepsis, were not in evidence, and neither the symptoms nor the ECG were consistent with myopericarditis.

Table 9.1 Causes of raised serum troponin. There is no clear correlation between the cause of troponin rise and the serum level of troponin. The problem is compounded by the availability of several different assays for troponin. In some cases, the raised troponin may correlate with an increased risk of morbidity or mortality

	Diagnosis	Mechanism
1. Demand ischaemia	Sepsis/systemic inflammatory response syndrome	Myocardial depression/supply–demand mismatch
	Hypotension	Decreased perfusion pressure
	Hypovolaemia	Decreased filling pressure/output
	Tachyarrhythmia	Supply–demand mismatch
	Left ventricular hypertrophy	Subendocardial ischaemia

Table 9.1 (continued) Causes of raised serum troponin. There is no clear correlation between the cause of troponin rise and the serum level of troponin. The problem is compounded by the availability of several different assays for troponin. In some cases, the raised troponin may correlate with an increased risk of morbidity or mortality

	Diagnosis	**Mechanism**
2. **Myocardial ischaemia**	Coronary vasospasm	Prolonged ischaemia with myonecrosis
	Intracranial haemorrhage or stroke	Imbalance of autonomic nervous system
	Sympathomimetic agents, e.g. ephedrine	Direct adrenergic effects
3. **Direct myocardial damage**	Cardiac contusion	Traumatic
	DC cardioversion	Traumatic
	Cardiac infiltrative disorders	Myocyte compression
	Chemotherapy	Cardiac toxicity
	Myocarditis	Inflammatory
	Pericarditis	Inflammatory
	Cardiac transplantation	Inflammatory/immune mediated
4. **Myocardial strain**	Congestive heart failure	Myocardial wall stretch
	Pulmonary embolism	Right ventricular stretch
	Pulmonary hypertension or emphysema	Right ventricular stretch
	Strenuous exercise	Ventricular stretch
5. **Renal impairment**	All sub-types	Unknown
6. **False positive**	Analytical interference	Several (see Table 9.2)

Table 9.2 Causes of false-positive troponin results due to analytical interference

Cause of analytical interference with cTn immunoassay
Fibrin clots and micro-particles in sample
Heterophile antibodies
Human anti-animal antibodies
Rheumatoid factor
Bilirubin
Haemolysis
Lipaemia
Elevated alkaline phosphatase
Immune complex formation
Analyser malfunction

7) **What is the most likely cause of the raised troponin and how can this be confirmed?**

Sherlock Holmes stated that 'when you have eliminated the impossible, whatever remains, however improbable, must be the truth'. After exclusion of possible diagnoses, the only plausible explanation for the raised cTnI is a false-positive result. False positives depend on the manufacturer, the analyser, and the definition of a positive result. Therefore, the prevalence of false-positive cTnI results cannot be inferred from the literature but various studies have reported up to 3%.

Serum cTn is raised but if CK, CK muscle and brain isoenzyme (CK-MB), aspartate transaminase (AST) and myoglobin are normal the raised cTn is likely to be a false-positive result. Cardiac stress testing can also be considered. If negative for ischaemia this is reassuring and also suggests a false-positive cTn result. A false-positive cTn may be due to analytical interference with the immunoassay used. Causes of analytical interference are listed in Table 9.2.

In this case, a reference laboratory detected heterophile antibodies in the patient's serum. These are weak antibodies against poorly defined antigens that can bind multiple sites. Heterophile antibodies against the immunoglobulins of the animal antibodies used in the immunoassay can cause cross-linking in the absence of cTnI. When the assay was repeated after blocking the heterophile antibodies the cTnI was negative (<0.01 μg/L). When a different assay was used the cTnI was also negative. Different manufacturers use antibodies from different species, so specific heterophile antibodies will not affect all cTn assays. This explains the different cTnI results from the DGH and the regional centre.

8) **How would you manage further admissions with chest pain?**

CK-MB and myoglobin assays should be performed on any subsequent admissions with chest pain. A copy of these instructions, with a discharge summary, should be given to the patient.

In this case, the chest pain was thought to be due to peptic ulcer disease. The patient's symptoms improved with high-dose proton pump inhibitors and a gastric motility stimulant (metoclopramide). He was discharged home with gastroenterology outpatient follow-up and has not been readmitted to hospital. See Case 36 for a discussion of non-cardiac chest pain.

Further reading

Burness CE, Beacock D, Channer KS. (2005). Pitfalls and problems of relying on serum troponin. *QJM*; **98**: 365–371.

Ismail, A (2009). Interference from endogenous antibodies in automated immunoassays: what laboratorians need to know. *J Clin Path*; **62**: 673–678.

Pernet P, Bénéteau-Burnat B, Hermand C, Vaubourdolle M. (2008). Point-of-care testing: false elevation of cardiac troponin I assayed in the emergency department. *Am J Emerg Med*; **26**: 969.e1–2.

Roongsritong C, Warraich I, Bradley C. (2004). Common causes of troponin elevations in the absence of acute myocardial infarction: incidence and clinical significance. *Chest*; **125**: 1877–1884.

Case 10

A 55-year-old man with chronic alcoholic liver disease presented with a 2-week history of increasing shortness of breath at rest, abdominal distension, and swollen legs. Although he regularly consumed half a bottle of vodka and 3 pints of beer a day he was asymptomatic until 2 weeks prior to this presentation. He had no other medical problems, had never smoked, and was not taking any prescribed medications.

On admission to hospital blood tests were as follows: haemoglobin (Hb) 9.6 g/dL, white blood cell count (WBC) 13.7×10^9 cells/L, platelets 105×10^{12} cells/L, creatinine 200 μmol/L, urea 16 mmol/L, bilirubin 200 μmol/L, AST 298 iu/L, alanine transaminase (ALT) 160 iu/L, gamma-glutamyl transferase (GGT) 410 iu/L, alkaline phosphatase 100 iu/L, international normalized ratio (INR) 2.5, albumin 18 g/L.

Abdominal ultrasound demonstrated a cirrhotic liver with mild splenomegaly and significant ascites but the renal tract was normal. The ascites was drained and diuretics (furosemide and spironolactone) were started. There was no evidence of spontaneous bacterial peritonitis (SBP) or malignancy in the peritoneal fluid.

There was no previous history of IHD. However, an ECG revealed LBBB with left-axis deviation. Echocardiography showed a markedly dilated left ventricle (7.3cm) with septal dyskinesia and moderately impaired systolic function (LVEF 35%).

He was discharged from hospital 1 month after admission as optimization of diuretic therapy was difficult. On discharge from hospital blood tests were as follows: Hb 10.6 g/dL, WBC 5.7×10^9 cells/L, platelets 300×10^{12} cells/L, creatinine 139 μmol/L, urea 9 mmol/L, bilirubin 40 μmol/L, AST 50 iu/L, ALT 60 iu/L, alkaline phosphatase 35 iu/L, INR 1.5, and albumin 28 g/L. Thyroid function tests were normal.

Over the next 6 months, despite remaining abstinent from alcohol and eating a low-salt diet, he was frequently readmitted for drainage of diuretic-resistant ascites. He was discussed with the regional transplant centre, who requested assessment of cardiac function prior to consideration for placement on the waiting list for liver transplantation.

Questions

1. What is a 'unit' of alcohol? Calculate the patient's weekly alcohol intake in units.
2. What are the recommendations for alcohol consumption in the UK?
3. What is the differential diagnosis for dilated cardiomyopathy (DCM) and what is the likely cause?
4. What are the effects of alcohol on the cardiovascular system?
5. What are the indications for cardiac resynchronization therapy? Is this indicated in this case?
6. What are the indications for implantable cardioverter defibrillator therapy? Is this indicated in this case?
7. How would you manage the DCM in this case? What is the prognosis?

Answers

1) **What is a 'unit' of alcohol? Calculate the patient's weekly alcohol intake in units.**

    Most guidelines on alcohol intake describe limits in terms of units or 'standard drinks'. In the UK one unit is equivalent to 8 g (10 mL) of ethanol.

    To calculate the number of UK units in an alcoholic beverage, the following formula can be used:

    volume of alcohol (L) × % alcohol by volume (mL/100mL) = units of alcohol

    Half a pint (284 mL) of beer (4%), a small glass (125 mL) of wine (8%), a single measure (25 mL) of spirits (40%), or a measure (50 mL) of fortified wine (20%) contain one unit of alcohol. A bottle (750 mL) of spirits (40%) contains 30 units and a bottle (750 mL) of wine (14%) contains 10.5 units.

    The patient reported that he consumed a half a bottle of vodka (approximately 15 units) and 3 pints of beer (6–9 units depending on strength) every day. His approximate weekly intake was 147–168 units. However, most patients will not report their true alcohol intake, so this figure should be considered conservative.

    Unfortunately, the definition of a 'unit' of ethanol varies between countries. For example, in USA one unit contains 15 g of ethanol. This should be considered when considering studies of alcohol use and guidelines for intake.

2) **What are the recommendations for alcohol consumption in the UK?**

    In the UK there are guidelines for both daily and weekly intakes. Men should drink ≤21 units and women ≤14 units per week. These amounts should not be consumed in one session; maximum daily intakes of 2–3 units (16–24 g) for women and 3–4 units (24–32 g) for men are advised. Binge drinking has been defined as episodic drinking of more than double the daily limit. Two alcohol-free days are recommended after heavy drinking.

3) **What is the differential diagnosis for DCM and what is the likely cause?**

    The causes of DCM are listed in Table 10.1. These should be excluded in any patient presenting with unexplained cardiac failure. Although ischaemia is one of the most common causes of heart failure, without a history of IHD or angina, ischaemic cardiomyopathy is unlikely. However, as the ECG is abnormal in this case, stress testing could be considered to screen for this. Alcohol-induced cardiomyopathy can cause regional wall motion abnormalities.

    As specific features to suggest another cause are absent and the patient has a significant alcohol history, alcohol-induced cardiomyopathy is the most likely diagnosis. However, in this case thiamine deficiency was excluded by measurement of red cell transketolase before administration of thiamine.

Table 10.1 Causes of DCM

Ischaemic heart disease
Hypertension
Toxic (e.g. alcohol, cocaine, chemotherapy, heavy metals)
Metabolic (e.g. nutritional deficiency, thyroid disease, diabetes, uraemia)
Infections (e.g. viral, bacterial, parasitic)
Vasculitis
Infiltrative (e.g. amyloidosis, sarcoidosis, haemochromatosis; see Case 28)
Hypertrophic cardiomyopathy and muscular dystrophy
Postpartum (see Case 11)
Genetic (familial)
Idiopathic

4) **What are the effects of alcohol on the cardiovascular system?**

Acute alcohol intake causes peripheral vasodilation and impairs myocardial contractility. The acute fall in BP, although small, results in a compensatory increase in cardiac output. Alcohol also enhances the exercise-induced increase in cardiac O_2 consumption. These acute effects may be deleterious to patients with cardiac pathology.

Arrhythmias (atrial or ventricular) occur in up to 60% of binge drinkers with or without other evidence of cardiac disease. An increased risk of atrial fibrillation has been reported among men with chronic heavy alcohol consumption. Most of the cases related to binge drinking occur over weekends or holidays, producing what has been termed 'holiday heart syndrome'.

There is no significant difference in the prevalence of the atrial arrhythmias and sustained or non-sustained ventricular tachycardia (VT) in patients with alcoholic cardiomyopathy in comparison to patients with idiopathic DCM. The most common manifestation is paroxysmal atrial arrhythmias, especially atrial fibrillation, but ventricular arrhythmias may also occur. Prolongation of the corrected QT interval, a major risk factor for ventricular arrhythmias, is found in a significant proportion of alcoholics compared with non-alcoholics. Hypomagnesemia and hypokalemia, which are common in chronic alcoholics, may contribute. Abstinence appears to reduce the frequency of arrhythmic events.

Drinking more than 3 units of alcohol per day results in a dose-dependent increase in BP. This usually returns to normal with abstinence. Chronic alcohol misuse is a significant cause of mild-to-moderate hypertension.

Chronic alcohol misuse can also cause arrhythmia (e.g. atrial fibrillation, atrial flutter, other supraventricular arrhythmias, and premature ventricular contractions), DCM, heart failure, and sudden death. Alcohol withdrawal is associated with stress-induced cardiomyopathy.

Alcohol-induced cardiomyopathy is a clinical diagnosis that should be considered in chronic alcohol misusers who present with heart failure and evidence of DCM.

Stigmata of alcohol abuse (e.g. parotid disease, telangiectasia or spider naevi, encephalopathy, and cirrhosis) may be present. Alcohol-induced hypertension may also contribute to LV dysfunction; this should be treated.

Chronic alcohol misuse causes up to a third of cases of DCM. Most alcohol misusers who develop alcoholic cardiomyopathy have been drinking over 80–90 g (10–11 units) of alcohol per day for over 5 years. However, alcoholic cardiomyopathy is uncommon in those under 40 years of age.

All patients presenting with heart failure should be asked about their alcohol intake. The risk of developing alcoholic cardiomyopathy is dose related. Mean daily intake, weekly maximum, duration of drinking, and lifetime consumption of alcohol are relevant.

Some studies suggest that light-to-moderate alcohol consumption (i.e. 1–2 drinks per day or 3–9 drinks per week) reduces the risk of IHD. For example, INTERHEART a standardized case–control study that screened all patients admitted for a first MI at 262 participating centres in 52 countries, suggested that consumption of alcohol ≥3 times per week was protective (see Table 5.1). However, heavy alcohol intake is associated with increased risk of IHD and cardiovascular moribidity and mortality.

Chronic alcohol misuse is associated with an increased risk of sudden death, which increases with age and alcohol intake.

5) **What are the indications for cardiac resynchronization therapy? Is this indicated in this case?**

Cardiac resynchronisation therapy should be offered to patients with NYHA class III–IV heart failure, LV ejection fractions <35% and QRS duration >120 ms who remain symptomatic after at least 3 months of optimal drug therapy for heart failure. During this trial period of medical therapy, symptoms and ventricular function may improve such that some patients may not require CRT. Longer periods may be required to recover from potentially reversible cardiomyopathies, such as alcohol-induced, acute MI, cardiac surgery, and tachycardia. CRT can be provided with or without an ICD but the evidence for the addition of an ICD to CRT for primary prevention is limited. However, this can be justified where disease progression is likely to lead to a stronger indication in the future.

6) **What are the indications for implantable cardioverter defibrillator therapy? Is this indicated in this case?**

Implantation of an ICD should be routinely considered for both primary and secondary prevention of life-threatening arrhythmias to reduce the risk of sudden cardiac death (SCD). Indications are listed in Table 10.2. Secondary prevention refers to the prevention of SCD in those patients who have survived a cardiac arrest or sustained VT (see Case 29). Patients with cardiac conditions associated with a high risk of SCD who present following unexplained syncope that is likely to be due to ventricular arrhythmias have a secondary indication. Primary prevention refers to the prevention of SCD in individuals without a history of cardiac arrest or sustained VT.

The ICD randomized controlled trials (RCTs) (MADIT I and II, SCD-HeFT) identified impaired LV function (ejection fraction <35%) as a key determinant of risk.

Other markers of risk not yet used in routine clinical practice include QRS duration (left bundle branch block (LBBB) - 50% increased risk), ventricular premature ectopic beats, non-sustained VT, late potentials, and microvolt T-wave alternans.

In the present case implantation of a biventricular pacemaker and ICD were considered for CRT and primary prevention of SCD. However, the echocardiogram performed after 9 months of abstinence showed a normal LV size with mildly impaired LV systolic function (LVEF 50%).

Table 10.2 Indications for implantation of an ICD

Secondary prevention

For patients who present, in the absence of a treatable cause, with:
- survival from cardiac arrest due to VT or VF
- spontaneous sustained VT causing syncope or significant haemodynamic compromise
- sustained VT without syncope/cardiac arrest with EF <35% and NYHA class II/III heart failure
- structural heart disease and spontaneous sustained VT
- symptomatic sustained VT in patients with congenital heart disease who have undergone haemodynamic and electrophysiological evaluation

---

Primary prevention

For patients with:
- previous myocardial infarction and all of the following:
  - non-sustained VT on Holter monitoring
  - inducible VT on electrophysiological testing
  - LV dysfunction with EF <35% and NYHA class II/III heart failure
- non-ischaemic DCM with EF <35% and NYHA class II/III heart failure
- a familial cardiac condition with a high risk of sudden death, including:
  - long QT syndrome
  - hypertrophic cardiomyopathy
  - Brugada syndrome
  - arrhythmogenic RV dysplasia
  - DCM
- recurrent syncope associated with complex congenital heart disease and advanced systemic ventricular dysfunction when thorough invasive and non-invasive investigations have failed to define a cause (see Case 48)

Patient groups in whom an ICD is usually not indicated

Syncope of undetermined aetiology and VT/VF not inducible

Incessant VT

VT amenable to surgical or catheter ablation

VT/VF due to transient or reversible cause

Significant psychiatric illness that may be aggravated by ICD or affect follow up

Terminal illness with poor prognosis (<6 months)

Patients with impaired LV function undergoing coronary artery bypass graft surgery, without spontaneous or inducible VT

Patients with NYHA class IV heart failure who are not candidates for heart transplantation

---

7) **How would you manage the DCM in this case? What is the prognosis?**

Complete abstinence from alcohol consumption is mandatory. Several small studies have reported recovery of cardiac function with abstinence. The largest study of the prognosis of alcoholic cardiomyopathy to date was reported in 1974. Of the 39 patients who continued to drink, only 4 patients improved. Of the 18 patients who abstained, 11 improved. However, the condition of 3 patients who stopped drinking continued to deteriorate.

Ensuring adequate calorific intake and supplemental minerals and vitamins (thiamine 200 mg daily, multivitamins, vitamin B12, and folate) are beneficial as alcohol misusers are often malnourished. Electrolyte abnormalities (e.g. hypokalemia, hypomagnesemia, and hypophosphatemia) should be corrected promptly because of the risk of arrhythmia.

Although anticoagulation may be beneficial to patients with severe LV dysfunction or AF, the risk:benefit ratio must be carefully considered in alcohol misusers. Treatment is otherwise identical to standard therapy for heart failure.

Further reading

Lucas DL, Brown RA, Wassef M, Giles TD (2005). Alcohol and the cardiovascular system: Research challenges and opportunities. *J Am Coll Cardiol*; **45**: 1916–1924.

Preedy VR, Richardson PJ (1994). Ethanol induced cardiovascular disease. *Br Med Bull*; **50**: 152–163.

Puddey IB, Rakic V, Dimmitt SB, Beilin LJ. (1999). Influence of pattern drinking on cardiovascular disease and cardiovascular risk factors–a review. *Addiction*; **94–5**: 649–663.

Guillo P, Mansourati J, Maheu B Etienne Y, Provost K, Simon O, Blanc JJ. (1997). Long-term prognosis in patients with alcoholic cardiomyopathy and severe heart failure after total abstinence. *Am J Cardiol*; **79**: 1276–1278.

Murray KF, Carithers RL Jr (2005). AASLD Practice Guidelines: Evaluation of the Patient for Liver Transplantation. *Hepatology*; **41**: 1–26.

Epstein AE, Dimarco JP, Ellenbogen KA Estes NA 3rd, Freedman RA, Gettes LS, Gillinov AM, Gregoratos G, Hammill SC, Hayes DL, Hlatky MA, Newby LK, Page RL, Schoenfeld MH, Silka MJ, Stevenson LW, Sweeney MO, Smith SC Jr, Jacobs AK, Adams CD, Anderson JL, Buller CE, Creager MA, Ettinger SM, Faxon DP, Halperin JL, Hiratzka LF, Hunt SA, Krumholz HM, Kushner FG, Lytle BW, Nishimura RA, Ornato JP, Page RL, Riegel B, Tarkington LG, Yancy CW; American College of Cardiology/American Heart Association Task Force on Practice Guidelines (Writing Committee to Revise the ACC/AHA/NASPE 2002 Guideline Update for Implantation of Cardiac Pacemakers and Antiarrhythmia Devices); American Association for Thoracic Surgery; Society of Thoracic Surgeons.(2008). ACC/AHA/HRS 2008 Guidelines for device-based therapy of cardiac rhythm abnormalities. A report of the American College of Cardiology/American Heart Association Task Force on Practice Guidelines (Writing Committee to Revise the ACC/AHA/NASPE 2002 Guideline Update for Implantation of Cardiac Pacemakers and Antiarrhythmia Devices) Developed in collaboration with the American Association for Thoracic Surgery and Society of Thoracic Surgeons. *J Am Coll Cardiol*; **51**: e1–e62.

Case 11

A 32-year-old woman who was 36 weeks into her second pregnancy presented to the labour ward in established labour. Her first pregnancy was uncomplicated. On admission the cardiotocograph demonstrated foetal bradycardia. Emergency (category 1) Caesarean section was performed under general anaesthetic. There were no complications during the 40-minute procedure; estimated blood loss was 600 mL and 1500 mL Hartmann's solution was administered. The patient was extubated and transferred to the recovery ward.

Within 20 minutes she was in severe respiratory distress and was tachypneoic (respiratory rate 35), tachycardic (rate 120; sinus rhythm) and hypotensive (80/50). Oxygen saturations dropped to 85% on 15 L/minute oxygen (pO$_2$ 7.5 kPa, pCO$_2$ 3.5 kPa). Examination revealed a third heart sound and bilateral fine inspiratory crepitations to the midzones. Her chest X-ray is shown in Fig. 11.1. She was reintubated and transferred to the intensive care unit (ITU), where dobutamine and noradrenaline infusions were started. Intravenous unfractionated heparin was started to treat a presumed pulmonary embolism (PE).

Her husband reported that over the preceding 3 weeks her shortness of breath and ankle swelling had increased significantly, severely limiting her exercise tolerance. Although her GP had requested a chest X-ray she had refused because of concerns about irradiation of the baby.

Renal function and a full blood count were unremarkable, urine dipstick detected a trace of proteinuria. ECG confirmed sinus tachycardia. Echocardiography demonstrated a dilated LV (6.5 cm) with global hypokinesia (ejection fraction 20%). There was no evidence of RV strain or pulmonary hypertension.

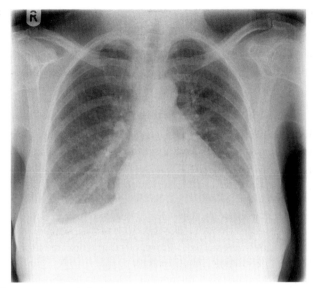

Fig. 11.1 Chest X-ray on admission.

Questions

1. When should dyspnoea in pregnancy be investigated?
2. How would you respond to a woman's concerns about irradiation during pregnancy?
3. Report the chest X-ray (Fig. 11.1).
4. What is the differential diagnosis?
5. What are pre-eclampsia and eclampsia and how are they diagnosed?
6. What are the echocardiographic features which characterize DCM?
7. What is peripartum cardiomyopathy (PCM)?
8. What is the prognosis of PCM and what are the common causes of death?
9. What medical therapy can be used to treat cardiac failure in the peripartum period?
10. What is the best mode of delivery of the foetus?
11. What advice should be given about breast feeding and subsequent pregnancies in PCM?

Answers

1) **When should dyspnoea in pregnancy be investigated?**

Breathlessness is common during pregnancy. Minute ventilation increases from the first trimester and is 20–40% above baseline at term. Alveolar ventilation increases by 50–70%. The tidal volume increases by 30–35% and the respiratory rate increases slightly. This increase in respiratory drive is due to increased CO_2 production and progesterone.

Up to 60% of women experience breathlessness on exertion but fewer than 20% are breathless at rest. Exercise tolerance is not significantly reduced and daily activities are not affected. Distinguishing pathological from physiological breathlessness is difficult but important. Investigation should be considered if exercise tolerance is significantly reduced or other symptoms and signs suggest a pathological cause.

In this case, urgent chest X-ray and echocardiography were indicated in view of the increasing breathlessness and markedly reduced exercise tolerance and signs of congestive cardiac failure.

2) **How would you respond to a woman's concerns about irradiation during pregnancy?**

Although there are risks to the foetus from radiation exposure, the chest X-ray is an important diagnostic test. Abdominal shielding is used so the dose to the foetus results from scatter of the X-ray beam through the mother, not direct exposure. Foetal exposure is about 0.005 rads (0.05 mGray). This is one-thousandth of the accepted limit of foetal exposure (5 rads; 50 mGray). The radiation dose increases in later pregnancy as the gravid uterus is closer to the source of the radiation. The radiation dose from a posteroanterior (PA) X-ray is less than that of an anteroposterior film because the distance from the uterus to the source of the radiation is greater in the PA position. However, in either case the overall doses are significantly less than those associated with foetal complications (see below). The risks to the foetus are therefore minimal.

The potential effects of irradiation on the foetus include prenatal death, growth restriction, congenital malformation, mental retardation, and increased risk of childhood cancer.

The sensitivity of a developing foetus to ionizing radiation varies with:

◆ gestational age

◆ dose

◆ duration of exposure.

Exposure to a total dose less than 5 rads during pregnancy has not been shown to affect the outcome of the pregnancy compared to controls exposed to background radiation (<0.1 rad over 9 months).

Exposure to 50–100 mGy (5–10 rads) before 2 weeks' gestation may cause prenatal death. At this stage of gestation the non-carcinogenic effects of radiation are unlikely.

Exposure to 50–100 mGy (20–25 rads) from 1 to 8 weeks' gestation may cause growth retardation. Exposures over 100 mGy from 8 to 25 weeks may cause mental retardation.

Exposure to over 1000 mGy (100 rads) after 26 weeks increases risks of stillbirth and neonatal death.

The dose from any single diagnostic procedure in current practice should not cause prenatal death, growth restriction, congenital malformation, or mental retardation. However, the risk of childhood cancer may be increased.

Most diagnostic procedures result in foetal doses of up to 1 mGy (0.1 rads). The associated risk of childhood cancer is less than 1:10000 (the natural risk is 1:500). This is considered acceptable in view of the potential benefits of imaging to the mother. However, some investigations result in foetal exposures over a few mGy. This may result in a significant increase in the risk of childhood cancer and should be avoided if possible. The most sensitive period is from 2 to 15 weeks, but the risk of childhood cancer may be increased by foetal irradiation at any stage of gestation.

3) **Report the chest X-ray**

The chest X-ray (Fig. 11.1) shows bilateral perihilar shadowing with vascular redistribution (upper lobe blood diversion) and cardiomegaly. There are bilateral pleural effusions. This suggests pulmonary oedema due to congestive cardiac failure. However, in pregnancy the colloid osmotic pressure is low (decreased serum albumin) so if capillary permeability is increased pulmonary oedema can occur despite normal cardiac filling pressures.

4) **What is the differential diagnosis?**

The causes of peripartum pulmonary oedema and respiratory failure are listed in Table 11.1. These should be considered in any woman presenting with unexplained cardiac failure in the peripartum period.

Table 11.1 Causes of pulmonary oedema in the peripartum period

Cardiac causes of pulmonary oedema	Non-cardiac causes of pulmonary oedema and respiratory failure
Ischaemic heart disease	Pre-eclampsia/eclampsia (diastolic dysfunction)
Aortic stenosis	Pulmonary embolism
Mitral stenosis	Aspiration pneumonitis
Malignant hypertension	Amniotic fluid embolism
Dilated cardiomyopathy	Sepsis (e.g. respiratory, urinary)
Restrictive cardiomyopathy	Drugs (e.g. cocaine, amphetamines, steroids, magnesium, tocolytics–salbutamol, residual neuromuscular blockade post-op)
Hypertrophic cardiomyopathy	Infectious, toxic, or metabolic disorders
	Transfusion reaction following blood transfusion for peripartum haemorrhage

5) **What are pre-eclampsia and eclampsia and how are they diagnosed?**

Pre-eclampsia is a multisystem disease with an incidence of 5% that occurs after 20 weeks of pregnancy. It is part of the spectrum of hypertensive diseases of pregnancy.

The characteristic features of pre-eclampsia are hypertension (systolic >140; diastolic >90), oedema, and proteinuria. However, the severity of these features is not proportional to the severity of the disease.

Pre-eclampsia may cause headaches, visual disturbances, abdominal pain, and swelling of the hands or face. Hypertension, hyperreflexia, clonus, right upper quadrant abdominal pain, and peripheral oedema may be present.

Pre-eclampsia is associated with creatinine >70 mmol/L, Hb >13 g/dL (unless there is associated haemolysis), elevated liver enzymes, thrombocytopenia, proteinuria (≥2+ on dipstick testing, >300 mg in 24-hour collection), and decreased 24-hour urine creatinine clearance (normally in pregnancy this is 150% above the non-pregnant level or approximately 150 mL/min).

Eclampsia is an acute life-threatening form of hypertensive encephalopathy characterized by tonic–clonic seizures and/or unexplained coma, usually in a patient with pre-eclampsia. Most cases of eclampsia present in the third trimester. About 80% of eclamptic seizures occur intrapartum or within 48 hours of delivery. However, eclampsia does rarely occur before 20 weeks' gestation and up to 23 days postpartum.

6) **What are the echocardiographic features which characterize DCM?**

The characteristic features of DCM include globally reduced LV function (EF <30%), LV dilatation (end diastolic diameter >2.7 cm/m^2), and mitral regurgitation (MR) due to dilatation of the mitral annulus. Mild pulmonary hypertension and an abnormal restrictive mitral inflow pattern are also seen. See Case 10 for further information on DCM.

7) **What is peripartum cardiomyopathy?**

Peripartum cardiomyopathy is a rare DCM of uncertain aetiology with an incidence of approximately 1 in 3000 gestations. It is a diagnosis of exclusion that should be considered if heart failure develops in the last month of pregnancy or within 5 months of delivery. Systolic dysfunction must be confirmed to prevent misdiagnosis as other conditions cause pulmonary oedema in pregnancy (see list of differentials). It is important to differentiate PCM from underlying DCM exacerbated by pregnancy.

Risk factors are not clearly defined and screening is not possible but PCM is more common in multiparous women, twin gestations, and pre-eclampsia.

8) **What is the prognosis of PCM and what are the common causes of death?**

Prognosis correlates with resolution of LV function, which should be reassessed 6 months postpartum. The systolic function often improves with time and returns to normal in up to 50% within 6 months.

However, heart failure may progress to the point that cardiac transplantation is required. Mortality rates of up to 50% have been reported, half of which occur within 3 months of delivery. The most common causes of death are cardiac failure, arrhythmia, and thromboembolism. Prophylactic anticoagulation with subcutaneous heparin should be started at diagnosis and continued for at least 6 weeks postpartum.

9) **What medical therapy can be used to treat cardiac failure in the peripartum period?**

When managing heart failure during pregnancy, the health of both the mother and the foetus should be considered. Management should be co-ordinated by obstetricians and cardiologists alongside a foetal and maternal medicine team with foetal heart monitoring.

Medical therapy during pregnancy includes loop diuretics, afterload reduction (hydralazine and nitrates) digoxin, and beta blockade (metoprolol or carvedilol). The risk of thrombosis is high. Anticoagulation should be considered if EF <30%.

Although beta-blockers are known to be beneficial in patients with heart failure, there are no studies in PCM. However, beta-blockers have been used in pregnant women with hypertension without any known adverse effects on the foetus.

Clearance of digoxin is increased and large doses may be required to maintain therapeutic levels during pregnancy. Digoxin crosses the placenta and is used to treat foetal arrhythmias. Although foetal heart block is unlikely, the foetus should be monitored by an obstetrician.

Angiotensin-converting enzyme inhibitors and angiotensin receptor blockers are teratogenic and so contraindicated in pregnancy. The teratogenic effects (foetal renal dysgenesis and death) are most common in the second and third trimester.

After delivery of the foetus, management is similar to that of non-pregnant women with DCM: ACE inhibitors or angiotensin receptor blockers (ARBs) should be started postpartum.

10) **What is the best mode of delivery of the foetus?**

Vaginal delivery is preferred because complications (oedema, effusions, endometritis, and pulmonary emboli) are more common after Caesarean sections. If the mother is stable it is best to allow spontaneous vaginal delivery. However, analgesia is important and epidural analgesia is ideal but may be prevented by anticoagulation.

If the patient does not respond to treatment or if obstetricians decide the foetus must be delivered, it is best to induce labour and proceed with vaginal delivery if possible. However, if the mother is decompensating, elective Caesarian with invasive haemodynamic monitoring should be considered.

After delivery of the foetus, metabolic activity is reduced but afterload increases (low-resistance placental bed is lost) and so the clinical condition of the mother may deteriorate. Admission to the ITU for monitoring and further management should be considered.

11) **What advice should be given about breastfeeding and subsequent pregnancies in PCM?**

Breastfeeding is generally discouraged because of associated metabolic demands and excretion of drugs in breast milk.

The risk of subsequent pregnancies depends on the patient's LV function. If LV function does not return to normal, subsequent pregnancies carry a high risk of progressive cardiac failure and should be discouraged. If LV function returns to normal, there is still a risk of possible recurrence, but in most cases successful pregnancy with delivery at term can be achieved with appropriate monitoring.

In this case, pulmonary embolism was excluded by computed tomography (CT) pulmonary angiography (CTPA). Peripartum cardiomyopathy was diagnosed on the basis of the history and exclusion of other causes of DCM. Ventilatory support was weaned after medical management of heart failure and she was extubated 3 days later then discharged home 1 week postpartum. Anticoagulation with warfarin was started but unfortunately despite this she developed a pulmonary embolism from a femoral deep vein thrombosis and was readmitted to intensive care for mechanical ventilation 2 weeks postpartum. She unfortunately died following cardiac arrest during femoral embolectomy and placement of an inferior vena caval filter.

Further reading

Damilakis J, Perisinakis K, Prassopoulos P, Dimovasili E, Varveris H, Gourtsoyiannis N. (2003). Conceptus radiation dose and risk from chest screen-film radiography. *Eur Radiol*; **13**: 406–412.

Sliwa K, Fett J, Elkayam U (2006). Peripartum cardiomyopathy. *Lancet*; **368**: 687–693.

Elkayam U, Akhter MW, Singh H, Khan S, Bitar F, Hameed A, Shotan A. (2005). Pregnancy-associated cardiomyopathy: clinical characteristics and a comparison between early and late presentation. *Circulation*; **111**: 2050–2055.

Kuklina EV, Callaghan WM (2010). Cardiomyopathy and other myocardial disorders among hospitalizations for pregnancy in the United States: 2004–2006. *Obstet Gynecol*; **115**: 93–100.

Case 12

A 60-year-old warehouse worker presented for routine preoperative assessment prior to elective right inguinal hernia repair. There was no past medical history of note but the report of a chest radiograph (Fig. 12.1) performed 2 weeks earlier suggested that further investigation was required. Although he had no cardiorespiratory symptoms he was referred to the admitting medical team. Trans-thoracic echocardiography was performed (Fig. 12.2) and this led the medical team to organize a contrast-enhanced CT scan of the chest (Fig. 12.3).

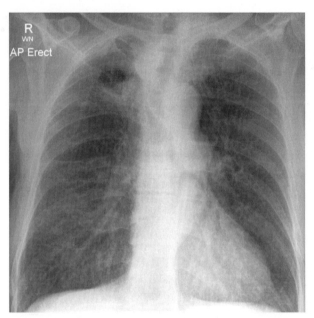

Fig. 12.1 Preoperative chest X-ray.

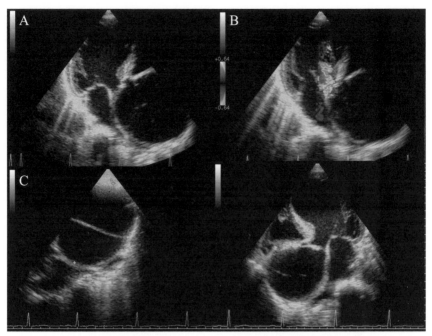

Fig. 12.2 Trans-thoracic echocardiogram: A, off-axis parasternal short-axis view; B, off-axis parasternal short-axis view with colour Doppler overlay; C, modified short-axis aortic root view; D, modified five-chamber view showing aortic root. (See colour plate 1)

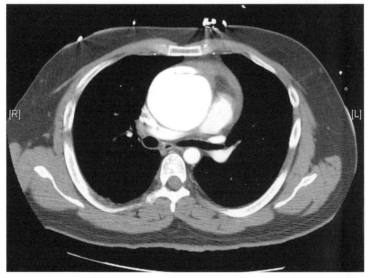

Fig. 12.3 Selected slice from contrast-enhanced CT chest at the level of the third thoracic vertebra.

Questions

1. Report the chest X-ray (Fig. 12.1).
2. What do the TTE images (Fig. 12.2) show?
3. What clinical signs may be present?
4. What does the CT scan (Fig. 12.3) show? Where anatomically does this lesion usually occur?
5. How is this condition classified?
6. What is the pathophysiology of this condition?
7. What definitive treatment, if any, would you recommend?

Answers

1) **Report the chest X-ray (Fig. 12.1).**

This is an anterior–posterior (AP) erect chest X-ray. The mediastinum is not widened but the aorta appears tortuous and dilated with some calcification of the aortic knuckle. There is reticular and possibly nodular shadowing in the right upper zone. The density of the right paratracheal strip is increased, which could be due to paratracheal lymphadenopathy. These appearances are probably secondary to previous exposure to tuberculosis (TB).

2) **What do the TTE images (Fig. 12.2) show?**

Figure 12.4 shows a 9.5-cm thoracic aortic aneurysm (Fig. 12.4A) with a dissection flap (Figs. 12.4A, C, and D) causing severe aortic regurgitation (Fig. 12.4B). Although not demonstrated in Fig. 12.4, blood flow was visualized in both the true and the false lumens, and no thrombus was seen.

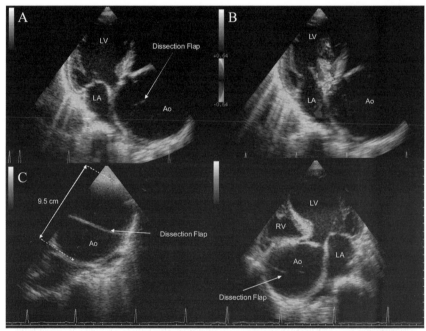

Fig. 12.4 Trans-thoracic echocardiogram demonstrating aortic dissection. A, off-axis parasternal short-axis view with dissection flap visible in aortic root; B, off-axis parasternal short-axis view with colour Doppler overlay demonstrating significant aortic regurgitation; C, modified short-axis aortic root view demonstrating a 9.5 cm aneurysm, D, modified five-chamber view showing aortic root demonstrating the dissection flap. (See colour plate 2)

3) **What clinical signs may be present?**

The patient may have signs of aortic regurgitation, such as a collapsing pulse, a widened pulse pressure, and an early diastolic murmur. An aortic systolic murmur may also be heard as a consequence of turbulent flow across the valve. Depending on the extent of the dissection and the branches of the aorta involved, physical signs of altered perfusion may also be apparent. These include:

- coronary ischaemia and infarction
- cerebrovascular phenomena and other neurological syndromes (e.g. anterior spinal artery syndrome)
- renovascular dysfunction with oligo/anuria
- peripheral ischaemia
- absent, reduced, or delayed pulses (radio-radial or radio-femoral delay)
- variation in BP measurement in the left and right arm.

In this case, the patient had a collapsing pulse and a grade IV early diastolic murmur but peripheral pulses were normal.

4) **What does the CT scan (Fig. 12.3) show? Where anatomically does this lesion usually occur?**

The CT image shows an aneurysmal ascending aorta with a normal descending thoracic aorta. The dissection flap is at the root of the aorta (Fig. 12.5). It is not possible to exclude involvement of the arch from Fig. 12.3. However, review of other images in the series excluded arch involvement. The most common site of dissection is the first 10 cm of the ascending aorta (90%). The second most common site is just distal to the left subclavian artery. In 5–10% of dissections an intimal tear is not seen.

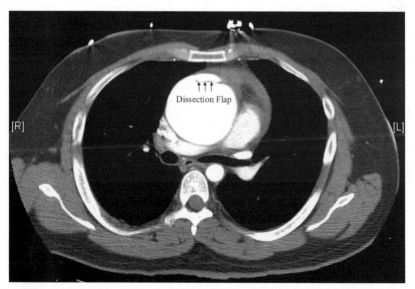

Fig. 12.5 Contrast-enhanced CT chest demonstrating dissection flap. Selected image from contrast-enhanced CT chest at the level of the third thoracic vertebra with dissection flap marked with arrows.

5) **How is this condition classified?**

Dissections can be classified either by how long they have been present or anatomically. If the time from the initial intimal tear, which normally coincides with the onset of symptoms, is less than 2 weeks then the dissection is acute. If, however, this period is greater than 2 weeks the dissection is defined as chronic.

Anatomical classification is based on whether there is involvement of the ascending aorta by the dissection (Table 12.1). This classification is clinically useful as management is primarily surgical if the ascending aorta is involved and conservative medical therapy if it is not. This is a chronic type A (Stanford) or type II (De Bakey) dissection as the chest X-ray was performed 2 weeks prior to the preoperative assessment, and the dissection is confined to the ascending aorta.

Table 12.1 Classification of aortic aneurysms by the Stanford and De Bakey systems

Anatomical position in aorta	The Stanford classification	The De Bakey classification
Ascending	Type A	Type II
Arch		Type I
Descending thoracic	Type B	
Abdominal		Type III

6) **What is the pathophysiology of this condition?**

Aortic dissection occurs as a result of aortic wall weakening initiated by destructive processes either in the intimal layer (most common) or the media of the vessel wall:

i. Aortic intimal weakening and damage occurs most frequently because of atherosclerosis but can be caused by other inflammatory processes within the vessel wall. This weakening can lead to tearing of this layer and bleeding into the media, which dissects it away from the adventitia as it propagates. Aortic dissection may also be caused by atherosclerotic plaque rupture, shearing forces secondary to rapid deceleration injury during road traffic accidents, or invasive catheter interventions and cardiac surgery (iatrogenic).

ii. Vessel media damage may be acquired through chronic repetitive trauma (e.g. long-standing hypertension) or inherited through defects in connective tissue components (Table 12.3). In both cases, damage can be caused to the vaso vasorum with intramural haemorrhage and haematoma formation. Further weakening of the arterial wall then occurs due to smooth muscle cell death (cystic medial necrosis). If the intima tears then further bleeding into the false lumen accelerates the process to acute dissection (21–47%). However, the haematoma may regress and can be reabsorbed (about 10%).

The European Society of Cardiology (ESC) has proposed a pathophysiological classification system for aortic dissection and wall disorders (Table 12.2), and importantly they highlight that the presence of intramural haematoma (ESC class 2) in the ascending aorta is an indication for urgent surgery as type A dissection may be imminent. However, distal intramural haematomas are recommended to be treated conservatively or by using some of the endovascular techniques that have been developed (see answer 7 below). Once dissection has occurred, the majority are progressive and life threatening, whilst some remain sub-clinical and present after a delay or incidentally. Unrecognized or untreated aortic dissection has a high mortality rate (25% at 24 hours; 90% at 1 month). However, 25% of patients have unrecognized dissections that are only diagnosed at postmortem.

Table 12.2 ESC classification of aortic dissection and wall disorders

Class	Definition
1	Classic dissection (intimal flap between true and false lumens)
2	Intramural haematoma/haemorrhage
3	Small dissection without haematoma
4	Plaque rupture/ulceration with surrounding haematoma
5	Trauma/iatrogenic dissection

Table 12.3 Some inherited defects in connective tissue

	Incidence	Inheritance/genetics	Pathophysiology
Marfan's syndrome	1 in 7000	Autosomal dominant Variable penetrance Genetic heterogeneity FBN-1 ≥150 mutations MFS-2 gene	Defective fibrillin in the extracellular matrix Elastolysis and cystic medial degeneration Elevated TGF beta
Ehlers–Danlos syndrome	Estimated at 1 in 5000	Aortic involvement primarily in Ehlers–Danlos syndrome type IV Autosomal dominant	Heterogeneous (11 types) Articular hypermobility Skin hyperextensibility Tissue fragility
Annulo-aortic ectasia and familial aortic dissection	Unknown	Sporadic or familial forms Autosomal dominant FBN-1 gene >5 mutations Loeys–Dietz syndrome	Similar to Marfan's syndrome Elastolysis and cystic medial degeneration No abnormalities of types I and III collagen or fibrillopathy TGF beta mutations

FBN-1, fibrillin-1 gene; MFS-2, Marfan's syndrome type 2; TGF, transforming growth factor

7) **What definitive treatment, if any, would you recommend?**

Urgent open surgical replacement of the aortic root and arch with aortic valve replacement and reimplantation of the coronary arteries are required. In the present case, the patient was transferred to the regional cardiothoracic centre where this was performed successfully 2 days later. The aetiology was not established. Three months later the right inguinal hernia was repaired.

The initial aims of immediate and definitive management of chronic aortic dissection and dilation are similar to the management of acute dissection (see Case 13). The main clinical concerns are the risk of rupture and complications associated with propagation of the dissection:

i. The conventional management of Stanford type A (De Bakey type I, II) is surgical because the risk of complications from propagation is high. The aim of surgery is to resect the intimal tear, prevent entry to the false lumen, and reconstruct the aorta. An interposition graft is used with either reimplantation or bypass of the coronary arteries, and resuspension of the native aortic valve. If the aortic valve leaflets are involved, valve replacement is also required with a composite valved prosthesis and coronary reimplantation. If the aortic arch (30%) or descending aorta are involved, resection of the intimal flap is not possible. Partial or total replacement of the arch may be required.

ii. Acute type B (type III) dissections are usually treated conservatively. Open surgical repair has no proven benefit over medical management. However, the use of endovascular techniques is increasing. Endovascular stent grafts reduce the risk of paraplegia from spinal artery occlusion (18% after open surgery). Stents seal entry tears, initiating thrombosis of the false lumen, improve flow in the distal true lumen and can potentially re-establish flow in side-branch arteries. However, indications for surgical repair include intractable pain and the prevention or treatment of life-threatening complications.

iii. An ascending aortic aneurysm ≥5.5–6 cm or a distal aortic aneurysm ≥6.0 cm generally warrants elective repair. The risk of mortality from the aneurysm is greater than that from the operation. An ascending aortic aneurysm ≥4.5–5.0 cm in a patient with Marfan's syndrome should be repaired electively.

Further reading

Erbel R, Alfonso F, Boileau C, Dirsch O, Eber B, Haverich A, Rakowski H, Struyven J, Radegran K, Sechtem U, Taylor J, Zollikofer C, Klein WW, Mulder B, Providencia LA; Task Force on Aortic Dissection, European Society of Cardiology. (2001). Diagnosis and management of aortic dissection: Task Force on Aortic Dissection, European Society of Cardiology. (2001). *Eur Heart J;* **22**: 1642–1681.

Khan IA, Nair CK. (2002). Clinical, diagnostic, and management perspectives of aortic dissection. *Chest*; **122**: 311–328.

Mastracci TM, Greenberg RK. (2009). Follow-up paradigms for stable aortic dissection. *Semin Vasc Surg*; **22**: 69–73.

Case 13

A 54-year-old accountant presented to his GP with a 1-week history of intermittent severe back pain that radiated to his chest. He also felt 'unsteady on his feet'. He had hypertension treated with ramipril 5 mg daily and smoked 20 cigarettes per day.

Observations were BP 170/80 mmHg (no postural drop) and HR 90 bpm. Further examination was unremarkable. He was reassured and advised to take simple analgesia.

Two hours later he collapsed whilst climbing the stairs at home. His wife called an ambulance. When the paramedics arrived he was conscious, with a GCS of 15, but short of breath and distressed, with severe abdominal pain. Observations were then BP 120/50 mmHg and HR 50 bpm.

He arrived at the ED 20 minutes later. The medical registrar was fast bleeped to assess him and an ECG was obtained (Fig. 13.1). He was semi-conscious, peripherally vasoconstricted, and in respiratory distress. The right radial pulse was impalpable. The BP was 80/40 mmHg in the right arm and 130/60 in the left. The JVP was raised above the earlobes bilaterally. The heart sounds were soft and crepitations were audible to the mid zones of both lung fields. The abdomen was distended and diffusely tender; bowel sounds were absent.

An AP semi-erect chest X-ray showed patchy alveolar shadowing in the mid and lower zones with upper lobe blood diversion, consistent with pulmonary oedema (Fig. 13.2). The heart size and cardiac contours appeared normal. The mediastinum did not appear to be significantly widened. There were no effusions. The medical registrar was unsure whether thrombolysis was indicated and so asked the cardiology registrar for an opinion. The cardiology registrar reviewed the patient and performed a bedside TTE (Fig. 13.3).

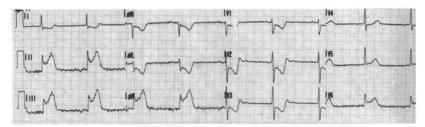

Fig. 13.1 Admission ECG.

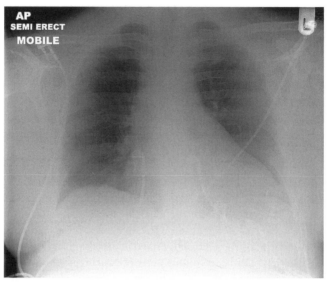

Fig. 13.2 This portable semi-erect AP chest X-ray demonstrates upper lobe blood diversion with bilateral alveolar shadowing in the mid and lower zones. The mediastinum does not appear to be significantly widened. There are no pleural effusions.

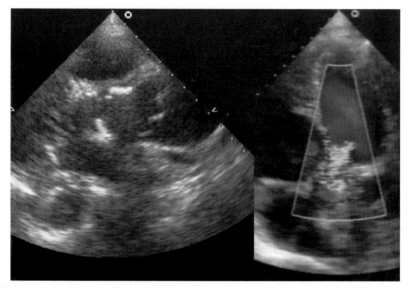

Fig. 13.3 Selected views from the bedside transthoracic echocardiogram: A, zoomed parasternal short axis view; B, apical five-chamber view with colour Doppler overlay. (See colour plate 3)

Questions

1. What does the ECG (Fig. 13.1) show?
2. What is the likely cause of the collapse? What would you do next?
3. Does the chest X-ray (Fig. 13.2) support the diagnosis?
4. What was the cause of his abdominal pain? How would you confirm this?
5. What is the mortality associated with this condition?
6. Did the delay of 2 hours make any difference?
7. What definitive procedure is required?
8. What follow-up is required?

Answers

1) **What does the ECG (Fig. 13.1) show?**

   The 12 lead ECG (Fig. 13.1) shows sinus bradycardia (50 bpm) with a normal QRS axis. There is widespread infero-lateral ST elevation (II, III, aVF, V6), with upwards concavity, anterior ST depression (V1–3), and biphasic T waves in I, aVL, and V2–3. There are no Q waves. Overall, these features are suggestive of acute inferior MI, even though the morphology of the ST elevation is reminiscent of pericarditis in some leads.

2) **What is the likely cause of the collapse? What would you do next?**

   The clinical signs (impalpable radial pulse and difference between the measured BP in the left and right arms) are consistent with acute aortic dissection complicated by aortic valve disruption, right coronary artery dissection (or secondary occlusion; suggested by the ECG findings - see above), and proximal extension into the pericardial space (suggested by the soft heart sounds and raised JVP). In this case the diagnosis was confirmed when TTE (Fig. 13.3) demonstrated a dissection flap in the proximal aorta, a pericardial effusion, and significant aortic regurgitation (Fig. 13.4).

   Although acute aortic dissection presents most commonly with chest pain (~70%) and/or back pain (~50%), it can also present with abdominal pain (~30%) or migrating pain (~15%). This pain is usually described as tearing or ripping in character (~50%), and severe or 'the worst ever pain' (~90%).

   Around 10% of patients present without pain; of these approximately 50% have neurological symptoms, which often delay diagnosis. Overall, around a third of acute dissections have neurological sequelae. These generally develop shortly after the dissection occurs and are commonly evanescent, resulting from arterial occlusion during propagation.

   There are four main types of neurological complications: persistent or transient ischemic stroke (15–30%); spinal cord ischaemia (<10%; e.g. anterior spinal artery syndrome and para/hemi-plegia), ischaemic neuropathy (10–20%), and hypoxic encephalopathy (<5%). Acute aortic dissection is associated with syncope (~10%), hypertension (~50%), hypotension (~8%), shock, and tamponade (~8%).

   The murmur of aortic regurgitation is heard in a third of patients. Pulse deficits are noted in around 20% at presentation.

   The immediate management of aortic dissection requires confirmation of the diagnosis if necessary, and prevention of further propagation, or intervening circulatory collapse. Urgent cardiothoracic surgical assessment is required to facilitate early definitive treatment with aortic root surgery. Thrombolysis is clearly contraindicated in aortic dissection as case reports usually associate this with a fatal outcome.

i. Drainage of a pericardial effusion causing tamponade usually improves haemodynamics. However, if the pericardial effusion is a complication of acute aortic dissection, drainage may accelerate bleeding and worsen shock. In addition, the hypotension resulting from tamponade may in fact limit, to a degree, further bleeding into the pericardial space. Hence, pericardiocentesis should only be attempted if complete circulatory collapse is imminent.

ii. Hypotension or normotension in a previously hypertensive patient, in the context of aortic dissection, may indicate continuing haemorrhage. Aggressive volume expansion, ideally with cross-matched blood, usually improves shock when LV function is preserved. Clinical judgements on fluid resuscitation more difficult in the context of right ventricular (RV) dysfunction or infarction because of right coronary artery dissection as the increased filling pressures required are reflected in a raised JVP. Furthermore, if LV function is compromised, any increases in intra-vascular volume could cause fluid overload, so caution is advised.

iii. Placement of an intra-aortic balloon pump (IABP) is contraindicated (see Case 46). Although an IABP could optimize diastolic coronary perfusion and ventricular function, there is a risk of exacerbating acute aortic insufficiency or entering the false lumen during insertion, thus propagating the dissection.

iv. Any conduction abnormalities should be recognized early and temporary transvenous pacing attempted if there is circulatory compromise or syncope.

v. Regardless of the exact aetiology, if haemodynamic status and consciousness are compromised, urgent anaesthetic assessment should be arranged. Endotracheal intubation and set-up of an extra-corporal circulation (cardiac bypass) may be required to stabilize the patient before surgery. However, rapid sequence induction of anaesthesia and laryngoscopy can cause sympathetic stimulation and an undesirable surge in HR and BP. The increased shear stress on the aorta could propagate the dissection and cause aortic rupture.

vi. If BP is normal or high it should be reduced along with force of ventricular ejection. This may delay or prevent further propagation of the dissection, whilst ensuring adequate cerebral, coronary, and renal perfusion. In previously normotensive patients the systolic BP target of 110 mmHg and a pulse of 60 bpm are usually achievable with adequate analgesia and beta-blockade. If beta-blockade is contraindicated (e.g. asthma, bradycardia, or heart failure) or insufficient, vasodilators and short-acting calcium channel blockers should be considered.

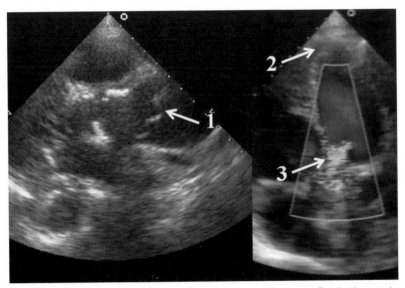

Fig. 13.4 Transthoracic echocardiogram demonstrating a dissection flap in the proximal aorta pericardial effusion and significant aortic regurgitation. The parasternal short-axis view (A) and five-chamber view with colour Doppler overlay. (B) These images demonstrate a dissection flap in the proximal aorta (1) suggestive of acute dissection. Aortic dissection has been complicated by pericardial effusion (2) and significant aortic regurgitation (3). (See colour plate 4)

3) **Does the chest X-ray (Fig. 13.2) support the diagnosis?**

The chest X-ray neither supports nor excludes the diagnosis of aortic dissection although the ascending aorta is prominent. The chest X-ray is only abnormal in half of all cases of aortic dissection.

4) **What was the cause of his abdominal pain? How would you confirm this?**

Although the intimal tear was visualized in the ascending aorta on TTE, the full extent of the dissection could not be determined. Clinical findings may suggest the distal limit of the dissection. For example, further bouts of pain suggest ongoing propagation. The extent of propagation of the dissection may be indicated by:

◆ changes in the location of the pain and pattern of radiation

◆ pulse deficits and limb ischaemia (aortic arch, femoral arteries)

◆ neurological signs (carotid, vertebral, and spinal arteries)

◆ oligo/anuria (renal arteries)

◆ abdominal signs (mesenteric circulation).

In the present case, the abdominal pain was probably due to involvement of the coeliac and mesenteric arteries, or intra-abdominal bleeding from aortic rupture. The cause of the pain could be determined by contrast CT aortography.

Transthoracic echocardiography can be used for point-of-care testing and can detect aortic regurgitation and pleural/pericardial effusions. However, the diagnostic accuracy for dissection involving the aortic root is low (sensitivity 60%; specificity 83%). The sensitivity of transoesophageal echocardiography (TOE) is higher. However, TOE is rarely available immediately and may not be tolerated by the patient without sedation. The diagnostic accuracy of contrast CT aortography is far better (sensitivity 83–100%; specificity 90–100%). It also provides the most complete anatomical assessment. Although this is the most commonly used imaging modality, the CT suite is an isolated site with limited facilities for resuscitation. The reduced level of consciousness and haemodynamic instability of patients with aortic dissection limits the utility of CT.

5) **What is the mortality associated with this condition?**

The mortality of acute aortic dissection is high, but can be reduced dramatically with appropriate medical and surgical therapy (Tables 13.1 and 13.2). An acute type A dissection, which involves the ascending aorta, is a surgical emergency. This should not be managed conservatively. The prognosis of type B dissections, which do not involve the ascending aorta, is generally better unless a malperfusion syndrome develops, when urgent surgery is also indicated.

Table 13.1 Mortality associated with acute aortic dissection

	Mortality			
	Acute type A		**Acute type B**	
Time from presentation	Medical management (%)	Surgical management (%)	Uncomplicated (%)	Malperfusion syndrome and medical management (%)
24 hours	20	10	—	—
48 hours	30	—	—	20
7 days	40	13	—	—
1 month	50	20	10	25

Table 13.2 Survival after acute aortic dissection (the De Bakey classification is described in Case 12)

De Bakey classification	1-year survival (%)	2-year survival (%)
I	52	48
II	69	50
III	70	60

6) **Did the delay of 2 hours make any difference?**

Delay in presentation significantly reduces the chance of survival. The mortality rate increases 1–2% per hour from the onset of symptoms.

7) **What definitive treatment is required?**

Aortic root surgery is the definitive treatment for type A aortic dissection, with the goal of operating prior to any life-threatening aortic rupture or tamponade (see Case 12). Medical management alone has a high mortality (20% at 24 hours, 30% at 48 hours). Endovascular stenting techniques are in their infancy and currently have no role. The surgical technique usually involves replacement of the aortic root and arch with aortic valve replacement and reimplantation of the coronary arteries. However, an interpositional aortic graft and aortic valve leaflet resuspension is an alternative in suitable patients. Long-term survival after emergency surgery for type A dissection is 80% at 30 days, 75% at 1 year, and 60% at 5 years.

In this case, the patient had tamponade and aortic rupture was suspected. Immediate surgery was mandatory. He underwent replacement of the aortic root and arch with an aortic valve replacement and reimplantation of the coronary arteries. Laparotomy confirmed ischaemic small bowel, which required resection. However, organ and limb perfusion improved significantly with realignment of the aortic intima, media, and adventitia. After a protracted admission to the cardiac ITU the patient was transferred to a general ITU for weaning of respiratory support. He was discharged home 7 weeks after presentation.

8) **What follow-up is required?**

Outpatient follow-up is required to ensure adequate BP control (<135/80 mmHg) and detect further dilation or dissection of the aorta. This can occur many years after the index event. Guidelines suggest serial imaging of the aorta at 3, 6, 9, and 12 months after discharge and annually thereafter.

Further reading

Golledge J, Eagle KA (2008). Acute aortic dissection. *Lancet*; **372**: 55–66.

Khan IA, Nair CK (2002). Clinical, diagnostic, and management perspectives of aortic dissection. *Chest*; **122**: 311–328.

Erbel R, Alfonso F, Boileau C, Dirsch O, Eber B, Haverich A, Rakowski H, Struyven J, Radegran K, Sechtem U, Taylor J, Zollikofer C, Klein WW, Mulder B, Providencia LA; Task Force on Aortic Dissection, European Society of Cardiology. (2001). Diagnosis and management of aortic dissection.: Task Force on Aortic Dissection, European Society of Cardiology. (2001). *European Heart Journal*. 2001; **22**: 1642–81681.

Case 14

A 60-year-old woman with permanent atrial fibrillation had a mechanical mitral valve replacement (MVR; 29-mm ATS Medical) implanted for rheumatic mitral valve disease. She was taking warfarin to maintain a target INR of 3.0.

Eighteen years later she presented to her GP 2 days after she developed a painful swollen left calf. Over-the-counter analgesics were not sufficient to control the pain. As she was allergic to penicillin, erythromycin was started for cellulitis and she was referred for an ultrasound scan of the left leg. Three days later the ultrasound revealed a calf haematoma and she was admitted to hospital. On admission to hospital INR was >11, activated partial thromboplastin time (APTT) 58s, thrombin time (TT) 14s, Hb 6.6 g/dL, WBC 13.7×10^9 cells/L, platelets 276×10^{12} cells/L, and CRP 90 mg/dL. Two units of blood were transfused and the coagulopathy was treated.

Two days after admission she developed abdominal pain and acute renal failure. She was hypotensive and anuric (serum creatinine 532 mmol/L; urea 50 mmol/L) and clinical examination suggested peritonitis. Although the patient was not febrile, blood was sent for microbial culture and intravenous cefuroxime and metronidazole started empirically.

Abdominal CT revealed free air and fluid within the peritoneal cavity. At laparotomy a section of perforated necrotic small bowel was excised and a defunctioning ileostomy was formed. Histological examination demonstrated cytomegalovirus ileitis with mucosal ulceration.

Twenty-four hours after the operation her temperature rose to 38°C and more blood was sent for culture. Blood tests revealed WBC 13.7×10^9 cells/L and CRP 159 mg/dL. Transthoracic echocardiography noted a dilated left atrium (6 cm) and a small mitral paraprosthetic leak, but was otherwise unremarkable. After 5 days of incubation, Candida was identified in one of the two blood culture bottles sent preoperatively. The following day the Candida were found to be non-albicans species.

Questions

1. Why was the clotting so deranged on admission?

2. Did the patient develop disseminated intravascular coagulopathy?

3. How would you have managed the anticoagulation initially? Would the onset of renal failure affect this? How would you manage the anticoagulation perioperatively?

4. Are there any risk factors for candidaemia in the present case? Is the candida isolated from blood cultures likely to be a contaminant?

5. Should the patient be treated with antifungal therapy and if so what should be started initially?

6. What further investigations are required?

7. What does the TOE (Fig. 14.1) show?

8. How would you manage the patient?

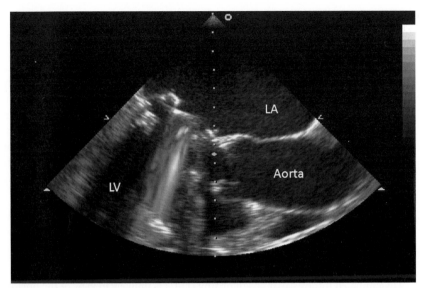

Fig. 14.1 Selected image from transoesophageal echocardiogram study

Answers

1) **Why was the clotting so deranged on admission?**

Several drugs interact with warfarin. Warfarin is metabolized by liver enzymes and in the present case erythromycin (inhibitor of cytochrome p450, particularly CYP3A4 isoenzyme) significantly increased the INR. Alteration in the vitamin K-dependent gut flora by antibiotics may also enhance the action of warfarin on the liver. Warfarin is highly protein bound and drugs such as non steroidal anti-inflammatory drugs (NSAIDs) (which may be present in over-the-counter analgesics) displace warfarin, increasing its effect. Any impairment of liver function, such as drug-induced hepatitis or congestion due to heart failure, may increase warfarin sensitivity.

Illness may also affect anticoagulation: warfarin requirement may increase as clotting factors increase in the acute phase response. Importantly, the dose may need to be reduced as the patient improves.

2) **Did the patient develop disseminated intravascular coagulopathy?**

Disseminated intravascular coagulopathy (DIC) is unlikely in view of the normal thrombin time and platelet count. Prolongation of the thrombin time suggests hypofibrinogenemia and the presence of fibrin degradation products. If DIC is suspected then fibrinogen and D-dimers should be measured directly and a blood film should be reviewed to exclude microangiopathic haemolytic anaemia.

3) **How would you have managed the anticoagulation initially? Would the onset of renal failure affect this? How would you manage the anticoagulation perioperatively?**

In the present case, vitamin K (5 mg intravenous) and fresh frozen plasma (FFP; 20 mL/kg) were administered. Six hours later the INR was 6 and more vitamin K (5 mg intravenous) was given. A factor concentrate was not administered as there was no active bleeding.

When the INR fell below 1.5, intravenous unfractionated heparin was started because the creatinine clearance was less than 30 mL/min. Low-molecular-weight heparin (LMWH) must be used with caution in renal failure as it can accumulate. If LMWH is used, the dose should be reduced and monitoring factor Xa levels can also be considered.

Perioperative management of anticoagulation?

The perioperative management of patients on anticoagulant therapy is a balance of the risks of thromboembolism and haemorrhage over the perioperative period. Patients with a mechanical heart valve who require emergency surgery are particularly problematic. Temporary discontinuation of anticoagulants increases the risk of valve thrombosis and embolism (see Case 50). However, continuing anticoagulation or restarting anticoagulants too early could result in significant haemorrhage.

There is no consensus on the management of anticoagulation in the perioperative period. However, a meta-analysis of RCTs involving patients with a mechanical heart valve, in which one group was not anticoagulated, reported that the risk of thromboembolism in these patients was 9% per year (Cannegieter *et al.*, 1994).

The risk of thromboembolism is affected by several valve and patient-related factors (Table 14.1). The American College of Cardiology guidelines suggest that even in the worst case scenario (a patient with a mechanical prosthesis with previous thromboemboli) the risk of a thromboembolism without anticoagulation is 10–20% per year. Theoretically, if anticoagulation were stopped completely in such a patient, the daily risk of thromboembolism would be 0.027–0.054%. Thus, some clinicians reserve perioperative intravenous heparin for high-risk patients (see Case 50). In the present case, the mitral valve position of the mechanical valve replacement, AF, dilated LA (>5 cm) and acute phase response to critical illness increase the risk of thrombosis significantly (Table 14.1).

Table 14.1 Factors which increase the perioperative risk of thromboembolism in patients with mechanical valve replacements

Operations for malignancy and infection
Another hypercoagulable state
More thrombogenic design of prosthesis
Mitral prosthesis
Prothrombotic intracardiac conditions (e.g. AF, left atrium (LA)>5 cm, impaired LV function)

The approach used in this case was to fully reverse the effects of warfarin before surgery and then start intravenous heparin. This was stopped 3 hours before surgery. Intravenous heparin and warfarin were restarted when surgical haemostasis had been achieved. Heparin was continued until the anticoagulant effect of warfarin was therapeutic. Heparin was continued for 2 days after the INR entered the therapeutic range because of the longer half-life of some of the vitamin K-dependent clotting factors. However, the risk of perioperative thromboembolism may be overestimated.

4) **Are there any risk factors for candidaemia in the present case? Is the candida in blood cultures likely to be a contaminant?**

Risk factors for candidaemia are listed in Table 14.2. In the present case, the risk factors include the change in flora induced by antibiotic treatment and the presence of the prosthetic heart valve, intravenous and urinary catheters, postoperative wound, and colitic bowel perforation.

Candida is a part of normal flora. Isolates from urine, sputum, or stool are often contaminants. Thus, it can be difficult to diagnose disseminated candidiasis as even the sensitivity of blood cultures is low. Although a Candida isolated from blood cultures may be a contaminant, the specificity of blood cultures is high, as is the mortality from candidaemia, so antifungal treatment must be considered if blood cultures are positive.

5) **Should the patient be treated with antifungal therapy and if so what should be started initially?**

There are no clear diagnostic criteria for systemic candidal infection. Treatment is often recommended for patients with risk factors for candidaemia with unexplained fevers. In the present case, antifungal treatment was started in view of the fever, positive blood cultures, and multiple risk factors.

Antifungal resistance among Candida species is uncommon, but some strains are resistant to fluconazole and may also be less sensitive to amphotericin B.

The standard treatment for systemic candidiasis is intravenous amphotericin B. Plain amphoteracin is nephrotoxic, which can narrow the therapeutic index if renal function is impaired, increasing toxicity. Lipid-based formulations are less toxic but expensive.

In this case, all intravenous lines were changed and oral fluconazole was started. However, this is only suitable in immune-competent patients and several species of candida are resistant to fluconazole. On classification of the Candida as a non-albicans species fluconazole was stopped and caspofungin was started.

The echinocandin caspofungin has fungicidal activity against Aspergillus and Candida. It affects fungal cell wall integrity by inhibiting $\beta(1,3)$-D-glucan synthase activity. Caspofungin is as effective as amphotericin B but has significantly fewer side effects. Capofungin is increasingly used first line for treatment of systemic candidiasis in view of the increasing resistance to fluconazole.

6) **What further investigations are required?**

Potential sources of candida should be identified and removed if possible. Intravenous catheters should be removed and the tips sent for culture. Blood and urine should be sent for culture prior to starting antifungal therapy. Transoesophageal echocardiography should be performed to assess the mitral valve for endocarditis. Opthalmological assessment is usually performed 1 week after detection of candidaemia to screen for endopthalmitis. The delay is required to allow fungal hyphae, if present, to grow to a sufficient size to allow detection.

7) **What does the TOE (Fig. 14.1) show?**

The TOE shows multiple, small vegetations on the atrial aspect of the mechanical mitral valve ring (arrowed in Fig. 14.2). In the present case, a diagnosis of definite endocarditis can be made using Duke's criteria [one major criterion (echocardiographic appearance consistent with endocarditis) and three minor criteria (fever, risk factors, and positive blood culture result not fulfilling a major criterion)].

Metal prostheses do not allow microorganisms to proliferate whilst free of thrombotic material. Mechanical prosthetic valve endocarditis generally develops on the sewing cuff or thrombi located near the sewing ring. Periprosthetic leaks, ring abscesses, and infection of adjacent tissue may be detected by TOE.

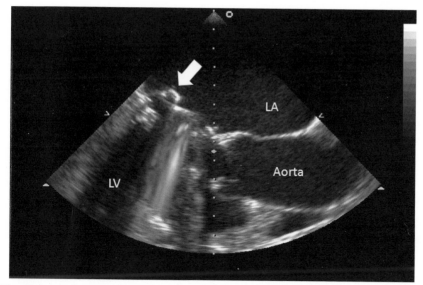

Fig. 14.2 A 2-dimensional transoesophageal long-axis echocardiogram demonstrating prosthetic valve endocarditis.

Candida species are an uncommon but increasing cause of infective endocarditis, accounting for up to 6% of cases. The increasing incidence of fungal endocarditis over the past 20 years has been ascribed to changes in drug therapy and placement of endovascular devices.

The mortality is high (>50%) despite treatment. However, candidaemia often develops in patients with multiple co-morbidities, so attributable mortality is difficult to assess. Optimal management requires a high index of suspicion and the prompt use of appropriate antifungal agents.

8) **How would you manage the patient?**

Daily electrocardiographic monitoring is useful to screening for the onset of heart block due to invasion of the cardiac conduction system. Outcomes are thought to be better when valve replacement is combined with antifungal therapy, particularly if a valve prosthesis is involved. However, there is no evidence from RCTs to support this. Close collaboration between cardiologists, microbiologists, and cardiac surgeons is useful to determine the best course of treatment.

In the present case, the patient was felt to be too unstable to undergo valve replacement and cure was attempted with drug therapy alone. This strategy was successful. Transoesophageal echocardiography performed 3 weeks after completion of a course of antifungal treatment demonstrated resolution of the vegetations and several sets of blood cultures over the following year were negative.

Table 14.2 Risk factors for candidiasis

Mechanical
Catheters (intravenous, urinary tract, peritoneal dialysis)
Wounds (burns and postoperative)
Prosthetic material (e.g. joints, valves, vascular grafts)
Nutritional
Obesity
Chronic acidosis
Chronic malnutrition
Alcohol and intravenous drug use
Total parenteral nutrition
Immunosuppression
Chemotherapy
Steroids
Organ transplantation
Neutropenia

References

Cannegieter SC, Rosendaal FR, Briet E (1994). Thromboembolic and bleeding complications in patients with mechanical heart valve prostheses. *Circulation*; **89**: 635–641.

Further reading

Rajendram R, Alp NJ, Mitchell AR, Bowler IC, Forfar JC. (2005). Candida prosthetic valve endocarditis cured by caspofungin therapy without valve replacement. *Clin Infect Dis*; **40**: e72–74.

Baglin TP, Keeling DM, Watson HG; British Committee for Standards in Haematology. (2006). Guidelines on oral anticoagulation (warfarin): third edition–2005 update. *Br J Haematol*; **132**: 277–285. http://www.bcshguidelines.com/pdf/oralanticoagulation.pdf.

Vahanian A, Baumgartner H, Bax J, Butchart E, Dion R, Filippatos G, Flachskampf F, Hall R, Iung B, Kasprzak J, Nataf P, Tornos P, Torracca L, Wenink A; Task Force on the Management of Valvular Hearth Disease of the European Society of Cardiology; ESC Committee for Practice Guidelines. Guidelines on the management of valvular heart disease: The Task Force on the Management of Valvular Heart Disease of the European Society of Cardiology. (2007). *Eur Heart J*; **28**: 230–268.

Bonow RO, Carabello BA, Chatterjee K, de Leon AC Jr, Faxon DP, Freed MD, Gaasch WH, Lytle BW, Nishimura RA, O'Gara PT, O'Rourke RA, Otto CM, Shah PM, Shanewise JS; American College of Cardiology/American Heart Association Task Force on Practice Guidelines. ACC/AHA VHD Guidelines: 2008 Focused Update Incorporated Into the ACC/AHA 2006 Guidelines for the Management of Patients With Valvular Heart Disease. A Report of the American College of Cardiology/American Heart Association Task Force on Practice Guidelines (Writing Committee to Revise the 1998 Guidelines for the Management of Patients With Valvular Heart Disease) (2008). *J Am Coll Cardio*; **52**: e1–142.

Case 15

A 16-year-old boy was referred to the cardiology clinic because his ECG was abnormal. The ECG had been performed at a voluntary pre-participation sports screening on joining the county athletics team after winning the 100 m sprint at a trial. He was otherwise well with no childhood illnesses of note. He attended the clinic with his parents and younger sister (aged 11 years). Observations were; HR 60 bpm and BP 120/80 mmHg. Venous pressure was not raised and a soft systolic murmur was audible at the left sternal edge. His ECG is shown in Fig. 15.1. After this was seen, ECGs were performed on the rest of his family (Figs. 15.2–15.4).

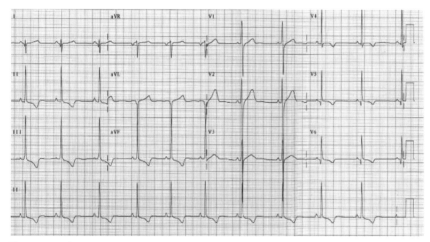

Fig. 15.1 Patient's ECG.

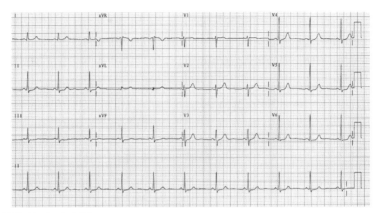

Fig. 15.2 Mother's ECG.

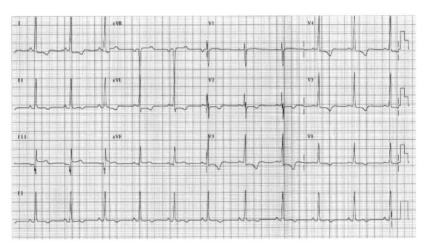

Fig. 15.3 Father's ECG.

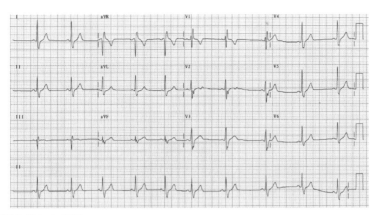

Fig. 15.4 Sister's ECG.

Questions

1. Report the patient's ECG (Fig. 15.1).
2. Report the ECGs of the other family members (Figs 15.2–15.4).
3. What is the inheritance of the ECG abnormalities and what is the likely diagnosis?
4. What is the next most useful investigation for the patient? What is it likely to demonstrate?
5. What further assessment is required for the patient's family?
6. What further assessment is required for the patient and what life style advice would you give?
7. How should the patient and his family be managed?

Answers

1) **Report the patient's ECG (Fig. 15.1).**

   The 12 lead ECG demonstrates sinus rhythm at a rate of 60 bpm with right-axis deviation. Voltage criteria for left ventricular hypertrophy (LVH) are met (see Case 16 for the Sokolow–Lyon index for LVH). There are prominent R waves in the anterior leads. There is infero-lateral T-wave inversion.

2) **Report the ECGs of the other family members (Figs 15.2–15.4).**

   The patient's mother's ECG (Fig. 15.2) is normal. However, his father's ECG is clearly abnormal (Figs. 15.3 and 15.4, respectively). The patient's father's ECG demonstrates LVH with pronounced global T-wave inversion and borderline inferior ST elevation. However, the QRS axis is normal. His sister has right bundle branch block (RBBB) and pronounced sinus arrhythmia with no evidence of LVH or T-wave abnormalities. Although sinus arrhythmia is almost always normal and right bundle branch block is a normal variant often found in young patients, this ECG should be viewed with suspicion.

3) **What is the inheritance of the ECG abnormalities and what is the likely diagnosis?**

   The presence of similar ECG findings in the patient and his father suggest an inherited abnormality, as shown in the pedigree in Fig. 15.5. A dominant mode of inheritance is likely as two consecutive generations of the family are affected but his mother does not display the ECG phenotype. If his sister's heart and ECG are also abnormal she may develop similar repolarization changes and LVH as she gets older. The inheritance would then be autosomal dominant.

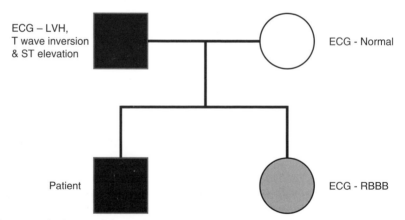

Fig. 15.5 Inheritance of the patient's ECG abnormality. LVH, left ventricular hypertrophy; RBBB, right bundle branch block.

The most likely cause of the gross LVH and repolarization changes seen on the ECGs of both father and son is hypertrophic cardiomyopathy. This is a disease of primary myocardial hypertrophy that is inherited as a Mendelian autosomal dominant trait. It is caused by mutations in several genes encoding protein components of the cardiac sarcomere (e.g. the actin–myosin complex and the regulatory troponin complex) and myocyte energy regulation.

4) **What is the next most useful investigation for the patient? What is it likely to demonstrate?**

In order to confirm the phenotype of hypertrophic cardiomyopathy (HCM), TTE can assess ventricular wall thickness, dimensions, and ventricular function, and determine the presence of an LV outflow tract (LVOT) obstruction. Outflow tract obstruction may be dynamic and require exercise provocation. It will also allow the detection of any aortic valve disease, which, along with systemic hypertension, could produce similar hypertrophy. Magnetic resonance imaging permits a more complete anatomical assessment. However, this has yet to become the first-line investigation of HCM.

Traditionally a wall thickness ≥15 mm was necessary for the diagnosis of HCM. However, the ability to make an absolute genetic diagnosis has lead to the recognition that any degree and distribution of LVH may develop with HCM. In the absence of genetic information, it may be difficult to distinguish mild HCM (wall thickness 13–14 mm) from physiological hypertrophy in athletes or hypertensive heart disease. However, ECG repolarization abnormalities and pathological Q waves may favour a diagnosis of HCM.

Echocardiographic data may allow the usually enlarged LV cavity of the athlete to be distinguished from the smaller one in HCM (assess the diastolic function, which is either normal or enhanced in athletes and impaired in HCM) and to measure the left atrial size (normal in athletes but often increased in HCM).

Although LVOT obstruction was once a defining feature of HCM, it is actually present only in around 25% and obstruction can occur at any level in the ventricle depending on the distribution of hypertrophy (mid-cavity or apical). However, subaortic obstruction is caused by a combination of physical obstruction from septal hypertrophy and systolic anterior motion (SAM) of the MV leaflets. Mid-systolic contact of the MV with the ventricular septum results from impedance to outflow, producing both a drag effect on the anterior leaflet and the Venturi phenomenon (increased fluid velocity through a constriction results in a decrease in pressure). The resulting mild–moderate MR is typically directed posteriorly with variation from this suggesting associated MV pathology.

In the present case, the echocardiogram demonstrated asymmetric LVH of more than 2 cm, particularly in the septum, with a small cavity and hyperdynamic flow (Fig. 15.6). Ventricular function was hyperdynamic but no significant LVOT obstruction was observed.

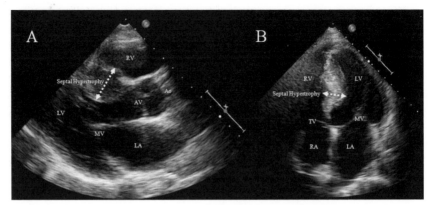

Fig. 15.6 Trans-thoracic echocardiogram demonstrating features of HCM. Septal hypertrophy of >2 cm is arrowed in both the para-sternal long axis view (A) and the apical four-chamber view (B).

5) **What further assessment is required for the patient's family?**

Current recommendations for the screening of relatives of patients with HCM are to perform an annual review from early adolescence. The clinical manifestations of HCM develop during pubertal growth. Pre-pubertal children should only be assessed if they are symptomatic, have a high-risk family history with incidents of SCD at an early age, or wish to participate in competitive sports. The absence of disease at physical maturity was previously considered to exclude HCM. However, as late-onset forms of HCM have been recognized, it is current practice to offer adult relatives of a patient with HCM evaluation every 5 years to reassess risk and document any developing symptoms. This assessment includes echocardiographic assessment of the degree of LVH and the presence of obstruction, prolonged Holter ECG recording to document any arrhythmias, and exercise testing to assess BP response and detect exercise-induced arrhythmias.

Echocardiography is not a perfect screening tool: around 25% of patients with a genetic mutation known to cause HCM do not fulfil conventional echocardiographic criteria for HCM even when ECG abnormalities are present. It would be theoretically possible to provide a perfect screening assessment if testing was conducted at the genetic level. It would not be necessary to await manifestation of the phenotype and pre-natal diagnosis would be possible. However, this would only be possible if either the genetic abnormality within the family is known (genetic diagnosis in an index case) or every mutation causing HCM was known (mutation screening). In reality, only 60% of causal mutations have been characterized so at present mutation screening would yield a 40% false-negative rate. Hence, index cases with a clinical diagnosis of HCM should be offered screening for a genetic diagnosis. If the presence of a mutation known to cause HCM were to be detected this would improve family screening.

6) **What further assessment is required for the patient and what lifestyle advice would you give?**

Once a diagnosis of HCM has been made the next issue is of risk stratification for the most serious complications of sudden death and heart failure. For this, distinguishing between obstructive or non-obstructive forms of HCM is important. Obstruction confers a two-fold increased risk of HCM-related death and about a four-fold increased risk of severe heart failure (NYHA class III or IV). The LVOT gradient can be present at rest or require provocation with exercise (Table 15.1).

Sudden cardiac death is most frequent in the minority of high-risk patients. These patients tend to be younger than 35 years of age and usually suffer a SCD after vigorous exertion. The aetiology of SCD is thought to be due to ventricular arrhythmias as non-sustained ventricular tachycardia (NSVT) is observed in around 20% of these patients undergoing 24-hour Holter ECG. Although such clinical markers are insufficient in identifying all those at risk of SCD, some have proven useful in identifying some of those at risk (Table 15.2).

Those not deemed to be high risk, particularly if they are asymptomatic, do not require treatment. They should be reassured and advised that they can lead an unrestricted lifestyle, but should avoid intense competitive sports. Hence, in this case the patient was advised not to join the county athletics team.

Table 15.1 Outflow tract gradient classification in HCM

Classification of outflow gradient	Continuous wave Doppler measurements
Obstructive	Gradient at rest ≥30 mmHg
Provocable	Gradient at rest <30 mmHg and >30 mmHg after treadmill or bicycle exercise
Non-obstructive	Gradient <30 mmHg at rest and after exercise

Table 15.2 High-risk markers for SCD in HCM

Prior cardiac arrest due to spontaneous sustained VT
Family history of a premature HCM-related SCD
Identification of a high-risk mutant gene (some troponin T and I mutations)
Unexplained syncope
Documented non-sustained VT (≥3 beats of at ≥120 bpm, duration < 30 seconds)
Attenuated BP rise or hypotension on exercise
Extreme LVH of ≥30 mm (present in 10% of HCM, carries 2% annual risk of SCD)

7) **How should the patient and his family be managed?**

Management goals include symptom control, prevention of complications, reducing the risk of SCD, and psychological and genetic counselling.

Medical therapy is indicated in the presence of symptoms or severe LVH. Asymptomatic patients with only mild LVH are thought not to require prophylactic drug therapy. The first-line agents include beta-blockers, which may reduce outflow tract obstruction and help to limit progressive muscle growth. Calcium antagonists such as verapamil or diltiazem have a negative chronotropic effect, reducing outflow obstruction, and also improve diastolic relaxation and function (positive lusitropic effect) through reducing intracellular calcium levels.

Those for whom medical therapy either fails to control symptoms or who have symptom progression can benefit from reducing the outflow gradient by surgical septal reduction or percutaneous alcohol ablation of the septum. Ventricular prexcitation achieved by permanent dual chamber pacing with short AV delay may reduce the LVOT gradient and improve symptoms in some patients.

Individuals with severe LVH, recurrent syncope, sustained and non-sustained ventricular tachyarrhythmias, a history of familial SCD, or a genetic phenotype for an increased risk of premature death should be offered an ICD (see Case 10). There is evidence of improved survival with amiodarone, but given the monitoring required and the risk of toxicity, particularly with prolonged administration, its use has declined with the advent of ICDs.

Further reading

Soor GS, Luk A, Ahn E, Abraham JR, Woo A, Ralph-Edwards A, Butany J.(2009). Hypertrophic cardiomyopathy: current understanding and treatment objectives. *J Clin Pathol*; **62**: 226–235.

Maron, BJ (2009). Distinguishing hypertrophic cardiomyopathy from athlete's heart physiological remodelling: clinical significance, diagnostic strategies and implications for preparticipation screening. *Br J Sports Med*; **43**: 649–656.

Bos JM, Towbin JA, Ackerman MJ.(2009). Diagnostic, prognostic, and therapeutic implications of genetic testing for hypertrophic cardiomyopathy. *J Am Coll Cardiol*; **54**: 201–211.

Maron BJ, McKenna WJ, Danielson GK, Kappenberger LJ, Kuhn HJ, Seidman CE, Shah PM, Spencer WH 3rd, Spirito P, Ten Cate FJ, Wigle ED; American College of Cardiology Foundation Task Force on Clinical Expert Consensus Documents; European Society of Cardiology Committee for Practice Guidelines. (2003). American College of Cardiology/ European Society of Cardiology Clinical Expert Consensus Document on Hypertrophic Cardiomyopathy. A report of the American College of Cardiology Foundation Task Force on Clinical Expert Consensus Documents and the European Society of Cardiology Committee for Practice Guidelines.(2003). American College of Cardiology/European Society of Cardiology Clinical Expert Consensus Document on Hypertrophic Cardiomyopathy. *Eur Heart J*; **24**: 1965–1991.

Case 16

A 28-year-old eastern European student was found to be hypertensive when he enrolled at a local gym, with a BP of 170/80 mmHg, and was asked to see his GP. He explained that he had wanted to start working out because he felt limited by occasional breathlessness on exertion and cramping pains in his legs when riding his new bicycle. He denied having any other medical history but did complain of frequent headaches. His GP heard a continuous systolic and diastolic murmur, performed a 12 lead ECG (Fig. 16.1), requested a chest X-ray (Fig. 16.2), started amlodipine 5 mg, and referred him to a cardiologist.

On examination in the cardiology clinic, his BP was noted to be raised in both arms at 180/70 mmHg, he had a regular pulse of 60 bpm, and the heart sounds were normal but a continuous murmur was audible throughout the praecordium that radiated to the back. Trans-thoracic echocardiography was performed (Fig. 16.3).

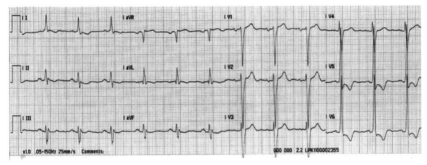

Fig. 16.1 12 lead ECG performed by GP.

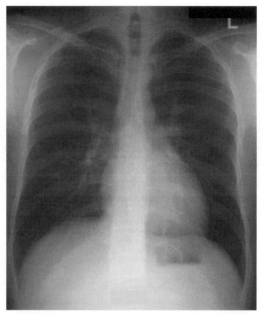

Fig. 16.2 Chest X-ray requested by GP.

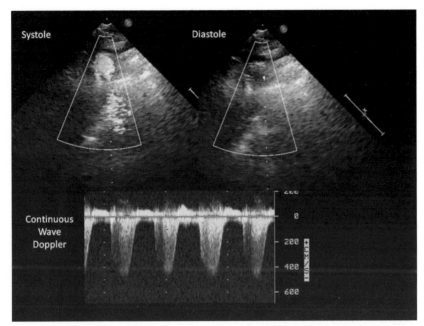

Fig. 16.3 A selected image from the TTE performed in the cardiology clinic showing systole and diastole. Underneath is a continuous wave Doppler tracing recorded along the path indicated by the dotted lines in the systolic and diastolic images. (See colour plate 5)

Questions

1. What could cause a continuous murmur?
2. Report the ECG (Fig. 16.1).
3. What does the chest X-ray (Fig. 16.2) show?
4. How was the echocardiographic (TTE) image (Fig. 16.3) obtained? What does it show?
5. What other clinical features may be present?
6. How could this condition be confirmed and managed?

Answers

1) What could cause a continuous murmur?

The causes of a continuous murmur are listed in Table 16.1. The most common cause in this age group is a persistent ductus arteriosus. However, as this does not cause hypertension it alone cannot explain all the clinical features of this case. Although coarctation of the aorta is less common (3% of congenital cardiac malformations) and initially causes a mid-systolic murmur, it would explain hypertension. Moreover, aortic coarctations that present in adulthood tend to be less severe and have had time to be compensated for by the development of inter-costal artery collaterals. Hence, as this collateral flow becomes more developed a continuous murmur may be heard over the praecordium and back.

Table 16.1 Causes of a continuous murmur

1. Persistent ductus arteriosus
2. Pulmonary arterio-venous fistula
3. Intercostal arterio-venous fistula (e.g. following trauma)
4. Venous hum
5. Ruptured Sinus of Valsalva aneurysm
6. Coarctation of aorta
7. Mammary soufflé – functional cardiac murmur heard over the breasts in late pregnancy and postpartum if lactating
8. Right-sided coronary-cameral fistula – communication between coronary artery and a cardiac chamber

2) Report the ECG (Fig. 16.1).

The 12 lead ECG shows sinus rhythm at a rate of 72 bpm. The QRS axis is within the normal range (0°). There is LVH, as defined by the Sokolow–Lyon index (Equation 1), with a strain pattern: asymmetric ST-segment depression and T-wave inversion in leads I, II aVL, V5, and V6.

The absence of ECG signs of hypertrophy do not exclude LVH (sensitivity <50%) but specificity is higher (75%) if voltage criteria are present (Equation 1). In addition, the diagnostic accuracy is improved further if a strain pattern is also present. Left ventricular strain is usually seen in the leads that assess the LV (I, aVL, V4–6). Echocardiography can be used to measure the actual thickness of the LV myocardium, and normal end diastolic thickness range between 0.6 and 1.1 cm, with LVH defined as a thickness greater than 1.1 cm.

The ECG therefore suggests that the hypertension detected at the gym was long standing as end-organ damage has occurred.

Equation 1 is the Sokolow–Lyon index for left ventricular hypertrophy. These criteria are only valid in those over 35 years old, having a 75% sensitivity and 75% specificity for LVH.

Equation 1

$$\text{S wave in V1} + \text{R wave in V5 or V6 (whichever is larger)} \geq 35 \text{ mm}$$

or

$$\text{R wave in aVL} \geq 11 \text{ mm}$$

3) **What does the chest X-ray (Fig. 16.2) show?**

The chest X-ray shows prominence of the left heart border and a double contour to the aortic knuckle strongly suggestive of aortic coarctation (Fig. 16.4). Notching of the lower margins of the ribs (Fig. 16.4), reflecting chronic expansion of the internal thoracic and intercostal arteries (functioning as collaterals), is just present (arrows).

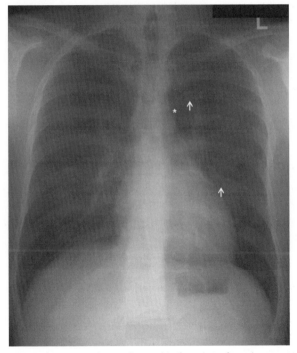

Fig. 16.4 Chest X-ray demonstrating radiographic features of aortic coarctation. This chest X-ray shows prominence of the left heart border and a double contour to the aortic knuckle (*) strongly suggestive of aortic coarctation. Notching of the lower margins of the ribs (arrowed), reflecting chronic expansion of the internal thoracic and intercostals arteries (functioning as collaterals), is just present (arrows).

4) **How was the TTE image (Fig. 16.3) obtained? What does it show?**

The TTE image with colour flow mapping in systole and diastole was obtained from the supra-sternal acoustic window. This view is used to image the aortic arch. The selected view (Fig. 16.3) is focused on the descending aorta. The colour flow mapping demonstrates turbulent flow during systole in the proximal descending aorta, just after the origin of the left subclavian artery (Fig. 16.5). This suggests the presence of an obstruction. The most common site for aortic coarctation to develop is distal to the left subclavian artery at the aorto-ductal junction (the site of the foetal ductus arteriosus). These findings are therefore consistent with a diagnosis of aortic coarctation. In the present case, aortic coarctation was initially suggested by the history of upper limb hypertension and lower limb claudication in a young patient.

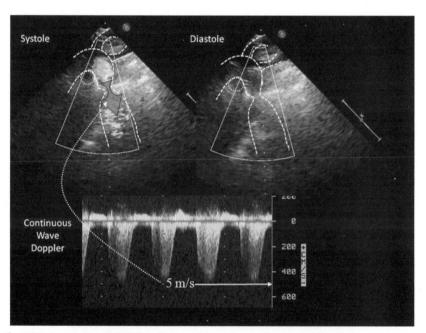

Fig. 16.5 Supra-sternal TTE showing an obstruction to flow in the descending aorta consistent with aortic coarctation. (See colour plate 6)

5) **What other clinical features may be present?**

These effects of coarctation depend on the severity of the stenosis. The most severe coarctations present in the neonatal period with cardiac failure and are associated with aortic stenosis and hypoplasia of the left ventricle. Less severe coarctation presents later in infancy with breathlessness or failure to thrive. The exact timing of presentation in later childhood and adulthood depends in part on the extent of the collateral circulation through the intercostal and internal thoracic arteries. In this age group, common symptoms include cold feet, claudication, or headaches. The diagnosis is usually made on routine medical examination, which reveals upper limb hypertension with delayed, reduced, or absent femoral pulses and/or a cardiac murmur. The continuous murmur of coarctation is usually best heard over the back. Commonly upper body muscular development is greater than the lower body from chronically reduced perfusion to the lower limbs. Occasionally, the first presentation is with aortic dissection or rupture.

6) **How could this condition be confirmed and managed?**

Non-invasive imaging (CT and MRI) can provide detailed anatomical information about the anatomy of the aortic arch and adjacent structures. MRI can also measure flow across a stenosis and grade functional severity. Cardiac catheterization and angiography allow pressure measurements and anatomical assessment of aortic coarctation.

The prognosis of coarctation of the aorta is less good in patients presenting in late childhood and as adults because of the increased persistence of hypertension despite anatomical relief of obstruction. Morbidity and premature death result from systemic hypertension, CAD, heart failure, renal impairment, and cerebrovascular disease. It is therefore important that hypertension be treated and preventative strategies adopted to reduce the risk of complications.

Specific intervention for the coarctation is required if there is a resting gradient over 30 mmHg with hypertension. Options include surgical resection and percutaneous stenting. The procedural success rate of stenting is high (>95%); however, around 25% of patients develop recurrent abnormalities, including aneurysm formation (≈10%). Long-term outcome data are lacking.

Hypertension may develop or persist despite relief of arch obstruction, especially if performed at an older age. Long-term follow-up is therefore required. Importantly, there should also be surveillance for aortic stenosis, as up to 75% of patients with coarctation of the aorta have a bicuspid aortic valve (and up to 25% with bicuspid aortic valves have aortic coarctation). There is an association with other vascular abnormalities, such as Berry aneurysms of the Circle of Willis that predispose to subarachnoid haemorrhage (see Table 16.2). Aortic coarctation is associated with non-cardiovascular conditions such as Turner syndrome (see Table 16.2), in which there is also an increased incidence of aortic dissection.

This patient had a percutaneous stent implanted successfully (Fig. 16.6) and is currently under annual follow-up.

Table 16.2 Abnormalities and syndromes associated with aortic coarctation

Intra-cardiac	Left-sided obstructive or hypoplastic defects	Bicuspid aortic valve (75%)
		Hypoplastic left heart syndrome
		Aortic arch hypoplasia
	Ventricular septal defects	
	Right-sided cardiac obstructive lesions (rare)	Pulmonary stenosis
		Pulmonary atresia
		Tetralogy of Fallot
Vascular	Berry aneurysms of the Circle of Willis (3–5%)	
	Right subclavian artery arising distal to the coarctation (5%)	
	Both subclavian arteries originate distal to the coarctation (rare)	
	Collateral arteries	Internal mammaries to external iliac arteries
		Spinal and intercostal arteries to the descending aorta
Non-cardiovascular	Turner syndrome (12–17%)	
	Musculoskeletal, genitourinary, gastrointestinal, or respiratory system abnormalities (~25% of children with coarctation)	

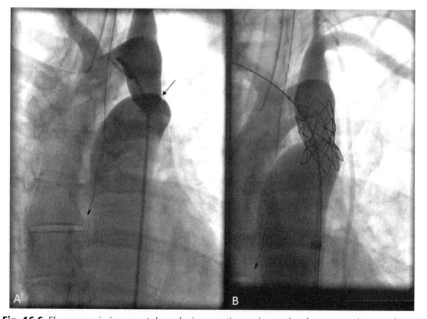

Fig. 16.6 Fluoroscopic images taken during aortic angiography demonstrating aortic coarctation (A, arrowed) and after placement of a stent across the coarctation (B).

Further reading

Deanfield J, Thaulow E, Warnes C, Webb G, Kolbel F, Hoffman A, Sorenson K, Kaemmer H, Thilen U, Bink-Boelkens M, Iserin L, Daliento L, Silove E, Redington A, Vouhe P, Priori S, Alonso MA, Blanc JJ, Budaj A, Cowie M, Deckers J, Fernandez Burgos E, Lekakis J, Lindahl B, Mazzotta G, Morais J, Oto A, Smiseth O, Trappe HJ, Klein W, Blömstrom-Lundqvist C, de Backer G, Hradec J, Mazzotta G, Parkhomenko A, Presbitero P, Torbicki A; Task Force on the Management of Grown Up Congenital Heart Disease, European Society of Cardiology; ESC Committee for Practice Guidelines. (2003). Task Force on the Management of Grown Up Congenital Heart Disease, European Society of Cardiology; ESC Committee for Practice Guidelines. *Eur Heart J*; **24**: 1035–1084.

Pewsner D, Jüni P, Egger M, Battaglia M, Sundström J, Bachmann LM.(2007). Accuracy of electrocardiography in diagnosis of left ventricular hypertrophy in arterial hypertension: systematic review. *BMJ*; **335**: 711.

Tanous D, Benson LN, Horlick EM. (2009). Coarctation of the aorta: evaluation and management. *Curr Opin Cardiol*; **24**: 509–515.

Case 17

A 38-year-old African woman with no previous medical history was brought to a walk-in centre by a friend. She had a 4-week history of generalized headache, dizziness, and blurred vision. Her GP had prescribed cyclizine 2 weeks previously but this had not improved the symptoms. The nurse consultant referred the patient to the medical registrar on call when the BP was found to be 250/140 mmHg. The patient was confused (GCS 14/15) so no further history was available. Fundoscopy demonstrated bilateral retinal haemorrhages and papilloedema.

Questions

1. What are the possible triggers for this patient's hypertensive crisis?
2. What investigations are required urgently?
3. What clinical features determine the urgency of management?
4. What is autoregulation of blood flow? How does failure of autoregulation result in end-organ damage?
5. Why is autoregulation important in the treatment of hypertensive emergencies?
6. What complications suggest acute end-organ damage from hypertension?
7. How would you manage this patient?
8. What is the incidence and long-term prognosis of hypertensive emergencies with treatment?

Answers

1) **What are the possible triggers for this patient's hypertensive crisis?**

The most common cause of a hypertensive emergency is a rapid idiopathic rise in BP on a background of chronic hypertension. In most cases treatment of chronic hypertension has been inadequate or patients have suddenly stopped medications. Other causes are listed in Table 17.1.

Table 17.1 Causes of hypertensive crises

Primary hypertension
Inadequately controlled chronic hypertension
Rebound hypertension after withdrawal of antihypertensive treatment
(e.g. beta-blockers, calcium channel blockers, ACE inhibitors, clonidine)
Secondary hypertension
Renal
Renal parenchymal disease (80% of secondary causes)
Renovascular disease
Collagen-vascular diseases (e.g. scleroderma, systemic lupus erythematosis)
Uraemia with fluid overload
Cardiovascular
Increased cardiac output (secondary to increase in vascular resistance)
Increased vascular resistance
Autonomic hyperactivity
Endocrine
Endocrine (e.g. pheochromocytoma, Cushings, hyperadosteronism)
Drugs
Drugs (e.g. cocaine, amphetamines, oral contraceptives, diet pills, cyclosporin, clonidine withdrawal, phencyclidine)
Drug interactions (e.g. monoamine oxidase inhibitors with tricyclics, antihistamines, or tyramine; serotonin syndrome)
Delirium tremens—withdrawal from benzodiazipines, barbiturates, chronic alcohol misuse
Neurological
Cerebrovascular (infarction, intracranial or subarachnoid haemorrhage)
Head injury
Pregnancy
Pre-eclampsia and eclampsia (pre- or postpartum)
Others
Perioperative hypertension; stress response to surgery

2) **What investigations are required urgently?**

In this case, all the investigations listed in Table 17.2 were performed. Of the investigations listed in Table 17.3 only a pregnancy test (negative) and CT brain (normal) were performed.

Table 17.2 Investigations required for all patients presenting with hypertensive emergencies

Investigations	Associated condition
Serum urea, electrolytes and creatinine	? Renal impairment
FBC ± blood film	? Microangiopathic anaemia
Urinalysis	
Dipstick urinalysis	? Haematuria or proteinuria
Urine microscopy	? Red blood cells (RBCs) or RBC casts
ECG	? Myocardial ischaemia
	? Left ventricular hypertrophy
Chest radiography	? Cardiac enlargement
	? Pulmonary oedema
	? Widened mediastinum

Table 17.3 lists investigations that should be considered in patients presenting with hypertensive emergencies.

Table 17.3 Investigations which may be required in hypertensive emergencies

Optional investigations	Indication
Toxicology screen	Cocaine, amphetamines
Pregnancy test	? Pre-eclampsia/eclampsia Pregnancy also affects medical treatment
Endocrine testing	Investigation of phaeochromocytoma, Conns, Cushings, etc.
CT head	Abnormal neurology
	? Intracranial bleeding
	? Cerebral oedema
	? Cerebral infarction
CT chest, TOE	? Aortic dissection

3) **What clinical features determine the urgency of management?**

A hypertensive emergency occurs if severely elevated BP [diastolic BP (DBP) often greater than 120 mmHg] is associated with acute or rapidly progressive end-organ damage. Immediate antihypertensive therapy to achieve controlled and progressive reduction in BP is required, with appropriate and careful monitoring.

Malignant hypertension is associated with retinal haemorrhages, exudates, and papilloedema. Distinguishing malignant and accelerated (only retinal haemorrhages or exudates are present) hypertension is not helpful as the prognosis and treatment are the same. Hypertensive encephalopathy refers to the presence of cerebral oedema caused by loss of cerebral autoreulation and severe and sudden rises in BP in malignant hypertension.

Most patients presenting with acutely elevated BP [systolic BP (SBP) >200 mmHg or DBP >120 mmHg] do not have symptoms or signs of end-organ damage (hypertensive urgency). These patients can be managed with oral antihypertensives and close outpatient follow-up.

4) **What is autoregulation of blood flow? How does failure of autoregulation result in end-organ damage?**

Autoregulation is a local regulation of blood flow and tissue perfusion. It is the ability of an organ to maintain constant blood flow despite changes in perfusion pressure. The initial response to mild–moderate increases in BP is arteriolar vasoconstriction. Blood flow initially increases but returns to normal over seconds to minutes. Higher BP is not transmitted to small, distal, more fragile vessels.

As BP rises, autoregulation eventually fails to compensate. The BP rises higher, damaging the vascular endothelium, allowing plasma into the walls of the arterioles and capillaries. The lumens of these vessels are then narrowed or obliterated, resulting in fibrinoid necrosis. Failure of cerebral autoregulation and vasodilatation in the brain results in cerebral oedema and hypertensive encephalopathy.

Although malignant hypertension is usually associated with diastolic BP above 120 mmHg, the BP at which fibrinoid necrosis occurs depends on the baseline BP. Chronic hypertension causes arteriolar hypertrophy, which reduces transmission of BP to the capillaries. However, in previously normotensive patients presenting with acute hypertension, hypertensive encephalopathy can be seen at diastolic BP as low as 100 mmHg. Patients with impaired autoregulation (e.g. following head injury) also develop hypertensive injury at relatively mild degrees of hypertension.

5) **Why is autoregulation important in the treatment of hypertensive emergencies?**

As hypertension is treated and BP falls, autoregulation maintains tissue perfusion via arterial and arteriolar vasodilatation. Flow is related to pressure divided by resistance. Blow flow is maintained if resistance to flow falls at the same rate as BP. Rapid reduction of BP outside the cerebral, renal, or coronary autoregulatory range markedly reduces organ perfusion. This could cause ischaemia or infarction. The arteriolar hypertrophy induced by chronic hypertension shifts the BP range for autoregulation upwards so hypoperfusion occurs at higher BP than in normotensive subjects.

Hypertensive emergencies should be treated with short-acting antihypertensive agents. These should be gradually withdrawn if the rate of reduction of BP is too rapid or symptoms of hypotension develop. It is important not to lower BP too quickly in this situation to avoid cerebral infarction at sites of critically reduced perfusion.

6) **What complications suggest acute end-organ damage from hypertension?**

Table 17.4 lists the complications of acute hypertension that suggest end-organ damage.

Table 17.4 Acute end-organ damage

Organ	Effect of end-organ damage
Brain	Hypertensive encephalopathy
	Cerebral infarction
	Intracranial haemorrhage
	Subarachnoid haemorrhage
	Retinopathy
	Eclampsia
Heart	Myocardial ischaemia/infarction
	Acute left ventricular dysfunction
	Acute pulmonary oedema
	Aortic dissection
Kidneys	Acute renal failure/insufficiency

7) **How would you manage this patient?**

The initial aim of management is control of BP. The cause of the hypertensive emergency should then be determined.

Differentiate primary malignant hypertension from secondary conditions (listed in Table 17.1) on the basis of history, examination, and the investigations listed in Tables 17.2 and 17.3. Differentiate global neurological symptoms and signs (headache, nausea, vomiting, restlessness, confusion, seizures, and coma) due to hypertensive encephalopathy from focal neurological symptoms and signs that may be due to cerebral haemorrhage or infarct. Exclude other hypertensive emergencies and acute end-organ damage (e.g. aortic dissection, acute pulmonary oedema, acute/impending myocardial infarction, cerebrovascular events, etc.).

This patient has hypertensive encephalopathy and requires admission for careful (usually parenteral) control of BP. The BP should be gradually lowered but *not* to normal levels. Lower the mean arterial pressure (MAP) by up to 20% of the MAP at presentation or lower the DBP to around 100–110 mmHg over a few hours. If the patient remains stable, the BP could then be lowered to around 160/100–110 mmHg over the next 12 hours.

These targets are best achieved by a continuous infusion of a short-acting, titratable, parenteral antihypertensive. Invasive arterial BP monitoring ($\pm$ central venous pressure) is often helpful. Antihypertensive therapy should be withdrawn temporarily if hypoperfusion occurs.

In hypertensive encephalopathy, agents with central nervous system side effects should be avoided (e.g. methyldopa, clonidine). Vasodilators such as GTN may increase cerebral perfusion and so should be used with caution. In this case, BP was controlled with intravenous labetalol. Her symptoms settled over 24 hours with control of BP. She was then started on oral antihypertensive agents and the labetalol was weaned over the next 48 hours. No secondary cause of hypertension was found in this case and so essential hypertension was diagnosed by exclusion.

8) **What is the incidence and long-term prognosis of hypertensive emergencies with treatment?**

As treatment of hypertension has improved, the incidence of hypertensive emergencies has fallen from 7% to 1% of patients with hypertension.

Effective antihypertensive therapy, including haemodialysis, is associated with 1- and 5-year survival rates of 90% and 80%, respectively. However, the outcomes of patients with renal impairment are generally worse. Despite effective treatment of malignant hypertension, some acute and chronic vascular damage persists and there is a risk of recurrence and ongoing risks of coronary, cerebrovascular, and renal disease.

Prevention of recurrence requires close outpatient follow-up. Lifestyle modification and compliance with medication are fundamental to survival. Before effective treatment was available (before 1950), life expectancy was under 2 years, and the 1- and 5-year survival rates were less than 25% and 1%, respectively. The most common causes of death are cardiovascular complications.

Further reading

Aggarwal M, Khan IA (2006). Hypertensive crisis: hypertensive emergencies and urgencies. *Cardiol Clin*; **24**: 135–146.

Amin A (2008). Parenteral medication for hypertension with symptoms. *Ann Emerg Med Mar*; **51**(3 Suppl): S10–5.

Barton JR (2008). Hypertension in pregnancy. *Ann Emerg Med Mar*; **51**(3 Suppl): S16–17.

Cheung AT, Hobson RW 2nd (2008). Hypertension in vascular surgery: aortic dissection and carotid revascularization. *Ann Emerg Med Mar*; **51**(3 Suppl): S28–33.

Diercks DB, Ohman EM (2008). Hypertension with acute coronary syndrome and heart failure. *Ann Emerg Med Mar*; **51**(3 Suppl): S34–36.

Hollander JE (2008). Cocaine intoxication and hypertension. *Ann Emerg Med Mar*; **51**(3 Suppl): S18–20.

Pancioli AM (2008). Hypertension management in neurologic emergencies. *Ann Emerg Med Mar*; **51**(3 Suppl): S24–27.

Slovis CM, Reddi AS (2008). Increased blood pressure without evidence of acute end organ damage. *Ann Emerg Med*; **51**(3 Suppl): S7–9.

Case 18

A 32-year-old woman was found to have high BP (155/90 mmHg) at the first antenatal appointment with her GP when 12 weeks pregnant. Hypertension was confirmed over the next week by two further clinic measurements and ambulatory BP monitoring. She was asymptomatic. There was no previous medical history or relevant family history. She did not smoke and had stopped drinking alcohol whilst pregnant. She did not take any regular medications and denied illicit drug use.

Clinical examination was unremarkable. Routine investigations were sodium 144 mmol/L, potassium 3.8 mmol/L, creatinine 50 µmol/L, and urea 3.0 mmol/L. Liver function tests were normal. Urine dipstick testing excluded haematuria and proteinuria. ECG was normal. Ultrasound demonstrated a normal foetus of 12 weeks' gestation.

Questions

1. In what position should pregnant women have their BP measured?
2. What are the Korotkoff sounds used for the measurement of BP?
3. Which Korotkoff sounds should be used to determine BP in pregnant women?
4. What are the indications for ambulatory BP monitoring?
5. How is hypertension classified in pregnancy?
6. Does this patient have pregnancy-induced hypertension?
7. When should investigation for secondary causes of hypertension be considered? What investigations should be performed?
8. In this patient, further investigations revealed:

    plasma aldosterone 712 pmol/L (normal range 28–445 pmol/L)

    plasma renin activity 0.2 ng/mL/h (0.7–5 ng/mL/h)

    plasma aldosterone concentration: renin activity ratio 3560 (normal <750).

    a. Interpret these results.
    b. What further investigations are required to determine the diagnosis?
    c. What BP targets are appropriate during pregnancy?
    d. How would you manage this patient during pregnancy?

Answers

1) **In what position should pregnant women have their BP measured?**

   Blood pressure should be measured whilst the patient is sitting. The cuff should be at the level of the heart. When a pregnant woman is supine, compression of the inferior vena cava by the uterus can reduce venous return and significantly reduce BP. Measurement of BP in the left lateral position may also be falsely low if measured in the higher arm, unless the cuff is at the level of the heart.

2) **What are the Korotokoff sounds used for the measurement of BP?**

   Korotkoff described five sounds:

   First sound – clear snapping sound first heard at the systolic pressure.

   Second sounds – murmurs heard for most of the area between the systolic and diastolic BP.

   Third sound – loud, crisp, tapping sound (rare).

   Fourth sound – described as muting of the sound. This occurs at pressures less than 10 mmHg above the diastolic BP.

   Fifth sound – silence as the cuff pressure drops below the diastolic BP. The disappearance of sound is considered DBP.

   The second and third Korotkoff sounds have little clinical significance.

3) **Which Korotkoff sounds should be used to determine BP in pregnant women?**

   Korotkoff sounds I (first sound) and V (disappearance of sound) should be used to determine systolic and DBP, respectively. In some pregnant women, the gap between the fourth (muffling) and fifth Korotkoff sounds is large. The fourth and fifth sounds should therefore be recorded (e.g. 160/95/50 mmHg; sound I/sound IV/sound V).

   Maternal systolic BP > 160 mmHg or DBP > 110 mmHg indicates severe hypertension. Depending on the gestational age and maternal health, delivery should be considered if hypertension in this range is sustained.

4) **What are the indications for ambulatory BP monitoring?**

   Although outcome trials are based on clinic measurements of BP, ambulatory monitoring is useful and can guide treatment decisions. Ambulatory BP monitoring is helpful in the diagnosis and assessment of hypertension in pregnancy. Other indications for ambulatory BP monitoring are listed in Table 18.1.

   In non-pregnant patients, ambulatory targets should be <130/80 (<130/75 in diabetics), but there is no evidence for true equivalence. Blood pressure targets in pregnant women are discussed below.

Table 18.1 Indications for ambulatory BP monitoring

BP is very labile
Guidance of treatment decisions in equivocal cases
BP remains high despite treatment with multiple agents
Assessment of the efficacy of BP control over 24 hours is required
Management of hypertension during pregnancy
Hypotension or white coat hypertension is suspected (e.g. young, women, non-smokers, normal BP at home)
Nocturnal or masked (reversed white coat hypertension) hypertension is suspected (e.g. alcoholics, smokers, high caffeine intake, physical inactivity, raised BP at home)

5) **How is hypertension classified in pregnancy?**

Hypertension is the most common medical problem in pregnancy, complicating 2–3% of pregnancies. Hypertensive disorders during pregnancy can be classified into four categories (Table 18.2).

Table 18.2 Classification of hypertensive disorders during pregnancy

1. Chronic hypertension
2. Pre-eclampsia–eclampsia
3. Pre-eclampsia with chronic hypertension
4. Gestational hypertension

Using population-based data, approximately 1% of pregnancies are complicated by chronic hypertension, 5–6% by gestational hypertension (without proteinuria), and 1–2% by pre-eclampsia.

6) **Does this patient have pregnancy-induced hypertension?**

Chronic hypertension is defined as BP above 140/90 mmHg before pregnancy or before 20 weeks' gestation. Hypertension identified before 20 weeks' gestation is rarely pregnancy induced. This patient is therefore most likely to have chronic hypertension as she was only 12 weeks pregnant when hypertension was diagnosed.

Pre-eclampsia must be excluded in women with new onset hypertension after 20 weeks' gestation. Pre-eclampsia occurs in 5% of all pregnancies, 10% of first pregnancies, and 20–25% of pregnant women with a previous history of chronic hypertension.

Gestational trophoblastic disease and/or molar pregnancy should be excluded if severe hypertension or pre-eclampsia are diagnosed before the second trimester.

Gestational (transient) hypertension occurs in late pregnancy without any other features of pre-eclampsia. Blood pressure returns to normal postpartum. It may be associated with chronic hypertension in later life.

Hypertensive disorders in pregnancy may cause maternal and foetal morbidity, and are a leading cause of maternal mortality.

7) **When should investigation for secondary causes of hypertension be considered What investigations should be performed?**

Hypertension is primary in 90–95% of patients. Investigation for secondary causes of hypertension should be considered for:

◆ young patients (aged <30 years)

◆ BP resistant to antihypertensive treatment

◆ family history of hypertension or stroke at age <50 years

◆ symptoms, signs, family history, or investigations suggesting a secondary cause.

A detailed social history, including alcohol intake and substance misuse (e.g. cocaine), may show reversible contributors to increased BP.

8) **In this patient, further investigations revealed:**

plasma aldosterone 712 pmol/L (normal range 28–445 pmol/L)

plasma renin activity 0.2 ng/mL/h (0.7–5 ng/mL/hour)

plasma aldosterone concentration: renin activity ratio 3560 (normal <750).

a) **Interpret these results**

These results suggest primary hyperaldosteronism. However, hyperaldosteronism and Cushings syndrome are difficult to diagnose during pregnancy as levels of cortisol normally increase.

Primary hyperaldosteronism is the most common cause of secondary hypertension, accounting for up to 5% of all hypertensive patients. Screening is based on measurement of plasma aldosterone concentration and renin activity.

Antihypertensive drugs (except spironolactone, eplerenone, amiloride, and beta-blockers) should not be stopped routinely before these investigations are performed but in some patients may contribute to false-positive and false-negative results.

In primary hyperaldosteronism the raised plasma aldosterone suppresses plasma renin so the ratio of plasma aldosterone concentration (pmol/L) to plasma renin activity (ng/mL/h) is high.

Only one-third of patients with primary hyperaldosteronism are hypokalaemic. As in this case, in the remaining two-thirds K^+ concentrations are usually at the lower end of the reference range and Na^+ concentrations at the upper end. Screening should therefore be considered in patients with normal plasma K^+.

b) **What further investigations are required to determine the diagnosis?**

If BP can be controlled, no further investigation is required until after delivery of the foetus. However, this patient will require referral to an endocrinologist to confirm the suspicion of primary hyperaldosteronism (usually by oral or intravenous Na^+ loading or fludrocortisone suppression test). Adrenal imaging (CT or MRI) and selective adrenal venous sampling is sometimes required to differentiate between the two main causes, which are Conn's syndrome (unilateral aldosterone-producing adenoma) and idiopathic hyperaldosteronism.

Less common causes include:

+ unilateral hyperplasia or primary adrenal hyperplasia
+ familial hyperaldosteronism type I (glucocorticoid-remediable aldosteronism)
+ familial hyperaldosteronism type II (familial aldosterone-producing adenoma or bilateral idiopathic hyperplasia or both)
+ aldosterone-producing adrenocortical carcinomas.
+ Ectopic aldosterone-secreting tumours (e.g. neoplasms in the lung, ovary or kidneys).

c) **What BP targets are appropriate during pregnancy?**

Aggressive BP reduction during pregnancy may be harmful to the foetus. One study reported that a 10 mmHg fall in MAP was associated with a 176 g decrease in birth weight. This effect was unrelated to the type of hypertension or choice of medication. Reasonable BP targets in pregnant women without end-organ damage are systolic BP 140–150 mmHg and DBP between 90 and 100 mmHg. However, in pregnant women with end-organ damage, the BP should be below 140/90 mmHg.

d) **How would you manage this patient during pregnancy?**

The main risk of chronic hypertension in pregnancy is pre-eclampsia. There is no evidence that treatment of mild hypertension reduces the risk of developing pre-eclampsia.

The course of hyperaldosteronism in pregnancy is variable. Mean arterial pressure normally drops 10–15 mmHg over the first-half of pregnancy as a result of the increased progesterone. Most women with mild chronic hypertension (SBP 140–160 mmHg, DBP 90–100 mmHg) do not require treatment during this period. However, when progesterone falls (within 24 hours of delivery), the effects of aldosterone manifest and require treatment.

However, DBP > 110 mmHg increases risk of placental abruption and intrauterine growth retardation, and systolic BP >160 mmHg increases risk of maternal intracerebral haemorrhage. These patients should be treated to targets of DBP < 105 mmHg and systolic BP < 160 mmHg.

Management options for mild chronic hypertension in pregnancy include:

1. If the woman is treated with an agent suitable for use in pregnancy, this may be continued.

2. If a woman is treated with an agent not suitable for use in pregnancy, this should be stopped or changed.

3. Antihypertensive medication may be withheld or discontinued. Blood pressure normally falls during pregnancy. However, this approach requires close monitoring of BP.

Women with chronic hypertension in pregnancy should be monitored for increasing BP and the development of pre-eclampsia. Perform investigations for pre-eclampsia if the BP increases or if signs or symptoms of pre-eclampsia develop.

Antihypertensive treatment during pregnancy

Antihypertensive medications recognized as safe for use during pregnancy include methyldopa and hydralazine. Other drugs commonly used to treat hypertension in pregnancy include nifedipine, labetalol, and clonidine. However, the safety of these drugs in pregnancy is less secure.

Diuretics prevent the volume expansion that normally occurs in pregnancy so are generally only used for volume-dependent hypertension (e.g. renal or cardiac disease). Beta-blockers, atenolol in particular, may be associated with some intrauterine growth restriction. Although long-term follow-up studies are lacking, use during pregnancy is best avoided unless alternatives are inappropriate.

Angiotensin-converting enzyme inhibitors should not be used as they are associated with a risk of foetal renal dysgenesis or death when used in the second and third trimesters. Angiotensin II receptor antagonists should also be avoided.

Spironolactone must not be used during pregnancy. Spironolactone crosses the placenta and can affect foetal genital development (i.e. feminise a male foetus). Only antihypertensive agents that are recognized to be safe for use during pregnancy should be prescribed.

Maternal and foetal monitoring

Antepartum assessment is directed towards early diagnosis of pre-eclampsia and foetal growth delay. This is best accomplished by frequent antenatal assessment for monitoring maternal blood pressure, proteinuria, and fundal growth, and by periodic estimation of foetal size by ultrasound. Over 85% of hypertensive women will have uncomplicated pregnancies.

In this case, no treatment was required during pregnancy. Three days after delivery of the foetus, a fludrocortisone suppression test confirmed primary hyperaldosteronism. There was no evidence of an adenoma on MRI.

Dietary sodium intake was reduced, weight loss and regular exercise were recommended, and spironolactone was started. The BP improved significantly (135/80 mmHg).

Further reading

Williams B, Poulter NR, Brown MJ, Davis M, McInnes GT, Potter JF, Sever PS, McG Thom S; British Hypertension Society. (2004). Guidelines for management of hypertension: report of the fourth working party of the British Hypertension Society, 2004—BHS IV. *J Hum Hypertens*; **18**: 139–185.

NICE guideline (2006). Hypertension: management of hypertension in adults in primary care. *NICE*. http://www.nice.org.uk/CG034.

Marik PE (2009). Hypertensive disorders of pregnancy. *Postgrad Med*; **121**: 69–76.

Funder JW, Carey RM, Fardella C, Gomez-Sanchez CE, Mantero F, Stowasser M, Young WF Jr, Montori VM; Endocrine Society. (2008). Case detection, diagnosis, and treatment of patients with primary aldosteronism: an endocrine society clinical practice guideline. *J Clin Endocrinol Metab*; **93**: 3266–3281.

Case 19

A 45-year-old non-smoker with a localized stage la T1N0M0 gastro-oesophageal junc-tion carcinoma underwent oesophagectomy and partial gastrectomy with no immedi-ate postoperative complications. Six months later he presented with sudden onset, 'excruciating', right-sided loin pain and macroscopic haematuria. He was normally independent but was not able to mobilize because of pain. He denied having any previous episodes of similar pain or renal stones. He was taking paracetamol 1 g and codeine 60 mg four times a day (qds) for the pain.

Observations: BP 114/66 mmHg, HR 61 bpm (sinus), respiratory rate (RR) 25 breaths/min, O_2 saturations 93% air, temperature 36.5°C.

On examination, JVP was not raised and heart and breath sounds were normal. The left-sided thoraco-laparotomy scar from the oesophagectomy had healed well. There was bilateral loin tenderness.

Investigations: Urine dipstick revealed blood (++) and protein (++) but no casts were seen on microscopy. Blood results: Hb 13.7 g/dL, white cell count (WCC) 13.3 × 10^9/dL (neutrophils 9.5 × 10^9/dL), platelets 305 × 10^{12}/dL), Na+ 137 mmol/L, K+ 4.0 mmol/L, creatinine 129 µmol/L (3 months previously 98 µmol/dL), amylase 35 iu/dL, CRP 235 mg/dL. The admission ECG is shown in Fig. 19.1; the preoperative ECG is Fig. 19.2. Troponin T <0.01 µg/L. Chest X-ray showed that the gastric air bubble was overlying the left lung field but was otherwise unremarkable.

Abdominal ultrasound was normal so CT abdomen was performed (Fig. 19.3A). This was reviewed immediately by a radiologist and after discussion with the surgical team a chest CT was performed (Fig. 19.3B). The patient was then referred to a cardi-ologist, who performed TTE and requested cardiac MRI (Fig. 19.4). Whilst awaiting these investigations the patient developed acute lower limb ischaemia with loss of all peripheral pulses below the femoral arteries in both legs. Aorto-femoral angiography was performed (Fig. 19.5).

Questions

1. Report the admission ECG (Fig. 19.1) and the preoperative ECG (Fig. 19.2). What does the troponin result imply?

2. What was found on CT (Fig. 19.3)?

3. What does the aorto-femoral angiogram (Fig. 19.5) show?

4. The patient has had, in the past, open repair and internal fixation for a tibial fracture, a laparoscopic cholecystectomy and an oesophagectomy and partial gastrectomy. Is MRI contraindicated?

5. What does the MRI (Figs 19.4A and 19.4B) show? What is the effect of gadolinium enhancement (Figs 19.4C and 19.4D)?

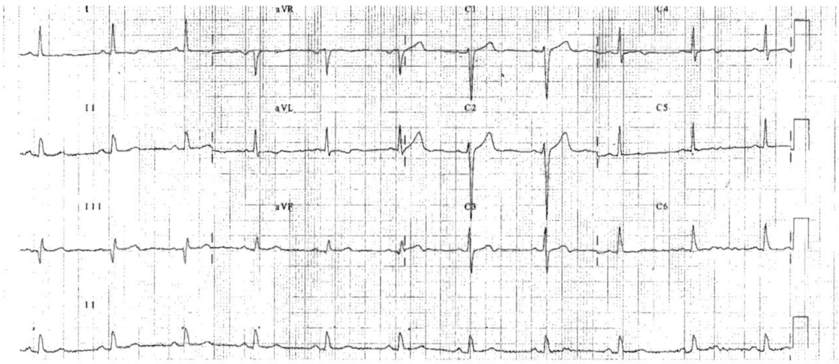

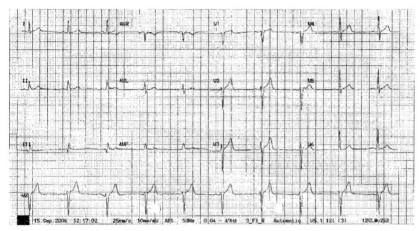

Fig. 19.1 Admission ECG.

Fig. 19.2 Preoperative ECG.

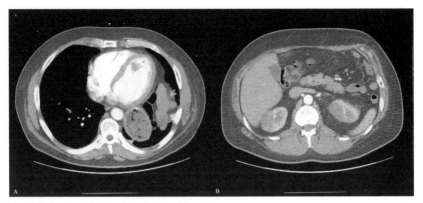

Fig. 19.3 CT chest (A) and abdomen (B).

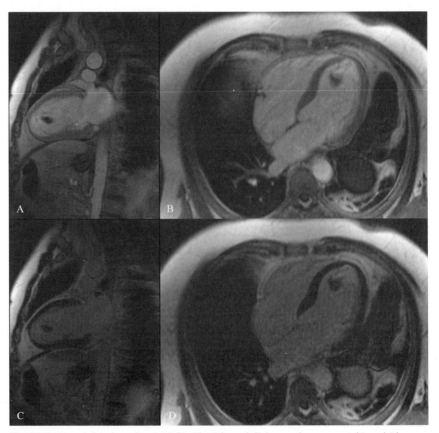

Fig. 19.4 T1-weighted cardiac MRI (A–D) with gadolinium enhancement (C and D).

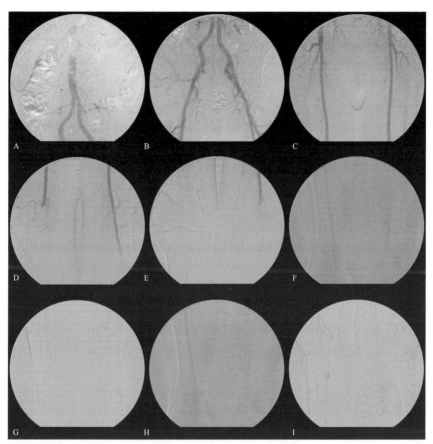

Fig. 19.5 Femoral angiogram.

Answers

1) **Report the admission ECG (Fig. 19.1) and the preoperative ECG (Fig. 19.2). What does the troponin result imply?**

The admission ECG shows sinus rhythm (rate 66 bpm). However, the T waves in V3–4 are biphasic, the T waves in V5–6 are flattened, and those in I and aVL are just inverted. The preoperative ECG is more normal, with upright T waves throughout the chest leads, including V1. The ECG has changed. The negative troponin suggests that the event resulting in these ECG changes occurred over a week previously or that the cause is extracardiac (see Case 6 for non-cardiac causes of T-wave inversion).

2) **What was found on CT (Fig. 19.3)?**

The contrast-enhanced CT of the abdomen (Fig. 19.3B) shows several areas of reduced perfusion in both kidneys, suggesting the presence of multiple small emboli (Fig. 19.6B). The CT chest (Fig. 19.3A) shows the stomach, pulled up into the chest, behind the heart. A large filling defect is present in the LV next to the septum (Fig. 19.6A).

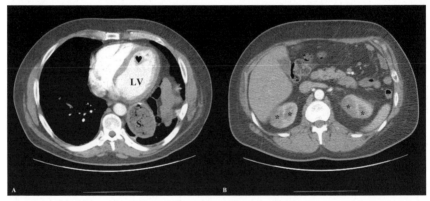

Fig. 19.6 Contrast-enhanced CT chest (A) and abdomen (B) demonstrating areas of reduced perfusion in the kidneys and an intracardiac filling defect. The CT abdomen (A) shows several areas of reduced perfusion (*) in both kidneys, suggesting the presence of multiple small emboli. The CT chest (B) shows the stomach (S), pulled up into the chest, behind the heart. A large filling defect (♥) is present within the left ventricle (LV) next to the septum.

3) **What does the aorto-femoral angiogram (Fig. 19.5) show?**

The aorto-femoral angiogram demonstrates multiple arterial emboli. Emboli are present within the right femoral artery at the adductor hiatus and in the left popliteal artery on the just proximal to the knee (Fig. 19.7). There is no significant distal run-off on either side.

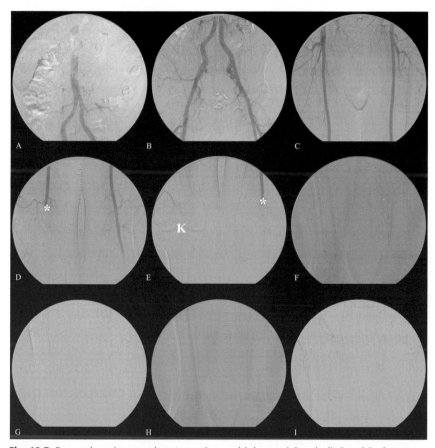

Fig. 19.7 Femoral angiogram demonstrating multiple arterial emboli. Panel D shows an embolus (*) within the right femoral artery at the adductor hiatus. Panel E shows an embolus (*) within the left popliteal artery just proximal to the knee (K). There is no significant distal run-off on either side.

4) **The patient has had, in the past, open repair and internal fixation for a tibial fracture, a laparoscopic cholecystectomy and an oesophagectomy and partial gastrectomy. Is MRI contraindicated?**

Implants and foreign bodies may malfunction, move, cause thermal injury, or cause imaging artefacts. Orthopaedic surgical implants are usually well anchored so should not move, but may be heated through induction. Unfortunately, image quality may be severely degraded. The radiographers should be informed of the presence of other metallic implants, such as surgical clips, etc. If magnetic, they may be hazardous, but fortunately most are not.

Patients with implants should provide information (manufacturer, model, serial number, and date of implantation) about all implants to the referring physician and radiographer before entering the room for MRI.

In the present case, the presence of these implants does not contraindicate MRI, but the radiographers should be informed.

Contraindications to MRI are listed in Table 19.1.

Table 19.1 Contraindications to MRI

Absolute contraindications	Relative contraindications
Electronically, magnetically, and mechanically activated implants	Cochlear implants
	Other pacemakers, e.g. for the carotid sinus
Ferromagnetic or electronically operated active devices, e.g. ICD	Insulin pumps and nerve stimulators
	Lead wires or similar wires (MRI safety risk)
Cardiac pacemakers[1]	Prosthetic heart valves (if dehiscence is suspected)
Metallic splinters in the eye[2]	
Ferromagnetic haemostatic clips in the central nervous system	Haemostatic clips (body)
	Non-ferromagnetic stapedial implants

[1]Highly specialized protocols have been developed to allow MRI of patients with some pacemakers.
[2]An orbital X-ray is required if there is any possibility that there may be small metal fragments in the eyes.

5) **What does the MRI (Figs 19.4A and 19.4B) show? What is the effect of gadolinium enhancement (Figs 19.4C and 19.4D)?**

This is a T1-weighted MRI. The sagittal two-chamber view (Fig. 19.4A) demonstrates the mass within the left ventricle (Fig. 19.8A). It has the same intensity as cardiac muscle. Figure 19.4B is a transverse four-chamber view also showing the mass (Fig. 19.8B). In the gadolinium-enhanced MRI (Figs. 19.4C and 19.4D) the mass is hypo-intense relative to cardiac muscle. The mass has not taken up gadolinium and is therefore more likely to be thrombus than tumour.

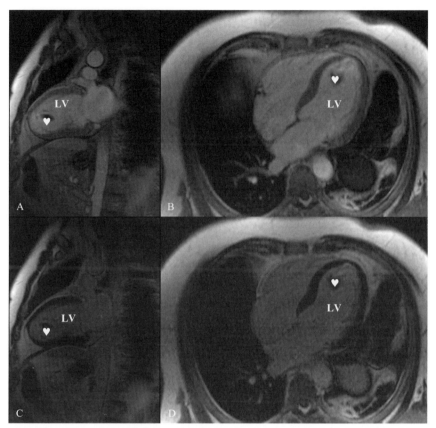

Fig. 19.8 T1-weighted cardiac MRI (A–D) with gadolinium enhancement (C and D) demonstrating intracardiac mass. The sagittal two-chamber view (A and C) demonstrates the mass (♥) within the left ventricle (LV). It has the same intensity as cardiac muscle. The transverse four-chamber view (B and D) also shows the mass. In the gadolinium enhanced MRI (C and D) the mass is hypointense relative to cardiac muscle. The mass has not taken up gadolinium and is therefore more likely to be thrombus than tumour.

The role of MRI in the investigation of cardiac masses

Echocardiography is the first-line investigation for the assessment of cardiac masses. However, the relationship of the mass to surrounding cardiac structures is best determined by MRI, which can also provide a better indication of the histological diagnosis. MRI can usually distinguish thrombus from tumour, particularly if contrast is used, which enhances tumour but not thrombus.

MRI can demonstrate pseudomasses. Some normal structures can be misinterpreted as masses on TTE (e.g. a moderator band in the right ventricle (RV) or a Chiari network). These can be shown to be normal variant anatomic structures by MRI. Large trabeculations, papillary muscles, and asymmetric ventricular hypertrophy can all emulate tumours. Cine MRI can confirm that these structures contract normally (not seen with tumours).

Lipomatous hypertrophy of the myocardium can occur in any location, but most often in the atrial wall or interventricular septum. This is commonly misdiagnosed as myxoma or thrombus on TTE but the characteristic signal intensity of fat makes diagnosis on MRI straightforward.

The Chiari network is an embryonic remnant of no clinical significance present in 2–3% of the population. It appears to be a web-like structure with a variable number of thread-like fronds. On echocardiography it is characterized by whip-like motion within the right atrium and attachment to the wall of the right atrium in close proximity to the entrance of the inferior vena cava.

A moderator band is a muscular ridge found only in the RV. It is present in the majority of normal individuals and contains fibres of the right bundle branch.

In this case, the patient was anticoagulated with warfarin. Embolic phenomena did not recur. The cardiac MRI was repeated 6 weeks later and demonstrated complete resolution of the cardiac mass. This was therefore assumed to be thrombus. Warfarin was discontinued after 6 months of anticoagulation and TTE confirmed that the thrombus had not recurred. Shortly thereafter the patient reported increasing breathlessness on exertion. Myocardial perfusion imaging demonstrated inducible ischaemia and subsequent coronary angiography demonstrated stenoses of the left anterior descending and circumflex arteries. These were treated with bare metal coronary stents and aspirin and clopidogrel were started. The left ventricular thrombus probably developed after a perioperative anterolateral MI.

Further reading

Hendel RC, Patel MR, Kramer CM, Poon M, Hendel RC, Carr JC, Gerstad NA, Gillam LD, Hodgson JM, Kim RJ, Kramer CM, Lesser JR, Martin ET, Messer JV, Redberg RF, Rubin GD, Rumsfeld JS, Taylor AJ, Weigold WG, Woodark PK, Brindis RG, Hendel RC, Douglas PS, Peterson ED, Wolk MJ, Allen JM, Patel MR. ACCF/ACR/SCCT/SCMR/ASNC/NASCI/SCAI/SIR (2006). Appropriateness Criteria for Cardiac Computed Tomography and Cardiac Magnetic Resonance Imaging. *J Am Coll Cardiol*; **48**: 1–23.

O'Donnell DH, Abbara S, Chaithiraphan V, Yared K, Killeen RP, Cury RC, Dodd JD. (2009). Cardiac tumors: optimal cardiac MR sequences and spectrum of imaging appearances. *Am J Roentgenol*; **193**: 377–387.

Waller BF, Grider L, Rohr TM, McLaughlin T, Taliercio CP, Fetters J (1995). Intracardiac thrombi: frequency, location, etiology, and complications: a morphologic review—Part I. *Clin Cardiol* Aug; **18**(8): 477–479.

Waller BF, Rohr TM, McLaughlin T, Grider L, Taliercio CP, Fetters J (1995). Intracardiac thrombi: frequency, location, etiology, and complications: a morphologic review—Part II. *Clin Cardiol*; **18**: 530–534.

Waller BF, McLaughlin T, Grider L, Rohr TM, Taliercio CP, Fetters J (1995). Intracardiac thrombi: frequency, location, etiology, and complications: a morphologic review—Part III. *Clin Cardiol*; **18**: 587–590.

Waller BF, Grider L, Rohr TM, McLaughlin T, Taliercio CP, Fetters J (1995). Intracardiac thrombi: frequency, location, etiology, and complications: a morphologic review—Part IV. *Clin Cardiol* **18**: 669–674.

Waller BF, Rohr TM, McLaughlin T, Grider L, Taliercio CP, Fetters J (1995). Intracardiac thrombi: frequency, location, etiology, and complications: a morphologic review—Part V. *Clin Cardiol* **18**: 731–734.

Case 20

A 72-year-old woman presented to the ED with a 4-week history of fever, cough, and mild wheeze. Her past medical history included treated hypertension, gastro-oesophageal reflux, and falls with transient loss of consciousness. After each fall she had regained consciousness rapidly on lying flat and so the syncope was thought to be vasovagal in origin. However, the falls had never been formally investigated. She was taking bendroflumethazide 2.5 mg once daily (od), amlodipine 5 mg od, omeprazole 30 mg od, and aspirin 75 mg od.

She initially presented to her GP 1 week after the symptoms began. Blood tests had revealed an Hb of 8.2 g/dL, WCC 5×10^9/dL, and an erythrocyte sedimentation rate (ESR) of 80 mm/hour. She was treated for suspected influenza with secondary bacterial infection and asthma with oral coamoxyclav, prednisolone, and a salbutamol inhaler. Her symptoms did not settle and so a chest X-ray was performed. The chest X-ray was reported to be normal. A second course of antibiotics (clarythromycin) was prescribed.

On examination she was short of breath at rest, her JVP was raised to the angle of the jaw at 45° but the apex beat was not displaced and normal in character. Although heart sounds were normal, an early diastolic murmur was heard. Fine inspiratory crepitations were present in both lung bases. There was no ascites or pedal oedema. Her pulse was regular at 90 bpm, with a BP of 110/60 mmHg and no postural drop. Blood O_2 saturations were 94% on air.

The chest X-ray performed on admission demonstrated upper lobe blood diversion and perihilar alveolar shadowing consistent with mild pulmonary congestion. The ECG confirmed sinus rhythm. She was treated with intravenous diuretics and antibiotics. The cardiology registrar was asked to perform a TTE to determine the cause of the diastolic murmur. After performing the TTE the cardiology registrar organized an urgent departmental TOE (Fig. 20.1).

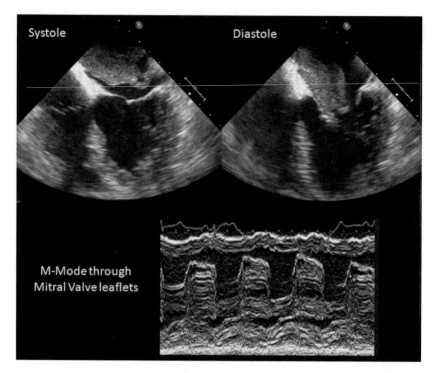

Fig. 20.1 Selected image from trans-oesophageal echocardiogram shown in systole and diastole (upper), with an M-mode tracing across the mitral valve obtained in the TTE below.

Questions

1. What do the TOE images (Fig. 20.1) show?
2. Can this explain the breathlessness and syncopal episodes?
3. What is the differential diagnosis?
4. What investigation would you request next?
5. What is the most likely diagnosis?
6. How should the patient be treated?

Answers

1) **What do the TOE images (Fig. 20.1) show?**

   The TTE shows a large mass prolapsing through the mitral valve in diastole both in the diastolic image from the TOE and on the M-mode tracing from the TTE (Fig. 20.2). The mass shows variable echogenicity and close apposition to the anterior mitral valve leaflet. Biventricular systolic function appears maintained.

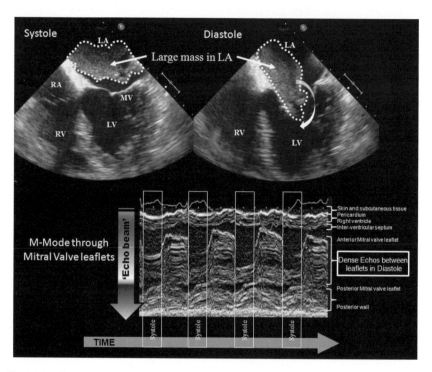

Fig. 20.2 Selected image from TOE shown in systole and diastole (above), with an M-mode tracing across the mitral valve obtained on TTE (below) demonstrating mass prolapsing through the mitral valve in diastole. The mass is seen in the left atrium in systole but prolapses into the LV in diastole. This is demonstrated on two-dimensional TOE (above) and transthoracic M-mode echocardiography (below).

2) **Can this explain the breathlessness and syncopal episodes?**

   Intra-cavity masses can disrupt blood flow by direct obstruction and secondary cardiac failure. The precise effects and resulting symptoms depend on location. Masses also impair valve function either by restricting opening or allowing regurgitation. Large myxomas can obstruct ventricular filling and cause syncope. These are more common on the left (75%) rather than the right (25%) heart.

   Friable left-sided masses can embolize widely, leading to a spectrum of presentation from mimicking vasculitis to embolic stroke. Right-sided masses can present with PE and pulmonary hypertension. Estimated clinical embolic event rates from left- and right-sided myxomas are 45–60% and 8–10%, respectively, possibly reflecting the more dynamic flow in the left heart although right-sided events are more likely to be asymptomatic.

Intra-mural ventricular masses can impair contractility, restrict diastolic function, and cause conduction abnormalities, ventricular arrhythmias, or sudden death. Intra-mural atrial masses can cause atrial arrhythmias.

Pericardial involvement can present with haemorrhagic effusion and tamponade or chest pain. Mediastinal and pleural spread, particularly for angiosarcomas, can lead to vena cava obstruction and respiratory symptoms. Distant metastases to lungs, mediastinum, vertebral column, brain, thyroid gland, bones, and other internal organs can also precipitate presentation.

Primary cardiac tumours also present with non-specific signs such as fever, weight loss, and tiredness. Myxomas increase synthesis of interleukin-6, which could explain constitutional symptoms (e.g. fever), raised inflammatory markers, and rheumatic symptoms. Cardiac para-gangliomas are extremely rare catecholamine-producing tumours that arise from intrinsic cardiac para-ganglial (chromaffin) cells and produce symptoms typical of phaeochromocytoma (arterial hypertension, headache, palpitations, and flushing).

Whilst cardiac masses may present with any of a multitude of possible symptoms, as described above, 20% of patients with cardiac myxomas are asymptomatic. Asymptomatic tumours are increasingly found incidentally as the use of non-invasive imaging expands.

3) **What is the differential diagnosis?**

An intra-cardiac mass could be thrombus, a vegetation (endocarditis), or a neoplasm (benign or malignant). Thrombus (see Case 19) is common in the context of impaired LV function, LA dilatation, AF and mitral stenosis. Right-sided thrombus is mostly embolic and retains the cast of the deep veins of its origin. The possibility of malignancy should always be considered.

Malignant cardiac lesions are most commonly secondary to either metastatic spread (3% of malignant tumours have cardiac metastases at autopsy) or result from direct invasion (e.g. thymoma, oesophagus, bronchial, and lymphoma). Metastasis occurs via lymphatic (e.g. epithelial malignancies and lymphoma) and haematological routes (e.g. melanoma, sarcoma, leukaemia, lymphoma, and renal cell). Cardiac metastases often present with large pericardial effusions and carry a poor prognosis (80% mortality). The mean survival after diagnosis of cardiac metastases is around 6 months. See Table 20.1 for a list of malignant cardiac tumours.

Primary tumours of the heart are comparatively rare (estimated prevalence 0.02%) and the majority are benign (75%). The most common benign tumours are myxomas (75%). The apparent incidence of primary cardiac tumours has risen with the increased use and improvements in the quality of non-invasive imaging. See Table 20.2 for a list of benign cardiac tumours.

Table 20.1 Malignant cardiac tumours

1. Sarcomas	Myxosarcoma
	Liposarcoma
	Angiosarcoma
	Fibrosarcoma
	Leiomyosarcoma
	Osteosarcoma
	Synovial sarcoma
	Rhabdomyosarcoma
	Neurofibrosarcoma
	Malignant fibrous histiocytoma
	Undifferentiated sarcoma
2. Lymphoma	

Table 20.2 Benign Cardiac Tumours

Benign Cardiac Tumours
Myxoma
Rhabdomyoma
Fibroma
Papillary Fibroelastoma
Haemangioma
Pericardial Cyst
Lipoma
Hamartoma

4) **What investigation would you request next?**

Although a chest X-ray should be performed as it may reveal a primary tumour or lymphadenopathy, it rarely provides diagnostic information for cardiac masses. Specifically, primary cardiac tumours rarely cause visible abnormalities on chest X-ray, but occasionally myxomas can calcify (litomyxoma).

Two-dimensional TTE is the first-line investigation for primary cardiac tumours. In most cases it is diagnostic, but it may be limited by acoustic windows. The use of micro bubble contrast may allow better definition of intra-cavity masses, allow assessment of their perfusion, and permit identification of the composition of the mass (tumour vs thrombus).

As some parts of the heart are difficult to visualize with TTE (e.g. atrial appendages), TOE may be useful. However, imaging anterior structures (i.e. aortic arch and pulmonary artery) is difficult with TOE and extra-cardiac spread is harder to detect than with TTE.

Cardiac CT or MRI is currently the imaging modality of choice as a complete assessment of the characteristics of the mass are possible. The most appropriate investigation will depend on availability and familiarity, but in this case cardiac MRI was performed. CT and MRI can be used to characterize suspected lesions, assess extra-cardiac spread and provide information for staging. See Case 19 for further discussion of the role of MRI in the assessment of cardiac masses.

5) **What is the most likely diagnosis?**

The most likely diagnosis given the clinical presentation and the features of the mass on imaging is an atrial myxoma.

Myxomas are the most common primary cardiac tumour and present most commonly in the 30- to 60-year age group with an equal sex distribution. Myxomas are polypoid, friable, pedunculated masses of endocardial origin up to 15 cm in size that commonly present with non-specific symptoms and raised inflammatory markers (e.g. elevated ESR and gamma-globulins). Myxomas mainly arise in the atria (95%: left, 75%; right, 15–20%) with a short broad attachment to the inter-atrial septum often around the fossa ovalis (90%). Myxomas rarely arise from cardiac valve tissue (usually fibroelastomas or myxoid fibrosarcomas).

Myxomas impair valve function by obstructing flow and may mimic mitral steno-sis. However, symptoms tend to be intermittent, develop suddenly, and may be positional. Sudden obstruction of blood flow may cause syncope from cerebral hypoperfusion. An early diastolic tumour plop may be audible if the tumour pro-lapses through the mitral valve and touches the ventricular wall. Presentations with pulmonary or systemic embolization, atrial arrhythmias, and congestive heart failure are also common.

Myxomas usually develop sporadically. Only 2.7% are associated with syndromes [e.g. LAMB (lentiginosis, atrial myxoma, mucocutaneous myxomas, blue naevi) and NAME (naevi, atrial myxoma, myxoid neurofibroma, ephelides)]. Patients with these syndromes tend to present earlier and have multiple right-sided myxo-mas. The inheritance is autosomal dominant with variable penetrance. A muta-tion in the gene encoding the R1a regulatory subunit of cyclic adenosine monophosphate-dependent protein kinase A (PRKAR1a) has been associated with a high risk of developing cardiac myxomas.

In the present case, a biopsy is not indicated as the diagnosis of myxoma is prob-able clinically. However, where diagnostic uncertainty exists a histological diagno-sis can affect management. Some tumours (e.g. rhabdomyoma in children) regress spontaneously whilst others respond to chemotherapy. Percutaneous endomyo-cardial biopsy can be used. Right-sided intra-cavity masses are accessible with the lowest risk. Left-sided lesions requiring a trans-septal atrial approach are associ-ated with a higher risk of embolism.

As atrial myxomas are the most common primary cardiac tumour, other diag-noses are only likely if intra-cardiac masses fail to conform to the characteristic features of myxoma.

Papillary fibroelastoma should be suspected (after exclusion of endocarditis and adherent thrombus) if the tumour arises from a heart valve in a patient over

60 years old. These may arise from the endocardium but occur most frequently on the aortic valve or the atrial aspect of the atrio-ventricular valves. They are the third most common primary tumour and are often present as incidental findings on echocardiography. They are benign hamartomas consisting of multiple delicate papillary fronds resembling normal chordae and may arise from prolonged mechanical wear. They are generally smaller than myxomas (<1 cm) but can embolize. They can develop thrombus or endocarditis.

Fibromas are the second most common benign cardiac tumour in adults, but present at much younger ages. Originating from fibroblasts, these commonly arise in the ventricles, and tend to be large (can be more than 10 cm) and locally invasive. Sudden death may follow extension into the conducting system. They can calcify and may be visible on the chest X-ray.

An intra-cardiac mass presenting below the age of 15 years is most likely to be a rhabdomyoma. These tumours are strongly associated with tuberous sclerosis (50% of cases). Rhabdomyoma can be asymptomatic, but commonly causes intra-cardiac obstruction with heart failure, and rhythm abnormalities. They rarely involve valves, tend to regress spontaneously in over 50%, and have a good prognosis.

Masses arising from the visceral (epicardium) and parietal pericardium are either pericardial cysts or lipomas. Common sites include the intra-atrial septum. This consists of an epicardial fat invagination, which can undergo lipomatous hypertrophy and enlarge to exceed 2 cm. Rhythm abnormalities and sudden death occur in a third.

Other rare tumours include haemangiomata, leiomyomas, neurofibromas, and endodermal heterotopia of the atrio-ventricular node and histiocytic cardiomyopathy.

Malignant tumours of the heart account for a quarter of all tumours, angiosarcomas (highest prevalence), rhabdomyosarcoma (second most common), mesotheliomas and fibrosarcomas being the most common. They cause symptoms of intra-cardiac obstruction and have a poor prognosis (median survival 10 months without resection). Primary cardiac lymphoma, although rare, accounts for 1% of primary cardiac tumours and 0.5% of extra-nodal lymphomas. It has been linked to AIDS, immuno-suppression, and cardiac transplantation.

6) **How should the patient be treated?**

The patient requires surgical resection of the atrial myxoma as it is causing life-threatening symptoms. However, for those tumours unlikely to cause symptoms, a conservative approach involving annual TTEs, anticoagulation, and monitoring for development of symptoms may be preferable to immediate surgery, especially where the patient presents a high operative risk.

Most myxomas are amenable to surgical resection and recurrence is unusual but well described. Recurrence rates are higher if resection is incomplete and in familial forms as multiple primary tumours are present. The results of surgical treatment of intra-cardiac benign tumours are good, regardless of their origins and number, in both the short and long term. In most patients TTE repeated at 1–2 yearly intervals should be sufficient to detect recurrence in most cases. More frequent screening should be considered in patients with multiple, familial, or atypical myxomas.

In this case, surgical resection of the tumour was performed. Histopathological analysis confirmed the clinical diagnosis of atrial myxoma. The patient will be followed up with 1–2 yearly echocardiograms to detect recurrence.

Further reading

Reynen K (1995). Cardiac myxomas. *N Engl J Med*; **333**: 1610–1617.

Roberts WC (1997). Primary and secondary neoplasms of the heart. *Am J Cardiol*; **80**: 671–682.

Butany J, Nair V, Naseemuddin A, Nair GM, Catton C, Yau T. (2005). Cardiac tumours: diagnosis and management. *Lancet Oncol*; **6**: 219–228.

Case 21

A 75-year-old lady with no previous medical history was brought to the ED by ambulance after being found collapsed at home by a neighbour. Her neighbour reported that the patient had not been well for the last week. Her oral intake had been poor and she had been bedbound.

On arrival she was confused and drowsy. There was pitting oedema at the ankles. Urine dipstick was positive (leukocytes +, nitrites +, blood ++, protein +) and she was started on intravenous antibiotics and fluid rehydration. Several hours later she was much more alert and asked for a commode. Whilst sitting on the commode she collapsed to the floor. She was caught by the attending nurse and did not hit her head. She was rapidly put back into bed and assessed.

She was unresponsive, struggling to breathe, sweaty, and peripherally shut down. The nurse noted a fast low-volume pulse and that her BP was unrecordable.

When attached to a cardiac monitor she had a sinus tachycardia of 130 bpm and O_2 saturations of 60% on 15 L/min O_2 via a non-rebreathe mask, with a respiratory rate of 30/min.

The medical registrar was called. Arterial blood gas analysis demonstrated PaO_2 6.4 kPa (O_2 saturations 85%), $PaCO_2$ 3.5 kPa. A 12 lead ECG confirmed sinus tachycardia (120 bpm) but was otherwise unremarkable. Portable chest X-ray was normal.

Questions – Part 1

1. What is the immediate management?
2. What is the differential diagnosis for the haemodynamic instability? What is the most likely cause?
3. What bedside test could narrow the differential?
4. What could cause the discrepancy between O_2 saturations measured by pulse oximetry and arterial blood gas (ABG) analysis?

Answers

1) **What is the immediate management?**

   Assessment and treatment of airway, breathing, and circulation should occur simultaneously:

   A – patent airway

   B – oxygenation and ventilation

   C – perfusion of the brain, heart, and kidneys

   Fluids and inotropes may be required to maintain the circulation. Although this may increase myocardial work, inadequate tissue perfusion increases morbidity and mortality. Once stability has been achieved, special investigations and treatments should be considered while continuing resuscitation.

2) **What is the differential diagnosis for the haemodynamic instability? What is the most likely cause?**

   Causes of cardiovascular collapse or shock (systolic BP <90 mmHg with reduced organ perfusion) can be classified as cardiac or non-cardiac.

     i. Cardiac

       a. Primary myocardial dysfunction (MI, LV failure, valve lesion, arrhythmia)

       b. Secondary myocardial dysfunction (PE, tamponade, tension pneumothorax)

     ii. Non-cardiac

       a. Reduced preload (loss of circulatory volume—haemorrhage, reduced pulmonary venous return).

       b. Reduced after load (reduced systemic vascular resistance—anaphylaxis, sepsis)

   In this case the most likely diagnosis is PE in view of the severe hypoxia, recent illness and reduced mobility, normal chest X-ray, and ECG demonstrating sinus tachycardia. Other possible causes of cardiovascular collapse in this case include anaphylaxis and sepsis.

3) **What bedside test could narrow the differential?**

   Bedside TTE can provide rapid and accurate assessment of:

     i. LV and RV structure and function

     ii. regional wall-motion

     iii. valve structure and function

     iv. pericardium (effusions and tamponade)

     v. volume status

If TTE is normal the cause of shock is most likely to be non-cardiac.

Echocardiographic assessment of the right heart should include:

i. Right atrial (RA) size

ii. Right ventricular size (end-diastolic diameter (30 mm – present in 25% of PE)

iii. assessment of RV function (PE can cause dyskinesia/akinesia of RV free wall)

iv. pulmonary and tricuspid valve structure and function

v. tricuspid regurgitation, pulmonary artery (PA) pressure, PA size and RV systolic pressure (RVSP)

vi. intra-ventricular septum motion (paradoxical/systolic movement to left as raised RV pressures)

vii. Dilation and flow reversal in the inferior vena cava.

Echocardiography has a sensitivity of around 60–70%. It cannot exclude PE and should not be used for diagnosis in haemodynamically stable patients. However, the absence of echocardiographic signs of RV dysfunction in hypotensive patients virtually excludes PE from the differential.

The combination of RV dysfunction and haemodynamic instability is almost pathognomonic for acute PE. Occlusion of more than 30–50% of the pulmonary arterial bed causes an abrupt increase pulmonary vascular resistance. If this is not overcome by increased RV systolic function, venous return to the LV is reduced. Systemic hypotension and syncope then occur with progression to shock with progressive RV failure.

However, signs of RV dysfunction may also be present if patients with chronic pulmonary disease develop haemodynamic instability from any other cause. The mode of presentation, history, and chest X-ray can be used to differentiate these.

4) **What could cause the discrepancy between O_2 saturations measured by pulse oximetry and ABG analysis?**

Peripheral pulse oximetry is less accurate in critically ill patients. The perfusion of the skin is often reduced and the probe may not detect a pulsatile signal. Vasoconstriction and hypothermia also reduce tissue perfusion. Arrhythmias interfere with the detection of a pulsatile signal and calculation of heart rate. Cardiac valve lesions (e.g. tricuspid regurgitation) or high airway pressures can cause venous congestion and pulsation; venous O_2 saturation may be reported. Nail varnish may also affect pulse oximetry. Furthermore, O_2 saturations below 70% are based on extrapolation from calibration data that are only available for the range 70–100%.

Other causes of inaccurate pulse oximetry readings include abnormal haemoglobins. Methaemoglobinaemia and carboxyhaemoglobin (produced in carbon monoxide poisoning) cause readings to approach 85% and 100%, respectively.

However, many ABG analysers report a calculated saturation that is less accurate than that provided by the pulse oximeter. To validate pulse oximeter readings perform ABG analysis using a CO-oximeter, which measures concentrations of Hb, deoxyhaemoglobin, carboxyhaemoglobin, and methaemoglobin to determine the actual O_2 saturation.

Questions – Part 2

5. How can the pre-test probability of PE be determined?
6. Can D-dimers be used to confirm or exclude venous thrombo-embolism (VTE) in this case?
7. What causes the hypoxia associated with PE?
8. What is the mortality associated with PE?
9. What definitive treatment is required?

Answers

5) **How can the pre-test probability of PE be determined?**

Several clinical prediction tools have been developed to determine the pre-test probability of PE, but only two have been validated. The Wells criteria (Table 21.1) were validated first and are widely used. However, the heavily weighted question 'Is an alternative diagnosis less likely than PE?' limits the objectivity of the Wells criteria. The revised Geneva rule (Table 21.1) only includes standardized clinical variables and is also validated.

These prediction tools stratify pre-test probability into low- (9%), moderate- (30%) or high-risk (68%) groups (Table 21.2). The results of further testing (D-dimer, CT, V-Q scan, venous Doppler) can then provide meaningful post-test risk assessment.

In this case, the Wells criteria suggested a high risk of PE (alternative diagnosis less likely, HR > 100 bpm, recent immobilization) as did the modified Geneva score (age 75, HR > 100 bpm, $PaCO_2$ 3.5 kPa, PaO_2 6.4 kPa).

Table 21.1 Comparison of the Wells and Geneva Scores for Risk stratification of suspected PE

Simplified Wells	Score	Geneva	Score
Alternate diagnosis less likely than PE	3.0	Age 60–79	1
Signs/symptoms of deep vein thrombosis (DVT), eg. leg swelling and pain on palpation of deep veins	3.0	Age >80	2
Heart rate > 100 bpm	1.5	Heart rate >100 bpm	2
Immobilization or surgery in last 4 weeks	1.5	Recent surgery	3
Previous DVT or PE	1.5	Previous DVT or PE	1
Haemoptysis	1.0	$PaCO_2$ < 4.8 kPa	2
Cancer treated actively in last 6 months	1.0	4.8–5.19 kPa	1
Risk: low <2, moderate 2–6, high >6		PaO_2 <6.5 kPa	4
		6.5–7.99 kPa	3
		8–9.49 kPa	2
		9.5–10.99 kPa	1
		Chest X-ray with plate atelectasis	1
		Chest X-ray with elevated hemidiaphragm	1
		Risk: low 0–4, moderate 5–8, high 9–16	

Table 21.2 Prevalence of PE in each risk stratum

Risk	Prevalence	Positive likelihood ratio
Low	8–20%	0.13–0.53
Moderate	25–45%	0.67–1.1
High	45–90%	12–1.9

6) **Can D-dimers be used to confirm or exclude venous thrombo-embolism in this case?**

No.

Clots form as a result of platelet activation and fibrin cross-linking. Simultaneous activation of endogenous fibrinolysis allows the release of D-dimers into the plasma. D-dimers can be measured by sensitive assays. However, D-dimers are non-specific markers of fibrin production and fibrinolysis. Levels can be raised by a multitude of pathological processes (Table 21.3). Levels also increase with age, probably because of reduced renal clearance, increased fibrinogen levels, and the presence of occult disease. The specificity and hence diagnostic utility of D-dimer measurements for excluding VTE is lower in older patients.

The positive predictive value is low so D-dimers cannot be used to confirm PE. A patient with a clinical presentation suggestive of PE, in the absence of another clear explanation, and a raised D-dimer requires further specific investigation. In the past ventilation–perfusion scintigraphy was commonly used. However, CT pulmonary angiography (CTPA) is probably now the investigation of choice (sensitivity 83%, specificity of 96%) although the radiation dose is higher. Guidelines suggest that a negative scan could exclude PE.

A negative D-dimer result has a high negative predictive value in patients with a low pre-test probability of PE. However, in this case the pre-test probability of PE was high and so D-dimers could not be used to exclude PE. Further specific testing was required. As the patient was haemodynamically unstable bedside TTE was performed.

Any diagnostic strategy should identify patients at high risk of PE. Unstable patients (presence of shock or hypotension) require echocardiography to exclude the differential diagnoses of cardiogenic shock, acute valvular dysfunction, tamponade, and aortic dissection, and confirm RV dysfunction and overload. If the patient can be stabilized with supportive treatment then a direct diagnosis should be sought by visualizing the pulmonary vasculature with CTPA.

In cases where there are no high-risk clinical features, measurement of D-dimer combined with clinical probability assessment allows exclusion of PE in around 30%, with CT used as a second-line test in the remainder.

Table 21.3 Causes of increased fibrin production and raised D-dimer

Cancer
Inflammation
Infection
Necrosis
Thrombosis
Dissection of the aorta

7) **What causes the hypoxia associated with PE?**

Pulmonary embolism causes ventilation–perfusion mismatch (increased dead space i.e. ventilated alveoli that are not perfused). If cardiac output is significantly reduced, the saturation of mixed venous blood will also fall as oxygen extraction in the tissues increases. Patients may also develop a right-to-left shunt through a patent foramen ovale (PFO; present in around 20% of the population), which is kept open by a reversed pressure gradient across the inter-atrial septum. A right-to-left intracardiac shunt could cause severe hypoxia and allows paradoxical embolization to occur. The presence of a PFO is an independent predictor of silent brain injury in patients with PE and cerebral embolic events may actually be more frequent than the apparent clinical neurological complication rate.

PE is generally associated with hypoxia, but 20% of patients with PE have a normal PaO_2, including those with large PEs. Pulmonary embolism is more likely to cause or exacerbate hypoxia in patients with pre-existing cardiac or pulmonary disease than in previously healthy patients.

8) **What is the mortality associated with PE?**

PE is fatal in 10% of patients within 1 hour of the onset of symptoms; shock or hypotension occurs in 5–10% of cases. The presence of RV dysfunction or myocardial injury identifies a population with a worse prognosis. In patients without RV dysfunction as assessed by echocardiography, in-hospital mortality is less than 1%. The mortality rises to 15% in patients with significant RV dysfunction, but stable systemic haemodynamics. If, as in this case, the systemic circulation is affected by right heart failure, the short-term mortality approaches 60%. Death is more likely if the diagnosis is missed; less than 10% of all deaths occur in patients treated for PE.

Stratification of patients with suspected PE by risk of early death allows identification and emergency treatment of high-risk cases which present with hypotension or shock (mortality >15%). Those with intermediate risk have at least one marker of RV dysfunction (RV dilation on echo or CT, with echo evidence of RV dysfunction–hypokinesia or pressure overload) and myocardial injury (raised troponin). Those at low risk have no evidence of RV dysfunction or myocardial injury (mortality <1%).

9) **What definitive treatment is required?**

Systemic thrombolysis can rapidly reduce obstructive thrombus and improve blood flow, allowing the RV to recover. However, the risk of bleeding is increased compared with anticoagulation (major haemorrhage 15%, fatal haemorrhage 1%). Only patients with haemodynamic instability secondary to proven RV dysfunction should be considered for thrombolysis. Thrombolysis of these patients is associated with a significant reduction in recurrent emboli and death. Thrombolysis is currently not indicated for haemodynamically stable patients with RV dysfunction, although some studies suggest it can improve the clinical course without affecting mortality.

Mechanical fragmentation of the thrombus with intra-pulmonary catheters may have a role. Emergency open-lung pulmonary thrombectomy should be considered if systemic thrombolysis fails to restore hemodynamic stability.

In this case, echocardiography confirmed RV dyskinesia and raised RVSP. The patient was thrombolysed and made a good recovery.

Further reading

Konstantinides S (2008). Clinical practice. Acute pulmonary embolism. *New Engl J Med*; **359**: 2804–2813.

Torbicki A, Perrier A, Konstantinides S, Agnelli G, Galiè N, Pruszczyk P, Bengel F, Brady AJ, Ferreira D, Janssens U, Klepetko W, Mayer E, Remy-Jardin M, Bassand JP. The Task Force for the Diagnosis and Management of Acute PE of the European Society of Cardiology (ESC) (2008). Guidelines on the diagnosis and management of acute PE. *Eur Heart J*; **29**: 2276–2315.

Brotman DJ, Segal JB, Jani JT, Petty BG, Kickler TS (2003). Limitations of D-dimer testing in unselected inpatients with suspected venous thromboembolism. *Am J Med*; **114**: 276–282.

Clergeau MR, Hamon M, Morello R, Saloux E, Viader F, Hamon M (2009). Silent cerebral infarcts in patients with pulmonary embolism and a patent foramen ovale: a prospective diffusion-weighted MRI study. *Stroke*; **40**: 3758–3762.

Case 22

A 62-year-old man was transferred to a regional cardiac centre for angiography 2 days after presentation with an NSTEMI. He had been woken from sleep with typical chest pain that lasted 45 minutes on the morning of admission. He was taken to the ED of his local district general hospital by ambulance.

The ECG performed on arrival at the ED showed deep anterior T-wave inversion. The 12-hour cTnI was raised (15 ng/mL). Observations were BP 128/75 mmHg and HR 68 bpm. Clinical examination was unremarkable. The symptoms settled partially with sublingual nitrate. However, a nitrate infusion and intravenous opiates were required to relieve the pain completely. Dual antiplatelet therapy and subcutaneous LMWH injections were prescribed.

He had been pain free for over 24 hours prior to transfer. He had no prior history of cardiovascular disease but had recently developed hypertension, for which he was receiving treatment.

Angiography demonstrated a significant stenosis in the proximal LAD coronary artery (Fig. 22.1A) and PCI with stent implantation was indicated. As LMWH had not been administered on the morning of the procedure, a weight-adjusted bolus dose of intravenous heparin and abciximab were administered. The LAD stenosis was crossed with difficulty using a balanced middle weight (BMW) wire. The wire was initially passed down a small first diagonal artery (Fig. 22.1B) unintentionally. The wire was then repositioned and passed into the distal LAD (Fig. 22.1C and D). The stenosis was first pre-dilated with a short compliant balloon and then stented with a 3.5-mm diameter drug-eluting stent. The patient experienced some transient chest pain during this procedure (Fig. 22.1E). The femoral sheath was removed in the catheter laboratory and the puncture site closed with a device that deployed an absorbable collagen plug.

The patient was transferred back to the recovery ward and remained in bed for the next 2 hours as per protocol. He then mobilized. There were no puncture site complications. However, 4 hours later he collapsed whilst getting out of his bed to go to the toilet. The nursing staff confirmed he was not in cardiac arrest and emergency paged the cardiology registrar to attend. When the cardiology registrar arrived, he found on the floor, semi-conscious (GCS 10/15; E2, V3, M5), with a systolic BP 50 mmHg, HR 120 bpm, and O₂ saturations 89% on air. There were clinical signs of pulmonary oedema. His abdomen was soft and there was no evidence of haematoma or bleeding from the site of femoral artery puncture. Echocardiography was performed (Fig. 22.2).

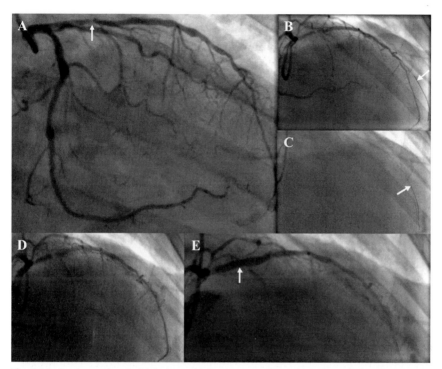

Fig. 22.1 Angiography. A, RAO view of left coronary artery demonstrating severe stenosis in proximal LAD (arrow) and an unobstructed circumflex artery. B, Initial position of angioplasty wire within small diagonal branch (arrow). C and D, Wire repositioned into LAD. E, Stent implanted in proximal LAD (arrow).

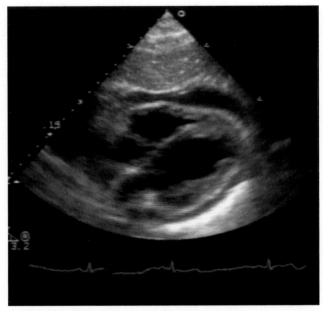

Fig. 22.2 Transthoracic echocardiogram: Subcostal view after patient collapsed post angioplasty.

Questions

1. What are the most likely causes of this man's collapse?
2. What does the TTE show?
3. What caused this complication?
4. What would you do next?
5. Describe how this procedure is performed and the potential complications.
6. What precautions should be taken?

Answers

1) **What are the most likely causes of this man's collapse?**

   Common causes of hypotension and pulmonary oedema during or after angioplasty include haemorrhage, cardiac tamponade, myocardial ischaemia and/or infarction, aortic dissection, and anaphylaxis.

2) **What does the TTE show?**

   The echocardiogram demonstrates a subcostal view of the heart with pericardial fluid visible anteriorly. As tamponade is likely the RV must be assessed for collapse.

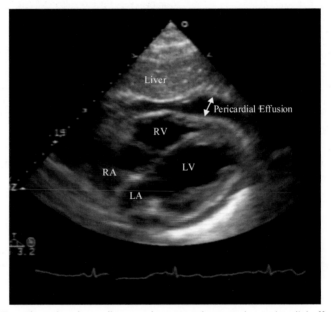

Fig. 22.3 Transthoracic echocardiogram demonstrating anterior pericardial effusion. The echocardiogram demonstrates a subcostal view of the heart with pericardial fluid visible anteriorly (arrowed). As tamponade is likely the right ventricle (RV) must be assessed for collapse. Right atrium (RA), left atrium (LA), left ventricle (LV).

3) **What caused this complication?**

   Reviewing the angiograms (Fig. 22.1) it can be seen that contrast began to appear in the pericardial space after the BMW wire was repositioned from the first diagonal into the LAD (Fig. 22.4). There was most likely a wire-related perforation of the diagonal, which resulted in pericardial bleeding and tamponade. Bleeding into the pericardial space is exacerbated by antiplatelet therapy and anticoagulation with heparin. Coronary perforations are a rare complication reported to occur in around 0.2–0.6% of cases. The risk of perforations is higher and and more common when more aggressive interventional devices are used (e.g. rotational atherectomy).

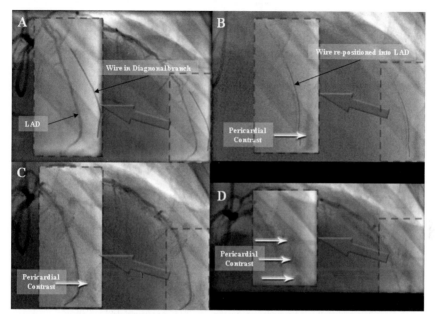

Fig. 22.4 Angiogram demonstrating contrast in the pericardial space. A, Initial wire position in diagonal branch. B and C, After placing the wire into the LAD, contrast is now visible in the pericardial space. D, At the end of the procedure contrast staining is more prominent.

4) **What would you do next?**

Pericardiocentesis should be performed immediately. The aim should be to remove enough blood from the pericardial space to restore ventricular filling, cardiac output, and BP. Definitive repair of the injury or reversal of the circumstances promoting bleeding are then required.

5) **Describe how this procedure is performed and the potential complications.**

Continuous monitoring (BP, HR, ECG, O_2 saturations) and full asepsis are required. Echocardiographic guidance is helpful.

A long needle (attached to a syringe containing saline) is inserted just to the left of the xyphoid process and advanced towards the tip of the left scapula. An approach from the apex of the heart may be preferred. Continuous negative pressure (suction) is applied with the syringe until the pericardial sac is entered and pericardial fluid aspirates freely. The haemodynamic status usually improves immediately. Confirmation of position within the pericardial space can be confirmed by injection of agitated saline visualized echocardiographically. A wire with a soft tip can be inserted through the needle into the pericardial space and a drainage catheter such as a pigtail catheter threaded over the wire (Seldinger technique) to allow continued aspiration as necessary.

There are numerous potential complications from this procedure, including trauma to the heart, liver, blood vessels, or lung, and infection. Occasionally, thrombus formation within the pericardial space limits percutaneous aspiration.

6) **What precautions should be taken?**

Whilst preparing for the procedure, protamine, FFP, and platelets should be organized to reverse the effects of unfractionated heparin (UFH), LMWH and antiplatelet therapy. Start the procedure as soon as possible. Do not wait for the blood products to be administered.

Cardiac tamponade as a complication of PCI. Cardiac tamponade is a rare complication that may present several hours after PCI. It is commonly due to coronary artery rupture or perforation and is life-threatening without prompt treatment. Some studies suggest a third require emergency surgical intervention to repair a coronary laceration or relieve tamponade if pericardiocentesis has failed. Alternative definitive treatments include use of covered intracoronary stents and coil embolization of distal perforations. The perforation can often be sealed by prolonged balloon inflation, with a perfusion balloon catheter to reduce myocardial ischaemia if necessary. Small leaks may stop with reversal of anti-thrombotic therapy alone, with platelet transfusion as necessary. Aggressive and early therapeutic intervention is important. Care with wire manipulation, balloon, and stent expansion, and true lumen confirmation help to prevent this complication.

This patient was transferred immediately to the CCU, where he received protamine and a pericardial drain was inserted under echocardiographic guidance. There was almost immediate haemodynamic improvement and he regained full consciousness. A total of 200 mL of blood was drained, which was seen to clot eventually. The drain was left in situ overnight and then removed. Serial echocardiograms failed to show any reaccumulation and he was eventually discharged home on day 7. No further angiographic procedure was needed.

Further reading

Holmes DR Jr, Nishimura R, Fountain R, Turi ZG. (2009). Iatrogenic pericardial effusion and tamponade in the percutaneous intracardiac intervention era. *JACC Cardiovasc Interv*; 2: 705–717.

Little WC, Freeman GL (2006). Pericardial disease. *Circulation*; 113: 1622–1632.

Maisch B, Seferovi PM, Risti AD, Erbel R, Rienmüller R, Adler Y, Tomkowski WZ, Thiene G, Yacoub MH; Task Force on the Diagnosis and Management of Pricardial Diseases of the European Society of Cardiology. (2004). Guidelines on the diagnosis and management of pericardial diseases executive summary; The Task force on the diagnosis and management of pericardial diseases of the European society of cardiology. *Eur Heart J*; 25: 587–610.

Case 23

A 27-year-old Nigerian woman was readmitted with a 4-week history of general malaise, low-grade fever, nocturnal sweating, increasing breathlessness, and non-productive cough.

She initially presented to hospital with similar symptoms 2 weeks prior to this readmission. She had lived in the UK for 5 years but had returned from a visit to Nigeria 2 months prior to the onset of her symptoms.

At the initial presentation examination was unremarkable. Full blood count revealed Hb 8.4 g/dL, mean cell volume 88 fl, WBC 7.8 × 10^9/L, and platelets 505 × 10^9/L. Liver function tests were mildly deranged (AST 74 iu/L; γ-G (gamma-glutamyl transferase) 43 iu/L, bilirubin 20 μmol/L, and albumin 25 g/dL). Urea, creatinine, and electrolytes were normal but CRP was raised (53 mg/L). Chest X-ray was normal. No sputum was produced but blood cultures were taken. There was no growth after 5 days of culture.

During the initial admission the patient was treated for presumptive *Mycoplasma* pneumonia with intravenous cefuroxime and clarythromycin on the basis of her symptoms. *Mycoplasma pneumoniae* immunoglobin (Ig)G antibody titres were 1:80 on agglutination (normal range <1:10). She was discharged home with oral antibiotics 5 days later. Her symptoms did improve with this treatment, but did not resolve completely.

On readmission 1 week after discharge the observations were BP 102/66 mmHg, HR 104 bpm (sinus), RR 25 breaths/min, O$_2$ saturations 98% on air, and temperature 37.3°C.

On examination; JVP was not raised. The heart sounds were soft but there were no added sounds and breath sounds were normal. ECG was normal. The results of laboratory blood tests were similar to the results of those performed at the initial presentation. The chest X-ray was repeated (Fig. 23.1) and echocardiography was performed (Fig. 23.2).

Questions

1. How is infection with *Mycoplasma pneumoniae* diagnosed and treated?
2. What do the chest X-ray and the echocardiogram (Figs. 23.1 and 23.2) show?
3. What may mimic this finding on the echocardiogram?
4. What is the differential diagnosis for these findings?
5. What is the most likely diagnosis?

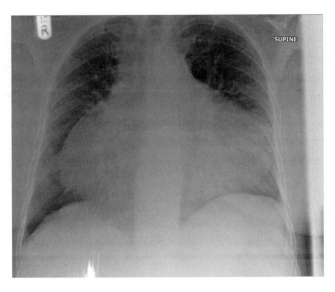

Fig. 23.1 Chest X-ray.

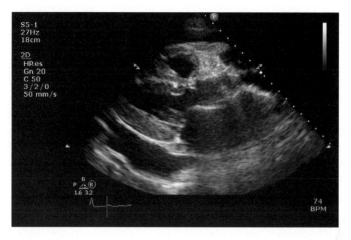

Fig. 23.2 Echocardiogram.

Answers

1) **How is infection with *M. pneumoniae* diagnosed and treated?**

   Infection with *Mycoplasma pneumoniae* is diagnosed by a four-fold rise in antibody titre between acute and convalescent sera and positive polymerase chain reaction (PCR) or growth in culture. However, isolating and culturing *Mycoplasma pneumoniae* is difficult so the sensitivity is very low. Cold agglutinin titres >1:64 support the diagnosis but are not specific. While immunoglobulin M (IgM) indicates recent infection, high titres of IgG may indicate previous, ongoing, or recurrent infections. However, antigenic cross-reactivity can lead to false-positive results. Measurement of serum levels too early or too late can lead to false-negative results.

   The low-grade fever, malaise, and dry cough combined with minimal physical findings are consistent with *Mycoplasma* pneumonia. However, macrolide antibiotics, although bacteriostatic, are highly effective against *Mycoplasma pneumoniae*. As the patient has failed to respond to this treatment alternative diagnoses should be considered. The raised *Mycoplasma pneumoniae* IgG may indicate previous subclincal infection.

2) **What do the chest X-ray and the echocardiogram (Figs. 23.1 and 23.2) show?**

   Gross globular cardiomegaly is present on the chest X-ray (Fig. 23.1), but there are no other abnormalities. Echocardiography (Fig. 23.2) shows an 'echo-free' space between the visceral and parietal pericardium (Fig. 23.3). This is consistent with a pericardial effusion.

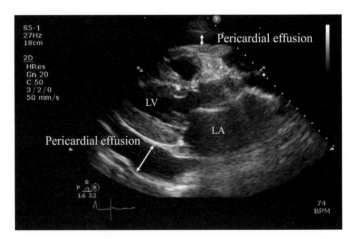

Fig. 23.3 Labelled echocardiogram.

3) **What may mimic this finding on the echocardiogram?**

   Pleural effusions, pericardial thickening, increased epicardial fat, atelectasis, and mediastinal lesions may also appear as an 'echo-free' space between the visceral and parietal pericardium. Epicardial fat is usually more prominent anteriorly but can be circumferential. However, pericardial fluid is echo-lucent and motionless, unlike fat, which is slightly echogenic and moves with the heart.

4) **What is the differential diagnosis for these findings?**

Any cause of pericarditis can cause a pericardial effusion. Common causes of pericardial effusions include infections (Table 23.1), neoplasia (often lung cancer, breast cancer, lymphoma, or leukaemia), and cardiac surgery. Less common causes are listed in Table 23.2.

Table 23.1 Infective causes of pericardial effusion

Common cardiotropic viruses
Enterovirus
Echovirus
Adenovirus
Cytomegalovirus (in immunocompromised patients)
Epstein–Barr virus
Herpes simplex virus
Influenza
Parvovirus B19
Hepatitis C
Human immunodeficiency viruses
Bacterial
Pneumococci
Streptococci
Staphylococci
Neisseria
Legionella
Mycoplasma
Tuberculosis
Fungal
Histoplasmosis
Coccidioidomycosis
Candida
Others
Syphilis
Protozoa
Parasites

Table 23.2 Less common causes of pericardial effusion

Uraemia
Myxedema/hypothyroidism
Severe pulmonary hypertension
Radiation therapy – usually months or years after initial exposure
Acute myocardial infarction and subsequent free wall rupture
Aortic dissection, haemorrhagic effusion in from leakage into pericardial sac
Trauma
Hyperlipidaemia
Chylopericardium
Familial Mediterranean fever
Whipple disease
Hypersensitivity or autoimmune related
Systemic lupus erythematosus
Rheumatoid arthritis
Ankylosing spondylitis
Rheumatic fever
Scleroderma
Wegener granulomatosis
Medications
Anticoagulants
Hydralazine
Isoniazid
Minoxidil
Methysergide
Phenytoin
Procainamide

5) **What is the most likely diagnosis?**

In view of the subacute presentation and the travel history, tuberculous pericarditis is the most likely cause of the pericardial effusion. *M. pneumoniae* can cause pericarditis. However, as discussed above infection with *Mycoplasma pneumoniae* is unlikely. Clarythromycin has some antituberculous activity and may explain the improvement after the initial presentation and subsequent deterioration when the clarythromycin was stopped.

Tuberculous pericarditis usually presents as a chronic slowly progressive febrile illness, but may be acute. It is frequently associated with an effusion (85% mortality if left untreated). Pericardial calcification is common and constriction can occur at any stage. When it presents as cardiac tamponade (common) or acute pericarditis (uncommon), the diagnosis is often delayed or missed.

Tuberculous pericarditis is almost always associated with extra-cardiac disease. Pericardial infection with *Mycobaterium tuberculosis* may occur via extension of infection from the lung or tracheobronchial tree, adjacent lymph nodes, spine, or sternum, or via miliary spread. In adults tuberculous pericarditis often represents reactivation of previous infection. The primary focus of infection is often not apparent in these patients.

Various therapeutic regimes of different durations have been trialled. A meta-analysis suggested that combination of steroids with anti-tuberculous treatment may be associated with fewer deaths and less frequent pericardiocentesis or pericardiectomy. Large doses of prednisone (1–2 mg/kg/day) may be required because of hepatic enzyme induction by rifampicin.

Tuberculosis and tuberculous pericarditis are common in developing countries. The increasing incidence in the West is driven by migration and the spread of HIV. The rise of multidrug-resistant (MDR) tuberculosis (defined as resistance to at least rifampicin and isoniazid) is particularly alarming. Nigeria is one of 27 countries which account for 85% of all MDR tuberculosis worldwide. The World Health Organisation estimates that 4000 or more cases of MDR tuberculosis occur in Nigeria annually.

In this case enzyme-linked immunospot (ELISPOT) assays identified T cells specific for antigens from *M. tuberculosis*, which suggested active infection with *M. tuberculosis*. Pericardial biopsy, drainage of the pericardial effusion, and pericardiectomy were performed. Histological examination of the pericardial biopsy revealed caseating granulomata with acid and alcohol fast bacilli. The patient was started on quadruple therapy (rifampicin, isoniazid, pyrazinamide, and ethambutol), pyridoxine and adjuvant corticosteroids for pericardial tuberculosis. Drug susceptibility testing excluded isoniazid resistance and culture of the pericardial fluid and biopsy confirmed *M. tuberculosis*. HIV testing was negative.

On review in clinic 3 months after discharge the patient's symptoms had resolved completely. Her weight increased and the anaemia had improved (Hb 11 g/dL). Ethambutol and pyrazinamide were stopped after 2 months of therapy but a total of 9 months of therapy with rifampicin and isoniazid was recommended.

Further reading

Little WC, Freeman GL *et al.* (2006). Pericardial disease. *Circulation*; **113**: 1622–3632.

Strang JI, Nunn AJ, Johnson DA Casbard A, Gibson DG, Girling DJ (2004). Management of tuberculous constrictive pericarditis and tuberculous pericardial effusion in Transkei: results at 10 years follow-up. *QJM*; **97**: 525.

Maisch B, Seferović PM, Ristić AD, Erbel R, Rienmüller R, Adler Y, Tomkowski WZ, Thiene G, Yacoub MH; Task Force on the Diagnosis and Management of Pricardial Diseases of the European Society of Cardiology. (2004). Guidelines on the diagnosis and management of pericardial diseases executive summary; The Task force on the diagnosis and management of pericardial diseases of the European society of cardiology. *Eur Heart J*; **25**: 587–610.

Case 24

A 22-year-old student was referred to the medical registrar on call. He described a 6-hour history of central chest pain radiating to the left shoulder. The constant dull ache was worse on inspiration and lying flat but eased on sitting forward. For 2 days prior to this presentation he had felt 'like he had the flu' and reported fatigue, mild breathlessness, myalgias, and low-grade fevers.

He smoked 20 cigarettes per day but drank less than 21 units of alcohol per week. There was no past medical history or relevant family history. There were no risk factors for IHD and the patient denied illicit drug use.

Observations and clinical examination were unremarkable. The chest X-ray was normal. The admission ECG, which was recorded whilst the patient was experiencing pain, is shown in Fig. 24.1. The CRP was 75 mg/dL and the serum cTnI and CK were elevated at 5 ng/mL and 1000 u/L, respectively. The full blood count and routine serum biochemistry (renal, liver, and bone profiles) were otherwise unremarkable.

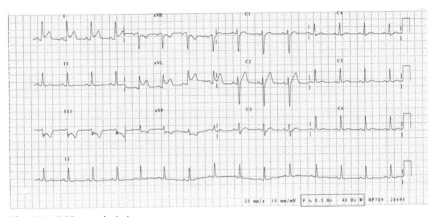

Fig. 24.1 ECG on admission.

Questions

1. Report the ECG (Fig. 24.1).
2. What is the differential diagnosis? What is the most likely diagnosis?
3. How would you investigate this patient initially?
4. How can the diagnosis be confirmed?
5. Cardiac MRI demonstrates LV thrombus. What treatment is required and what is the potential risk from treatment?

Answers

1) **Report the ECG (Fig. 24.1).**

The ECG shows sinus rhythm (90 bpm). There is 1–2 mm of antero-lateral ST elevation with a concave upwards pattern predominantly in leads I and aVL. The ST segments are depressed in leads III, aVF and aVR. The PR segments are depressed in leads I and aVL. The PR segments are elevated in aVR and III.

The significance of PR-segment depression and elevation

The baseline of the ECG is measured from the TP segment. Atrial repolarization begins during the PR segment. Depression of the PR segment relative to the TP segment may be a normal variant (<0.8 mm). Significant PR-segment depression (>0.8 mm) most commonly results from atrial damage or inflammation. Causes include pericarditis, atrial infarction (rare), trauma, and atrial tumours.

Acute pericarditis often causes an atrial current of injury. This is reflected by elevation of the PR segment in lead aVR and depression of the PR segment in other limb leads and V5–6. In acute pericarditis, PR and ST segments usually change in opposite directions. In aVR, the PR segment is elevated and the ST segment is usually depressed. Other leads may also show PR depression and ST elevation (Fig. 24.1).

Although PR-segment depression can occur in the absence of any other ECG features of pericarditis, atrial infarction must be considered. However, other ECG changes suggestive of MI are almost always present if atrial infarction has occurred.

2) **What is the differential diagnosis? What is the most likely diagnosis?**

The history of chest pain and the PR-segment depression and concave upward pattern of ST segment elevation in I and aVL are characteristic of pericarditis. However, the reciprocal changes of ST depression in III and aVF do not occur in isolated pericarditis and suggest myocardial injury. The significantly elevated cTnI and CK are also consistent with this. Although pericarditis can increase cTn, the level is usually below that taken to be diagnostic of MI in a patient with an ACS <1.5 ng/mL (see Case 43). Furthermore, increases in CK are also less common in pericarditis. Thus, in view of the combination of pericardial and myocardial disease the differential diagnosis in this case should include:

◆ pericarditis
◆ myocarditis with associated pericarditis (i.e. perimyocarditis or myopericarditis)
◆ pericarditis after a silent MI
◆ acute ST-elevation MI presenting with atypical chest pain.

In this case, the most likely diagnosis is an overlap syndrome of myocarditis with associated pericarditis. The features which favour this diagnosis over IHD include the patient's age, the absence of risk factors for ischaemic heart disease, and the viral prodrome.

Both pericarditis and myocarditis are often caused by cardiotropic viruses so it is not surprising that acute pericarditis and myocarditis can occur together. If both are present, the resulting clinical syndrome reflects the dominant process. Perimyocarditis is myocarditis with some pericardial inflammation but in myopericarditis, which is more common, the features of pericarditis are dominant. However, these terms are often used interchangeably.

The precise clinical presentation of perimyocarditis and myopericarditis is determined by the degree of pericardial and myocardial inflammation. This may be focal or diffuse and affect one or more cardiac chambers.

Symptoms include those associated with myocarditis and/or pericarditis, and a prodrome of fever, malaise, and myalgia is common. Many cases are subclinical and subtle cardiac symptoms may be masked by the viral infection. However, a severe diffuse myocarditis can cause an acute DCM and may present with cardiac failure. Other potential complications include arrhythmias and AV node block.

The positive predictive value of a raised cTn for myocarditis is around 80% (sensitivity 35%; specificity 90%).

In this case, the focal ST elevation with reciprocal ECG changes and level of elevation of cTn and CK suggest that the myocarditis is the dominant pathological process. Perimycarditis is the most likely diagnosis.

However, as is often the case, the presentation is difficult to distinguish from that of coronary ischaemia. The symptoms, signs, ECG changes, and laboratory findings of myocarditis in particular can simulate an acute coronary syndrome. A thorough and a detailed assessment is required to avoid misdiagnosis.

3) **How would you investigate this patient initially?**

The most important initial investigations are serial recordings of 12 lead ECGs and bedside TTE.

Monitoring the development of ECG changes on serial recording of 12 lead ECGs at 15–30 minute intervals may demonstrate progression of ECG changes.

T waves can invert while the ST segment is still elevated in STEMI. In pericarditis, T waves invert only after resolution of the ST-segment elevation, days to weeks later. However, in this case the ST-segment changes remained focal and did not progress.

Urgent bedside TTE may identify features that may suggest pericarditis (e.g. pericardial effusion). However, both myocarditis and MI can cause regional wall motion abnormalities and impair LV systolic function.

In this case, the TTE was normal. There was no pericardial effusion or regional wall motion abnormality. Biventricular systolic function was normal.

In this case, although the presentation was atypical the ECG and TTE findings could not exclude STEMI and so coronary angiography was performed. The coronary arteries were normal.

CT coronary angiography, which has a very high negative predictive value for excluding CAD, is a non-invasive alternative, but was not immediately available in this case.

In one series of 45 patients with a typical history of MI but normal coronary arteries, 35 had evidence of myocarditis (17 diffuse, 18 focal; Sarda et al., 2001).

4) **How can the diagnosis be confirmed?**

It is difficult to establish the diagnosis of perimyocarditis as there is no established non-invasive gold standard investigation for myocarditis.

Confirmation of myocarditis classically requires histological confirmation with an endomyocardial biopsy reported according to the Dallas criteria. However, because myocarditis may be patchy the sensitivity of blind biopsy is low (<35%).

Endomyocardial biopsy should be considered to detect fulminant myocarditis in patients without a clear cause of acute cardiac failure that causes haemodynamic compromise. Endomyocardial biopsy may also be helpful if heart failure with a dilated LV or new high-grade AV block or ventricular arrhythmia does not respond to treatment (see Case 28).

However, in this case endomyocardial biopsy is not indicated as there are no symptoms of heart failure or evidence of LV systolic dysfunction.

Cardiovascular MRI (CMRI) can be useful in this setting. The sensitivity and specificity of CMRI for myocarditis are around 75% and 95%, respectively. Late gadolinium enhancement of the myocardium occurs in most cases of acute myocarditis. The distribution of this enhancement is characteristically patchy and does not conform to any particular coronary artery territory. It is also usually subepicardial and not subendocardial, further differentiating it from MI.

Thus, myopericarditis and perimyocarditis can be differentiated from simple pericarditis and acute MI by contrast-enhanced CMRI. However, if the diagnosis remains in doubt, the CMRI findings can be used to target endomyocardial biopsy.

In this case CMRI demonstrated normal biventricular mass, volumes, and systolic function (EF 60%). There were no regional wall motion abnormalities. However, late gadolinium imaging revealed subepicardial hyperenhancement in the lateral myocardial wall, which also involved the pericardium (Fig. 24.2).

Myocarditis should be 'strongly suspected' if any two of the three features listed below are present.

1. Compatible clinical symptoms.

2. Cardiac structural and/or functional defect or myocardial damage in the absence of regional coronary ischaemia.

3. Regional delayed contrast enhancement or increased T2 signal on CMRI.

In this case, the presence of myocarditis was 'highly probable' as all three of the features listed above were present. As CMRI also demonstrated pericardial involvement this patient was diagnosed with perimyocarditis.

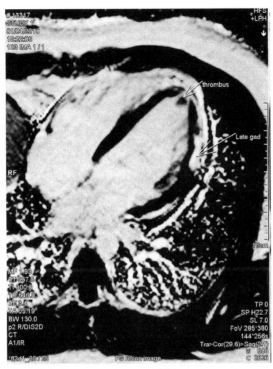

Fig. 24.2 A transverse four-chamber view from a contrast-enhanced CMRI. Late gadolinium imaging reveals subepicardial hyperenhancement in the lateral myocardial wall, which also involves the pericardium (arrowed). A small thrombus (0.9 × 0.7 cm) was also identified at the apex the left ventricle. This did not enhance with contrast.

5) **Cardiac MRI demonstrates LV thrombus. What treatment is required and what is the potential risk from treatment?**

Ventricular thrombus occurs in 15% of patients with myocarditis studied with echocardiography. In this case, anticoagulation is required to reduce the risk of embolization from LV thrombus (see Case 19). However, this may precipitate the development of a haemorrhagic pericardial effusion in patients with perimyocarditis. This raises a relatively common but difficult decision. Should anticoagulation be given to a patient at risk of bleeding?

The decision is potentially life saving and yet potentially life threatening. However, there is little guidance from published literature.

No large studies have assessed the risk:benefit ratio of long-term anticoagulation in patients with perimyocarditis associated with LV thrombus. In a recent study of 274 consecutive cases of idiopathic or viral acute pericarditis 40 (15%) were found to have myopericarditis (Imazio *et al.*, 2008). The presentation mimicked MI in 17 patients (6 had a final diagnosis of pericarditis, 11 had a final diagnosis of myopericarditis). However, in these patients neither myopericarditis nor the use of heparin, oral anticoagulation, and glycoprotein IIb/IIIa inhibitors were associated with an increased risk of cardiac tamponade or recurrences during follow-up.

Data from these 17 patients are not sufficient to conclude that anticoagulation is safe in patients with pericarditis, myocarditis, or the overlap syndromes. However, more guidance can be obtained by extrapolating data from a similar situation. Haemorrhagic pericarditis and tamponade has been described in patients receiving anticoagulation after MI but large studies have demonstrated that there is no significant increase in the incidence of these complications if patients are treated with anticoagulants.

The use of anticoagulants is not contraindicated if pericarditis develops after MI. In the Gruppo Italiano per lo Studio della Streptochinasi nell'Infarto Miocardico (Italian: Italian Group for the Study of the Survival of Myocardial Infarction (GISSI) trials the incidence of pericardial effusion in patients who received thrombolysis and heparin was lower than in those who did not. The rate of in-hospital mortality of patients who received thrombolysis did not increase if pericarditis developed.

How accurately the risk of bleeding after MI reflects the risk in patients with inflammatory myocarditis or pericarditis is unknown. However, the relatively low incidence of bleeding in these patients suggests that the risk in acute perimyocarditis is also likely to be low.

However, even a small risk of a potentially life-threatening complication should not be taken lightly. To decide whether it is appropriate to expose this patient to the risk of anticoagulation requires assessment of the potential risk of embolisation from LV thrombus and the potential reduction of risk with anticoagulation.

Although not specifically assessed in patients with acute perimyocarditis, risk of embolization from LV thrombus that develops after MI is around 30% without anticoagulation but can be reduced to about 7% with anticoagulation.

On the assumption that the risks of embolization and potential benefit are similar in acute perimyocarditis the risks of anticoagulation were considered less than the risks of not anticoagulating the patient in this case. The patient was anticoagulated with warfarin after discussion of the potential risks. The CMRI was repeated 6 weeks later and demonstrated complete resolution of the cardiac mass. The late gadolinium enhancement of the myocardium had reduced, but had not resolved completely. Warfarin was discontinued after 6 months of anticoagulation.

In this case, anticoagulation would still have been recommended if the patient had had a pericardial effusion at presentation. However, echocardiography would have been performed to assess the size of the effusion at least weekly. The risk:benefit ratio of anticoagulation would have been re-evaluated in the presence of a pericardial effusion that increased in size.

Reference

Imazio M, Cecchi E, Demichelis B, Chinaglia A, Ierna S, Demarie D, Ghisio A, Pomari F, Belli R, Trinchero R. (2008). Myopericarditis versus viral or idiopathic acute pericarditis. *Heart*; **94**: 498.

Sarda L, Colin P, Boccara F, Daou D, Lebtahi R, Faraggi M, Nguyen C, Cohen A, Slama MS, Steg PG, Le Guludec D. (2001). Myocarditis in patients with clinical presentation of myocardial infarction and normal coronary angiograms. *J Am Coll Cardiol*; **37**: 786–792.

Further reading

Blauwet LA, Cooper LT (2010). Myocarditis. *Prog Cardiovasc Dis*; **52**: 274–288.

Galve E, Garcia-Del-Castillo H, Evangelista A, Batlle J, Permanyer-Miralda G, Soler-Soler J (1986). Pericardial effusion in the course of myocardial infarction: incidence, natural history, and clinical relevance. *Circulation*; **73**: 294–299.

Case 25

A 38-year-old lecturer consulted his GP with a 10-day history of dry cough productive of clear sputum. There was no previous medical history and he did not take any regular medication. He was a non-smoker and was married with two children. He usually cycled to work but admitted he was becoming breathless whilst cycling uphill and had instead started driving 1 month ago.

The GP heard a grade 3 systolic murmur on auscultation of the heart and referred the patient to the medical registrar on call with a suspected diagnosis of endocarditis.

On admission to the medical assessment unit observations were temperature 37.5°C, O_2 saturations 99% on air, BP 110/60 mmHg, and HR 60 bpm. An ECG (Fig. 25.1) and a chest X-ray were performed (Fig. 25.2). Full blood count was normal (Hb 15 g/dL, WBC 7.5×10^9 cells/L, platelets 300×10^{12} cells/L). The results of serum biochemistry were serum sodium 140 mmol/L, potassium 4.8 mmol/L, creatinine 90 μmol/L, urea 7 mmol/L, bilirubin 70 μmol/L, albumin 35 g/L, ALT 34 u/L, alkaline phosphatase 63 iu/L, gammaglutamyltransferase 35 u/L, and CRP <5 mg/L. Urine dipstick was negative.

The cardiology registrar on call was asked to review the patient and performed a TTE (Fig. 25.3). Right- and left-heart catheterization was then arranged, the main results of which are shown in Table 25.1.

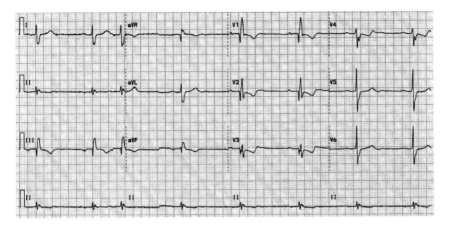

Fig. 25.1 12 lead ECG.

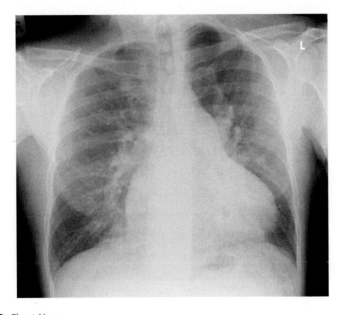

Fig. 25.2 Chest X-ray.

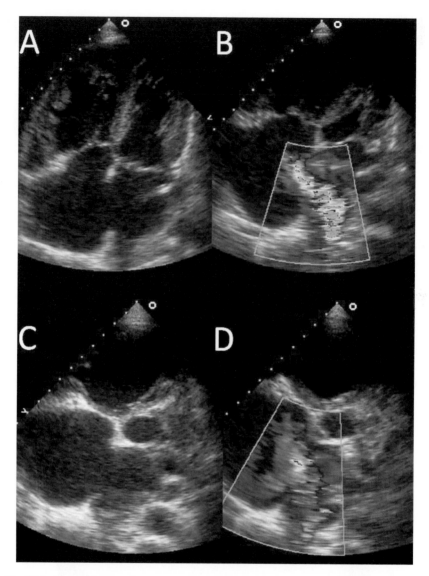

Fig. 25.3 Selected images from the transthoracic echocardiogram. The views shown are the two-dimensional apical four-chamber views (A and B) and short-axis parasternal views at the level of the aortic valve (C and D). Colour Doppler overlays on the apical four-chamber view (B) and short-axis parasternal view at the level of the aortic valve (D) are also shown. (See colour plate 7)

Questions

1. Report the ECG in Fig. 25.1.
2. Report the chest X-ray in Fig. 25.2.
3. What do the selected images in Fig. 25.3 demonstrate?
4. What are the characteristic features of the heart sounds and murmurs associated with this condition?
5. What investigations are required?
6. Report the data in Table 25.1.
7. How should this patient be managed?

Table 25.1 Haemodynamic data from catheterization of left and right sides of the heart

Left heart pressures (mmHg)		Right heart pressures (mmHg)		O_2 saturations (%)	
LV systolic	164	RA mean	7	SVC	76
LV EDP	11	RA V wave	12	IVC	85
Aorta systolic	175	PA systolic	51	RA	89
Aorta diastolic	79	PA diastolic	16	RV (mid)	92
Aorta mean	116	PA mean	29	PA	92
		LA mean	9	LA	97
				Aorta	97

Coronary angiogram
Incidental finding of 90% stenosis mid right coronary artery

Answers

1) **Report the ECG in Fig. 25.1**

   The 12 lead ECG shown in Fig. 25.1 demonstrates sinus bradycardia 45 bpm with an atrial ectopic beat. There is RBBB, borderline right axis deviation, and first-degree heart block. These findings suggest trifasicular conduction block. The tall R waves seen in leads V1 and V2 are consistent with some RV hypertrophy.

2) **Report the chest X-ray in Fig. 25.2**

   The PA chest X-ray in Fig. 25.2 shows cardiomegaly with a dilated RA. The pulmonary trunk and proximal pulmonary arteries are enlarged. These findings suggest pulmonary plethora and possible pulmonary hypertension. The lungs fields are clear.

3) **What do the selected images in Fig. 25.3 demonstrate?**

   Apical four-chamber views (Fig. 25.3A and 25.3B) and short axis parasternal views (level of AV; Fig. 25.3C and 25.3D) demonstrate a large defect in the interatrial septum [atrial septal defect (ASD); Fig. 25.4]. The defect is in the centre of the septum between the right and left atrium; an ostium secundum defect. Colour Doppler overlay demonstrates a broad jet of flow from LA to RA (Fig. 25.4B and 25.4D).

   Systemic-to-pulmonary shunting can be caused by defects in the interatrial or interventricular septum. Symptoms from ASDs include mild exercise intolerance and atrial arrhythmias (AF or flutter). However, pulmonary hypertension or paradoxical embolism does occur occasionally. ASDs may be diagnosed on further investigation of an abnormal ECG [right-axis deviation, left axis deviation (ostium primum), RV hypertrophy, incomplete RBBB] or an asymptomatic cardiac murmur (pulmonary ejection systolic flow murmur with fixed splitting of the second heart sound or tricuspid regurgitation).

   ASDs comprise 7% of all congenital heart defects and can occur in several sites within the atria (Fig. 25.5) but most commonly involve the foramen ovale (ostium secundum ASD). Ostium secundum ASDs result from a deficiency in the flap valve that normally ensures the fossa is fenestrated or incompletely covered during development. The defect can occur in isolation or as part of more complex congenital structural malformations. It has been suggested that up to a fifth of ostium secundum ASDs present in adulthood, but there is no evidence that these patients are at increased risk of endocarditis. Defects can occur in other parts of the septum (Fig. 25.5).

   Ventricular septal defects (VSDs) are the most common congenital heart defects (32%). They can occur in any of the four areas of the ventricular septum [membranous (most common) or muscular (inlet, trabecular, and outlet)]. The clinical effects are determined by the size and pulmonary vascular resistance, which determine the systemic to pulmonary shunt. Most VSDs are small, haemodynamically insignificant (Maladie de Roger), and eventually close spontaneously without intervention. There is an increased risk of endocarditis associated with larger VSDs, and there is a risk of developing Eisenmenger's syndrome. Management options include surgical closure, banding of the pulmonary trunk (multiple VSDs), and trans-catheter closure.

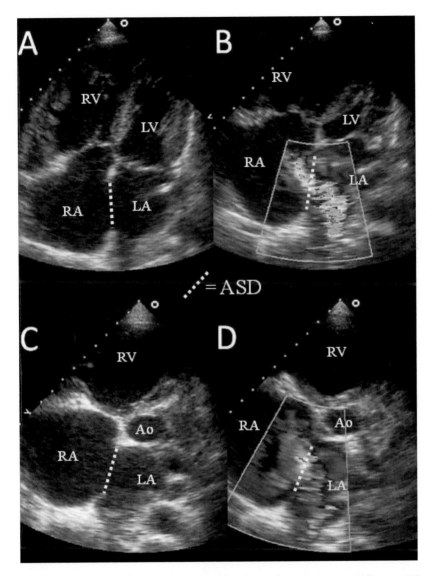

Fig. 25.4 Selected views from the transthoracic echocardiogram demonstrating an ASD. The apical four-chamber views (A and B) and short-axis parasternal views at the level of the aortic valve AV (Ao; C and D) demonstrate a large defect in the interatrial septum (ASD). The defect is in the centre of the septum between the right and left atrium; an ostium secundum defect. Colour Doppler overlay demonstrates a broad jet of flow from LA to RA (B and D). (See colour plate 8)

Ostium primum ASD (1)

This is an atrioventricular septal defect. These are the second most common ASD (3% of all congenital heart disease). Associated with trisomy 21 (Down's syndrome). May disrupt atrio-ventricular valve structure and function causing heart failure. Closure may require complex surgery.

Ostium secundum ASD (2)

The most common type of ASD (6–10% of all congenital heart disease). Usually arises from an enlarged foramen ovale, inadequate growth of the septum secundum, or excessive absorption of the septum primum.

Most secundum ASD are asymptomatic to early adulthood. 70% are symptomatic before 40 years. Symptoms include breathlessness, reduced exercise tolerance, palpitations and syncope.

Complication of an uncorrected secundum ASD include PH, RV failure, AF or flutter, stroke, and Eisenmenger's syndrome.

While PH is rare under 20 years of age, it is present in 50% of those over 40 years old. Progression to Eisenmenger's occurs in 5 – 10% late in the disease process.

Coronary sinus ASD (3)

This develops in the part of septum that includes the coronary sinus orifice. and are At least part of the common wall that separates the coronary sinus and the left atrium is absent.

Sinus venosus ASD (4&5)

These ASD involve either the SVC (superior; 4) or the IVC (inferior; 5). Superior sinus venosus ASD which are located at the junction of the SVC and RA comprise 2 – 3% of all ASD. Superior sinus venosus ASD are often associated with anomalous drainage of the right-sided pulmonary veins into the RA instead of the LA.

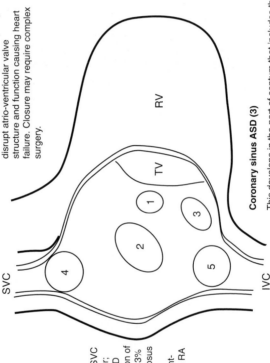

Fig. 25.5 Schematic diagram of ASD. The view is into an open IVC, SVC and RA. 1, ostium primum ASD; 2, ostium secundum ASD; 3, defect involving coronary sinus; 4, superior sinus venosus ASD; 5, inferior sinus venosus ASD.

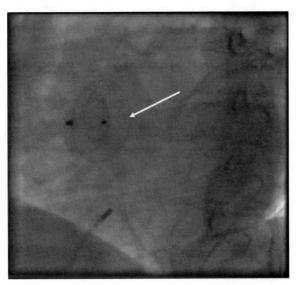

Fig. 25.6 Fluoroscopic image taken after closing the ASD with a helix septal occluder device (arrowed).

4) **What are the characteristic features of the heart sounds and murmurs associated with this condition?**

When an ASD is present, the LA pressure initially exceeds RA pressure with greater RA compliance so blood flows as a left-to-right shunt through the ASD, hence increasing the volume that flows into the right ventricle. The consequent increase in flow through the pulmonary valve causes the systolic flow murmur loudest in the pulmonary area (2nd intercostal space, left sternal edge). Tricuspid regurgitation may also develop and a tricuspid diasolic flow murmur may be present if the left-to-right shunt is large. The increased RV volumes also cause wide fixed splitting of the second heart sound (S2) as more time is required to eject blood from the RV, thus delaying closure of the pulmonary valve. As inspiration does not affect the pressure difference between atria, which equilibrates via the ASD, the delay in pulmonary valve closure remains constant or fixed with respiration. In contrast, physiological splitting of S2 occurs during inspiration when increased venous return transiently increases RV end diastolic volume.

5) **Why is cardiac catheterisation required? What other investigations may be required?**

Cardiac catheterization is useful to confirm the diagnosis of an ASD to assess the shunt fraction, pulmonary artery (PA) pressures, and vascular resistance. If the PA pressure >75% systemic pressure, reversibility studies with PA vasodilators should be performed (see Case 27). Patients over 40 years old usually also require coronary angiography.

In most cases the ASD size, position, and suitability for device closure can be assessed with TTE. However, in this case TOE was required because the ASD was so large. TOE is required before device closure of ASD if:

◆ TTE images are inadequate

◆ the ASD is large (>3 cm)

◆ there is doubt about possible contraindications.

6) **Report the data in Table 25.1**

In the present case, the cardiac catheter data demonstrate moderately increased PA pressure (mean 29 mmHg). However, this is only a quarter of mean systemic arterial pressure (116 mmHg). A left-to-right shunt has been defined with significant increase in blood O_2 saturation between two right-sided vessels/chambers: Table 25.1 documents higher blood O_2 saturation in the RA than in the IVC and superior vena cava (SVC), suggesting a left-to-right shunt at atrial level.

The shunt fraction (Qp:Qs) is 3.8:1 (Equation 1). This is a large (Qp:Qs > 2) left-to-right shunt. Desaturation at LA level (not present in this case) would have suggested bidirectional shunting at atrial level The pulmonary arterial resistance (0.8 Wood units; 64 dyn s/cm⁵) and total pulmonary vascular resistance (1.16 Wood units; 92 dyn s/cm⁵) were normal despite elevation of pulmonary artery (PA) pressure (Equations 3 and 4).

Equation 1 Calculation of the pulmonary (Qp) to systemic (Qs) blood flow ratio (Qp/Qs) using the Fick principle from invasive oximetry data:

Equation 1

$$\frac{Qp}{Qs} = \frac{Sat\,Aorta - Sat\,MV}{Sat\,PV - Sat\,PA}$$

where Sat Aorta is aortic saturations, Sat MV is mixed venous saturations, Sat PV is pulmonary venous saturations, and Sat PA is pulmonary arterial saturations. This assume isolated L→R shunting

Equation 2 shows the calculation of Sat MV.

Equation 2

$$Sat\,MV = \frac{(3 \times Sat\,SVC) + (1 \times Sat\,IVC)}{4} = \frac{(3 \times 76) + (1 \times 85)}{4} = \frac{228 + 85}{4} = 78$$

where Sat SVC is superior vena caval saturations and Sat IVC is inferior vena caval saturations.

In the present case, pulmonary venous saturation must be the same as arterial saturation as there is no right-to-left shunting (Sat Aorta = 97%)

$$\frac{Qp}{Qs} = \frac{97 - 78}{97 - 92} = \frac{19}{5} = 3.8 : 1$$

Equation 3 The calculation of total pulmonary vascular resistance (PVR) and Equation 4 shows the calculation of pulmonary arterial resistance (PAR):

Equation 3

$$PVR = \frac{mean\,PA\,pressure}{pulmonary\,blood\,flow}$$

(normal range 67 ± 25 dyn s/cm^5)

Equation 4 Calculation of pulmonary arterial resistance (PAR):

$$PAR = \frac{(mean\,PA\,pressure\, - \,mean\,LA\,pressure}{pulmonary\,blood\,flow}$$

(normal range 205 ± 50 dyn s/cm^5)

In order to calculate PVR, pulmonary blood flow must be determined. In the normal heart pulmonary and systemic blood flow are the same. However, in the presence of an intracardiac shunt if systemic blood flow is known, pulmonary blood flow can be determined using the shunt fraction. The Fick principle can be used to estimate systemic blood flow or pulmonary blood flow.

Estimation of systemic blood flow using the Fick principle

Oxygen uptake at rest is assumed to be approximately 220 mL/min (120 mL/min/m^2).

Oxygen content = Hb × 1.34[1] × O_2 saturation, where 1.34 is Huffners constant, the O_2 carrying capacity of normal Hb.

O_2 content of systemic arterial blood = 15 × 1.34 × 0.97 = 19.5 mL/dL

O_2 content of mixed venous blood = 15 × 1.34 × 0.78 = 15.7 mL/dL

Systemic arterio-venous concentration difference of O_2 = O_2 content arterial blood – O_2 content venous blood

Systemic arterio-venous concentration difference of O_2 = 19.5–15.7 = 3.8 mL/dL = 38 mL/L

Systemic blood flow = O_2 uptake/systemic arterio-venous concentration difference of O_2

Systemic blood flow = 220/38 = 5.9 L/min

Indirect estimation of pulmonary blood flow using the shunt fraction (assumed O_2 uptake)

Pulmonary blood flow = shunt fraction × systemic blood flow

Pulmonary blood flow = 3.8 × 5.9 = 22.41 L/min

Alternative indirect estimation of pulmonary blood flow (assumed O_2 uptake)

O_2 content of pulmonary arterial blood = 15 × 1.34 × 0.92 = 18.5 mL/dL

O_2 content of pulmonary venous blood = O_2 content of LA blood = 15 × 1.34 × 0.97 = 19.5 mL/dL

Pulmonary arterio-venous concentration difference of O_2 = O_2 content arterial blood – O_2 content venous blood

Pulmonary arterio-venous concentration difference of O_2 = 19.5 – 18.5 = 1 mL/dL = 10 mL/L

Pulmonary blood flow = O_2 uptake/pulmonary arterio-venous concentration difference of O_2

Pulmonary blood flow = 220/10 = 22 L/min

Estimation of pulmonary arterial resistance

$$PAR = \frac{(\text{mean PA pressure} - \text{mean LA pressure})}{\text{pulmonary blood flow}}$$

$$= 29 - 8/22.4 = 0.94 \text{ Wood units} = 75 \text{ dyn s/cm}^{5*}$$

*To convert Wood units to dyn s/cm^5 multiply by 80.

Estimation of total pulmonary vascular resistance

$$PVR = \frac{\text{mean PA pressure}}{\text{pulmonary blood flow}}$$

$$= 29/22.4 = 1.29 \text{ Wood units} = 104 \text{ dyn s/cm}^5$$

In this patient, pulmonary vascular resistance is normal and the elevation of mean pulmonary pressure can be attributed to the large increase in pulmonary blood flow through the ASD.

7) **How should this patient be managed?**

The aim of the management of patients with mimimally symptomatic but large systemic to pulmonary shunts is to prevent the onset of significant PH, which may be progressive and ultimately result in shunt reversal and the Eisenmenger syndrome. This syndrome causes cyanosis and progressive exercise intolerance is associated with a reduced life expectancy (50 years). Pregnancy is contraindicated as the risk to both mother and child is unacceptably high. The timing of the onset of PH depends on the size and type of defect present. When pulmonary blood flow and pressure are first increased the pulmonary vascular resistance remains unchanged, and even after medial hypertrophy and intimal proliferation develop a degree of reversibility exists. However, pulmonary hypertension is irreversible once plexiform lesions and arteritis develop, and this obliteration of the pulmonary vascular bed increases vascular resistance. Shunt reversal occurs if pulmonary vascular resistance increases above systemic vascular resistance. This can be prevented if the defect is corrected early.

A second potential indication for defect closure is to reduce the likelihood of progressive right atrial and ventricular dilatation over time, which may result in impaired exercise capacity and persistent atrial arrhythmias, particularly atrial fibrillation.

Methods of ASD closure include surgical and percutaneous techniques. For surgical closure, an atrium must be opened to allow patching or suture under direct vision. At present, percutaneous closure is limited to small- and medium-sized defects with a defined circumferential rim. Indications and contraindications for percutaneous closure of ASD are listed in Table 25.2.

Closure of an ASD before the age of 25 years has a low risk of complications and subsequent life expectancy is comparable to a healthy age-matched population. The management of asymptomatic 25–40-year-old patients with clinically significant shunts is less clear. However, closure of the ASD probably prevents progression of PH and cardiac failure.

Perioperative mortality from surgical closure of an ASD is lowest if performed before significant PH is present (systolic PA pressure <40 mmHg). After the onset of cyanosis, the procedural risk is high regardless of the method of closure and is often inappropriate. Individuals with a pulmonary vascular resistance >7 Wood units may show regression of symptoms (including NYHA functional class).

If PVR >15 Wood units the mortality associated with closure of the ASD is increased. Closure of the ASD may cause immediate RV failure as the after load against the RV suddenly increases.

In this case, the pulmonary vascular resistance was normal and the defect suitable for percutaneous closure. The patient noticed a significant clinical improvement in his symptoms when reviewed in the clinic 3 months after the defect was successfully closed with a large Helix device (Fig. 25.6).

Table 25.2 Indications and contraindications for percutaneous closure of ASD

Indications for percutaneous device closure of ASD

I. Secundum ASD ≤ 40 mm (stretched diameter) with left-to-right shunt Qp:Qs > 1.5
II. Significant right-heart volume overload (RA and RV dilatation)
III. Paradoxical embolisation

Contraindications to percutaneous device closure of ASD

I. ASD > 40 mm (stretched diameter)
II. Insufficient rim (<5 mm) – occlusion device could obstruct SVC, IVC, tricuspid valve or mitral valve
III. Ostium primum, sinus venosus, coronary sinus defect, or anomalous pulmonary drainage
IV. Other conditions that require cardiac surgery
V. Intracardiac thrombus, sepsis or decompensated heart failure
VI. Pulmonary hypertension with net right-to-left shunt and systemic desaturation

---

Further reading

Rao PS (2009). When and how should atrial septal defects be closed in adults? *J Invasive Cardiol*; **21**: 76–82.

Deanfield J, Thaulow E, Warnes C, Webb G, Kolbel F, Hoffman A, Sorenson K, Kaemmer H, Thilen U, Bink-Boelkens M, Iserin L, Daliento L, Silove E, Redington A, Vouhe P, Priori S, Alonso MA, Blanc JJ, Budaj A, Cowie M, Deckers J, Fernandez Burgos E, Lekakis J, Lindahl B, Mazzotta G, Morais J, Oto A, Smiseth O, Trappe HJ, Klein W, Blömstrom-Lundqvist C, de Backer G, Hradec J, Mazzotta G, Parkhomenko A, Presbitero P, Torbicki A; Task Force on the Management of Grown Up Congenital Heart Disease, European Society of Cardiology; ESC Committee for Practice Guidelines. (2003). Management of Grown Up Congenital Heart Disease–ESC guidelines. *Eur Heart J*; **24**: 1035–1084.

Wilkinson JL (2001). Congenital heart disease: Haemodynamic calculations in the catheter laboratory. *Heart*; **85**: 113–120.

Case 26

A 31-year-old man with spina bifida presented with acute shortness of breath and right-sided pleuritic chest pain. He denied cough, sputum, haemoptysis, wheeze, or palpitations but reported a 9-month history of gradually increasing breathlessness on exertion. He was usually able to transfer independently and mobilize with a wheelchair, but was finding this increasingly difficult.

The meningomyelocele was corrected when the patient was 7 months old. At the age of 8 months he required a ventriculoatrial (VA) cerebrospinal fluid (CSF) shunt for progressive hydrocephalus. The VA shunt was revised twice at the age of 3 years and 10 years. An ileocutaneous urostomy was formed at the age of 8 years. He performed intermittent self-catheterization and developed recurrent urinary tract infections.

On admission, observations were RR 30 breaths/minute, BP 85/30 mmHg, HR 130 bpm (sinus), and temperature 36.5°C. O_2 saturations were 90% on air but improved to 98% on high-flow oxygen. Examination of the chest and abdomen revealed a kyphoscoliosis and signs of PH. Neurological examination demonstrated paraparesis and absent sensation below the waist. There was no evidence of deep vein thrombosis.

Full blood count, renal, liver, and bone profile were unremarkable. D-dimer and CRP were raised (3234 µg/L and 64 mg/L, respectively). Arterial blood gas (ABG) analysis on air revealed pO_2 6.7 kPa, pCO_2 2.7 kPa, pH 7.55, and HCO_3^- 18 mmol/L.

An ECG (Fig. 26.1) and a chest X-ray (Fig. 26.2) were performed. Echocardiography revealed right heart dilatation with RV hypertrophy and severe tricuspid regurgitation (TR). The peak velocity of the TR was 5 m/s. Left heart size and function was within normal parameters, all valves were structurally normal, and there was no evidence of intracardiac shunt or thrombus. Computed tomographic pulmonary angiogram was performed (Figs. 26.3 and 26.4).

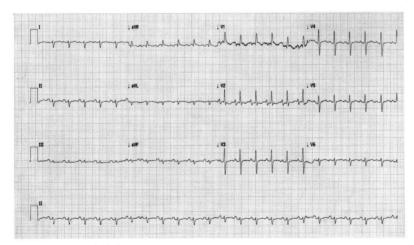

Fig. 26.1 ECG on admission.

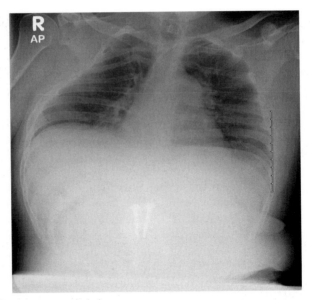

Fig. 26.2 Chest X-ray on admission.

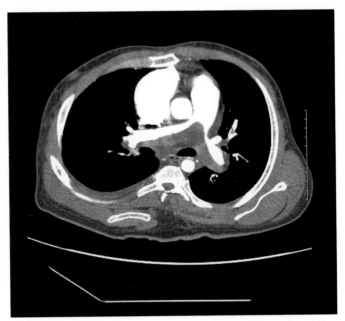

Fig. 26.3 CTPA image viewed on mediastinal windows at the level of the bifurcation of the pulmonary trunk.

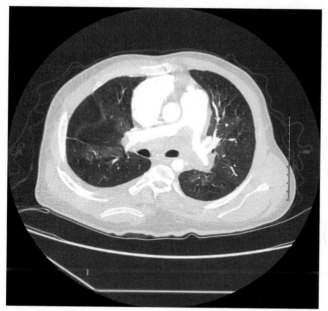

Fig. 26.4 CTPA image viewed on lung windows at the level of the bifurcation of the pulmonary trunk.

Questions

1. Interpret the ABG.
2. What does the ECG (Fig. 26.1) show?
3. What does the chest X-ray (Fig. 26.2) show?
4. Calculate the RVSP. Is it raised?
5. How reliable is the Doppler estimate of PA pressure?
6. What does the CTPA (Figs. 26.3 and 26.4) show? What is the cause of the PH?
7. What is the pathophysiological mechanism resulting in PH?
8. What are the risk factors for developing this condition?
9. What is the treatment of choice?
10. What other treatments are available?

Answers

1) **Interpret the ABG.**

The arterial blood gas demonstrates type I respiratory failure. The alveolar arterial pO_2 gradient is approximately 10 kPa (Equation 1). There is an alkalaemia due to a respiratory alkalosis. The reduced bicarbonate may reflect renal compensation but is more likely to be due to the ileal urinary conduit, which causes a hyperchloraemic (normal anion gap) metabolic acidosis.

Equation 1

$$\text{Alveolar arterial PO}_2 \text{ gradient} = pAO_2 - paO_2$$

The estimation of pAO_2 is shown in Equation 2.

Equation 2

$$pAO_2 \approx FiO_2(\text{Patm} - pH_2O) - paCO_2 / R$$

where pAO_2 is the alveolar partial pressure of oxygen, FiO_2 is the fraction of inspired gas that is oxygen, Patm is the atmospheric pressure (101 kPa at sea level), pH_2O is the saturated vapour pressure of water at body temperature at Patm (6 kPa), $paCO_2$ is the arterial partial pressure of carbon dioxide, and R is the respiratory quotient (the ratio of the amount of CO_2 produced to the amount of O_2 consumed during metabolism, which depends on the relative proportions of carbohydrate, fat, and protein being metabolized but is usually 0.8 at rest).

In this case:

$$pAO_2 \approx 0.21(101 - 6) - 2.7 / 0.8 \approx 20 - 3.4 \approx 16.6$$
$$pAO_2 - paO_2 = 16.6 - 6.7 = 9.9 \text{kPa}$$

2) **What does the ECG (Fig. 26.1) show?**

The ECG shows sinus tachycardia (rate 132 bpm), RBBB pattern conduction delay, marked right-axis deviation, sharp biphasic P waves in V1–2, and RV hypertrophy (R-to-S wave ratio >1 in lead V1 and S wave in V6).

3) **What does the chest X-ray (Fig. 26.2) show?**

The AP chest X-ray shows cardiomegaly, dilated proximal pulmonary arteries, and peripheral pruning. The patient is kyphotic and the VA shunt and metalwork in the lumbar spine are visible.

4) **Calculate the RVSP. Is it raised?**

Calculation of the RVSP pressure (Equation 3) using the modified Bernoulli equation (Equation 4) is 100 mmHg + right atrial pressure (RAP). This RVSP is extremely high (normal range 15–25 mmHg), in keeping with chronic PH.

Equation 3 is the modified Bernoulli equation:

$$\Delta P = 4v^2$$

Where v is the velocity of tricuspid regurgitation (TR) jet (m/s).

Equation 4

$$RVSP = \Delta P + RAP$$

where ΔP is the pressure difference as determined by the modified Bernoulli equation (Equation 3).

5) **How reliable is the Doppler estimate of PA pressure?**

Doppler echocardiography is the most reliable non-invasive method of measuring PA pressure. It depends on the detection and measurement of the TR jet to estimate RVSP using the modified Bernoulli equation above. In the absence of pulmonary valve disease or RVOT abnormalities RVSP and PA systolic pressure are the same.

TR can be detected in >90% of patients with severe PH and grouped mean data suggest excellent correlation with direct measurement. However, there are several sources of error in this assessment, including visualization of the TR jet, Doppler transduction, and the choice of peak velocity profile.

Doppler echocardiography is useful for long-term follow-up, but confirmation of PH often requires cardiac catheterization. Cardiac catheterization also provides left-heart pressure measurements and cardiac output and can help to exclude diastolic LV dysfunction.

6) **What does the CTPA (Fig. 26.3) show? What is the cause of the PH?**

The CTPA confirmed acute PE (filling defect; Fig. 26.5) in the lobar arteries of the left lung. A chronic organized saddle embolus is also seen within the posterior wall of the pulmonary trunk and extending into the main pulmonary artery (Fig. 26.5). The proximal pulmonary arteries are dilated.

The PH is probably due to acute PE on a background of chronic thromboembolic pulmonary hypertension (CTEPH). However, the kyphosis is likely to cause a restrictive lung disease, which would contribute to the PH.

CT features of CTEPH include complete occlusion of pulmonary arteries, eccentric filling defects consistent with organized thrombi, recanalization, stenoses, and a mosaic pattern of perfusion (Figs 26.4 to 26.6).

CTEPH results from single or recurrent pulmonary thromboemboli. PE usually resolves completely, with restoration of normal pulmonary haemodynamics. However, in some cases, for reasons which remain unclear, the PE does not resolve but forms endothelialized obstructions of the pulmonary vasculature. This results in CTEPH, which occurs after 0.1–0.5% of acute non-fatal PE.

Exertional dyspnoea develops months to years after the initial PE. In some cases the initial PE is asymptomatic, and diagnosis of CTEPH therefore requires a high index of suspicion in patients presenting with unexplained breathlessness. Diagnosis is made by ventilation perfusion scan, CTPA, and/or pulmonary angiography.

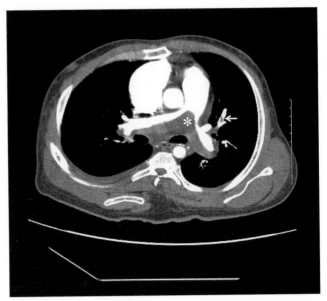

Fig. 26.5 CTPA demonstrating acute PE and chronic pulmonary thromboembolism. The proximal pulmonary arteries are dilated and there is an excentric filling defect within the pulmonary trunk that extends into the left and right pulmonary arteries (*). The lumen arterial is irregular. These features are consistent with chronic pulmonary thromboembolism. There is also evidence of acute PE (filling defect; arrowed) in the lobar arteries of the left lung.

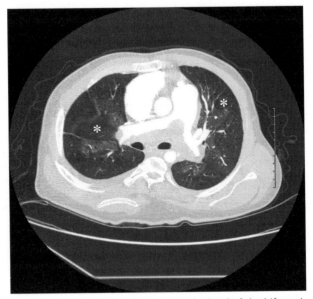

Fig. 26.6 CTPA image viewed on lung windows at the level of the bifurcation of the pulmonary trunk demonstrating mosaic pattern of perfusion. There are bilateral areas of decreased attenuation and vascularity (two examples marked *). This mosaic appearance results from redistribution of blood flow.

7) **What is the pathophysiological mechanism resulting in PH?**

PH in CTEPH is due to hypoxic vasoconstriction and chronic obstruction of the pulmonary vasculature by thrombus. When the PA pressure begins to rise, over 60% of the total pulmonary vasculature has already been lost. A mild-to-moderate increase in mean PA pressure occurs with acute PE. However, peak systolic PA pressures rarely rise above 50 mmHg, and generally return to normal with treatment. Recurrent PE can cause progressive PAH.

8) **What are the risk factors for developing this condition?**

The risk factors for CTEPH include:

◆ previous PE

◆ chronic inflammatory diseases (e.g. inflammatory bowel disease)

◆ immobility

◆ presence of a VA shunt

◆ splenectomy (mechanism unclear).

In patients with a VA shunt, PE and PH are clinically recognized in 0.3% and 0.4%, respectively. However, at autopsy, the incidence of these complications in children is much higher (around 60% and 6%, respectively). The incidence in adults is uncertain. The use of ventriculo-peritoneal (VP) CSF shunts has considerably reduced the extent of this problem. However, VA shunts remain an alternative treatment for hydrocephalus if the placement of a VP shunt is not possible.

9) **What is the treatment of choice?**

Pulmonary endarterectomy (rather than embolectomy), although high risk, can improve symptoms and restore more normal pulmonary pressures. An endarterectomy of all the affected lung vasculature is needed to reopen the pulmonary vasculature. The procedure involves cardiopulmonary bypass, circulatory arrest, and systemic cooling. The patients usually require life-long anticoagulation thereafter.

A large case series of thromboendarterectomy for CTEPH reported the outcomes of 743 patients between 1999 and 2004. The patients were divided into two groups on the basis of preoperative systolic PA pressures: >100 mmHg (group 1) and <100 mmHg (group 2). The overall survival was slightly lower in group 1 (89%) than in group 2 (96%). The reduction in pulmonary vascular resistance was similar, therefore even patients with advanced PH can benefit from endarterectomy.

The decision to proceed to surgery depends on the extent and location of the thrombi and the severity of PH. Surgery is best for proximal thrombi as distal obstructions may not be so amenable to endarterectomy. Successful surgery returns pulmonary haemodynamics close to normal. Operative mortality is 5–10% depending on the severity of the PAH. However the 5-year survival of patients with CTEPH and PA pressure >50 mmHg is poor and in some series less than 10%.

10) **What other treatments are available?**

Long-term anticoagulation with warfarin is required for CTEPH. Other medical treatments for PH can be applied to inoperable distal CTEPH (see Case 27). However, there are no clear data on efficacy and attempts at medical management often delays referral for thromboendarterectomy. Lung transplantation can also be performed for advanced cases.

In the present case, the patient was treated with LMWH and warfarin. Although he was referred for pulmonary endarterectomy he had an asystolic cardiac arrest whilst awaiting surgery. Cardiopulmonary resuscitation was attempted but was not successful.

Further reading

Thistlewaite PA, Kemp A, Lingling D, Madani MM, Jamieson SW (2006). Outcomes for pulmonary endarterectomy for treatment of extreme thromboembolic pulmonary hypertension. *J Thoracic Cardiovasc Surg*; **131**: 307–313.

Bonderman D, Jakowitsch J, Adlbrecht C, Schemper M, Kyrle PA, Schönauer V, Exner M, Klepetko W, Kneussi MP, Maurer G, Lang I. (2005). Medical conditions increasing the risk of chronic thromboembolic pulmonary hypertension. *Thromb Haemost*; **93**: 512–516.

Kluge S, Baumann HJ, Regelsberger J, Kehler U, Koziej B, Klose H, Greinert U, Kreymann G, Meyer A. (2009). Development of Pulmonary Hypertension in Adults after Ventriculoatrial Shunt Implantation. *Respiration*; **78**: 30–35.

Jensen KW, Kerr KM, Fedullo PF, Kim NH, Test VJ, Ben-Yehuda O, Auger WR. (2009). Pulmonary hypertensive medical therapy in chronic thromboembolic pulmonary hypertension before pulmonary thromboendarterectomy. *Circulation*; **120**: 1248–1254.

Case 27

A 48-year-old man was referred to the medical registrar on call with a 5-day history of gradually increasing breathlessness on minimal exertion and ankle swelling. The onset of the symptoms had coincided with his stopping smoking. Six months before, he had developed a chronic dry cough. His current exercise tolerance was less than 50 yards and he had lost over 10 kg in weight over 3 months. He had been dieting but also reported loss of appetite. Treatment with inhaled salbutamol and becotide, several courses of oral antibiotics, and furosemide (20 mg daily) had failed to improve the symptoms.

There was no relevant family history but his male partner had died from a severe chest infection 6 months prior to this presentation. He had been advised to have an HIV test by the clinicians looking after his partner; this was negative. He denied having any relationships after this. He also denied illicit drug use.

On admission, observations were HR 105 bpm (sinus), BP 104/76 mmHg, RR 28 breaths/min, and temperature 36.6°C. O_2 saturations were 83% on air but improved to 99% with high-flow oxygen.

Examination of the cardiovascular and respiratory systems revealed signs of a parasternal lift and a loud second heart sound suggestive of PH. There were no signs of deep vein thrombosis.

Full blood count, renal, liver, and bone profile were unremarkable. D-dimer and CRP were normal (100 µg/L and <5 mg/L, respectively). Arterial blood gas analysis on air revealed pO_2 6.9 kPa, pCO_2 5.0 kPa, pH 7.44, and HCO_3^- 26 mmol/L.

An ECG showed sinus rhythm (rate 100 bpm) with RBBB. Chest X-ray was reported as normal. Echocardiography revealed right-heart dilatation with RV hypertrophy and severe TR. The peak velocity of the TR was 4 m/s. Left-heart size and function were normal, and all valves were structurally normal. There was no evidence of intracardiac shunt or thrombus. Computed tomographic pulmonary angiogram excluded acute PE and CTEPH. Lung function tests were normal.

Questions

1. Define PH.
2. How is PH classified?
3. What symptoms and signs are associated with PH?
4. How would you investigate the patient?
5. What causes of secondary PAH should be specifically considered in this case?
6. How should the patient's previous HIV test results be interpreted?
7. What is the prognosis if the PH is left untreated?
8. How is this condition staged?
9. What treatment is available for PAH?

Answers

1) **Define PH.**

   PH is defined as:

   ◆ mean PA pressure >25 mmHg at rest or

   ◆ mean PA pressure >30 mmHg on exertion.

   Mean PA pressures of 8–20 mmHg at rest are considered normal. The significance of mean PA pressures in the range 21–24 mmHg at rest is uncertain. Increases in pulmonary blood flow, pulmonary vascular resistance, or pulmonary venous pressure can all increase PA pressure.

2) **How is PH classified?**

   Simply classifying PH as primary or secondary is inadequate. Some forms of secondary PH are similar to primary PH in their histopathological features, natural history, and response to treatment. It is therefore more useful to classify PH clinically (Table 27.1) or by haemodynamic data (Table 27.2).

Table 27.1 World Health Organisation classification of pulmonary hypertension

Group 1. Pulmonary arterial hypertension[1]	Group 2. Pulmonary venous hypertension[2]
Idiopathic (primary)	Left-heart disease or chronic untreated systemic hypertension increase left-sided cardiac filling pressures, pulmonary venous pressures and PAH develops to maintain blood flow.
Familial	
Secondary:	
◆ connective tissue disease	**Group 3. PH associated with hypoxia**
◆ congenital systemic-to-pulmonary shunts (see Case 25)	Several chronic lung diseases cause hypoxia, including COPD and interstitial lung diseases.
◆ portal hypertension	
◆ HIV infection	
◆ drugs and toxins (e.g. fenfluramine)	**Group 4. Chronic thromboembolic PH**
◆ other (thyroid disorders, glycogen storage disease, hereditary haemorrhagic telangiectasia, haemoglobinopathies, significant myeloproliferative disease, splenectomy)	See Case 26
◆ venous or capillary involvement	**Group 5. Miscellaneous**
◆ pulmonary veno-occlusive disease	For example sarcoidosis, histiocytosis X, and lymphangiomatosis
◆ pulmonary capillary haemangiomatosis	

[1]Group 1 is a heterogenous collection of diseases with similar presentation, haemodynamic features, pathophysiological mechanisms, and response to treatment of PH.
[2]The most common cause of PH in patients with cardiovascular disease.

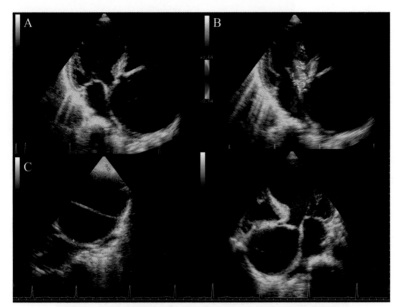

Plate 1 Trans-thoracic echocardiogram: A, off-axis parasternal short-axis view; B, off-axis parasternal short-axis view with colour Doppler overlay; C, modified short-axis aortic root view; D, modified five-chamber view showing aortic root. (See Fig. 12.2 p 84)

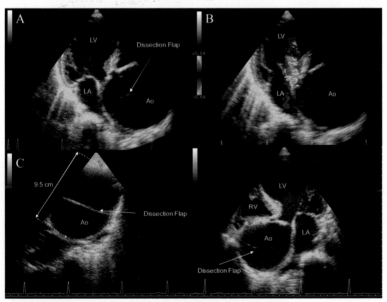

Plate 2 Trans-thoracic echocardiogram demonstrating aortic dissection. A, off-axis parasternal short-axis view with dissection flap visible in aortic root; B, off-axis parasternal short-axis view with colour Doppler overlay demonstrating significant aortic regurgitation; C, modified short-axis aortic root view demonstrating a 9.5 cm aneurysm, D, modified five-chamber view showing aortic root demonstrating the dissection flap. (See Fig. 12.4 p 86)

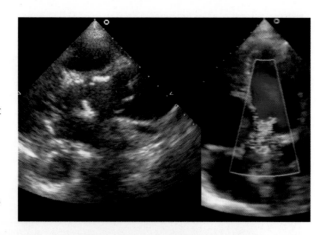

Plate 3 Selected views from the bedside transthoracic echocardiogram: A, zoomed parasternal short axis view; B, apical five-chamber view with colour Doppler overlay. (See Fig. 13.3 p 92)

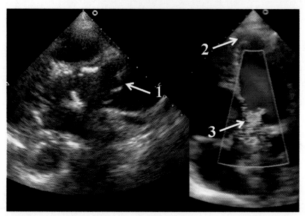

Plate 4 Transthoracic echocardiogram demonstrating a dissection flap in the proximal aorta pericardial effusion and significant aortic regurgitation. The parasternal short-axis view (A) and five-chamber view with colour Doppler overlay. (B) These images demonstrate a dissection flap in the proximal aorta (1) suggestive of acute dissection. Aortic dissection has been complicated by pericardial effusion (2) and significant aortic regurgitation (3). (See Fig. 13.4 p 96)

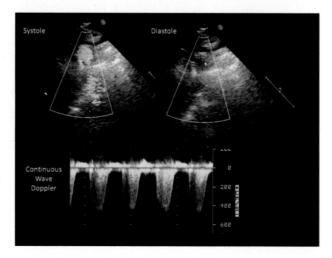

Plate 5 A selected image from the TTE performed in the cardiology clinic showing systole and diastole. Underneath is a continuous wave Doppler tracing recorded along the path indicated by the dotted lines in the systolic and diastolic images. (See Fig. 16.3 p 177)

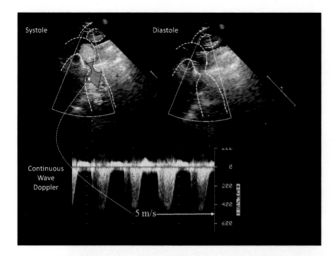

Plate 6 Suprasternal TTE showing an obstruction to flow in the descending aorta consistent with aortic coarctation. (See Fig. 16.5 p 120)

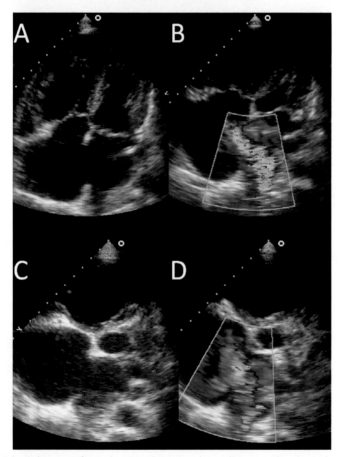

Plate 7 Selected images from the transthoracic echocardiogram. The views shown are the two-dimensional apical four-chamber views (A and B) and short-axis parasternal views at the level of the aortic valve (C and D). Colour Doppler overlays on the apical four-chamber view (B) and short-axis parasternal view at the level of the aortic valve (D) are also shown. (See Fig. 25.3 p 190)

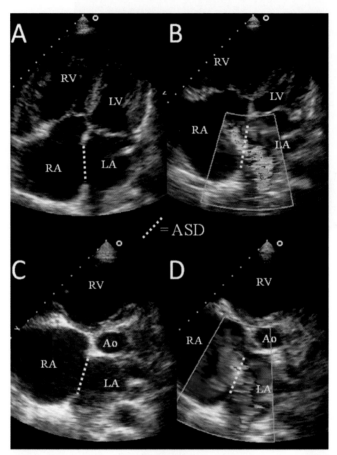

Plate 8 Selected views from the transthoracic echocardiogram demonstrating an ASD. The apical four-chamber views (A and B) and short-axis parasternal views at the level of the aortic valve AV (Ao; C and D) demonstrate a large defect in the interatrial septum (ASD). The defect is in the centre of the septum between the right and left atrium; an ostium secundum defect. Colour Doppler overlay demonstrates a broad jet of flow from LA to RA (B and D). (See Fig. 25.4 p 193)

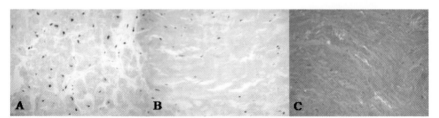

Plate 9 Cardiac biopsy. A, Haematoxylin and eosin (H&E) stained section of normal cardiac muscle. B, H&E stained section of cardiac biopsy showing eosinophilic infiltrate. C, Congo red stained section of cardiac biopsy photographed under polarized light showing apple-green biorefringence. (See Fig. 28.5 p 226)

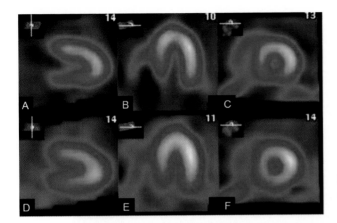

Plate 10 Myocardial perfusion scan. (See Fig. 29.4 p 230)

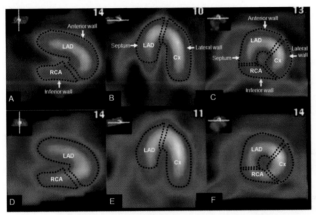

Plate 11 Myocardial perfusion scan demonstrating reversible perfusion defect in the distribution of the RCA. These images from the myocardial perfusion scan show a moderate-to-large perfusion defect in the inferior and inferoseptal walls (A–C) in the distribution of the RCA. The defect is completely reversible (D–F), indicating inferior inducible ischaemia and myocardial viability. (See Fig. 29.6 p 232)

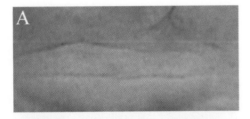
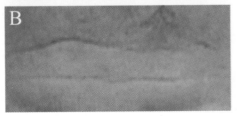

Plate 12 Intermittent changes in facial appearance. Photograph of patient's forehead demonstrating pallor (A) and flushing (B). (See Fig. 35.1 p 266)

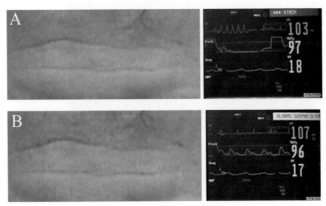

Plate 13 Photographs demonstrating association of facial pallor with ventricular tachycardia. A, The facial pallor was associated with ventricular tachycardia. B, The facial flush was associated with spontaneous cardioversion to sinus rhythm. (See Fig. 35.3 p 269)

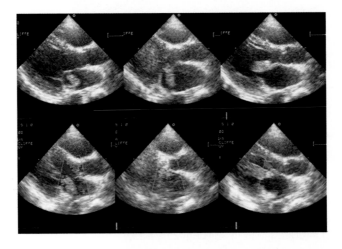

Plate 14 TTE. Selected sequential images with corresponding colour flow beneath. (See Fig. 40.4 p 307)

Plate 15 TOE. Selected sequential images with corresponding colour flow beneath. (See Fig. 40.5 p 307)

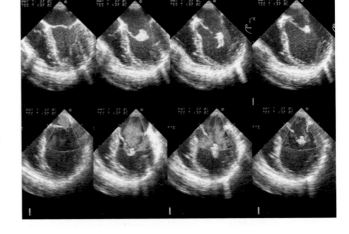

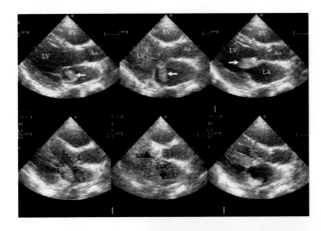

Plate 16 TTE demonstrating a vegetation on the mitral valve (white arrow) and MR (black dotted arrow). (See Fig. 40.8 p 309)

Plate 17 TOE demonstrating vegetation (white arrow) on mitral valve and MR (black dotted arrows). A valvular and a para-valvular jet are visible. (See Fig. 40.9 p 310)

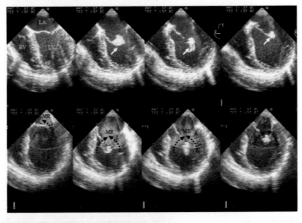

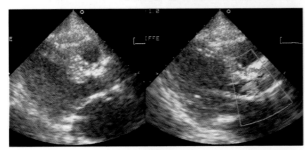

Plate 18 Transthoracic echocardiogram: parasternal long-axis view with colour flow Doppler over the aortic valve prosthesis. (See Fig. 41.2 p 318)

Plate 19 TOE short axis AVR views. Arrows indicate the extent on the abcess cavity. (See Fig. 41.3 p 321)

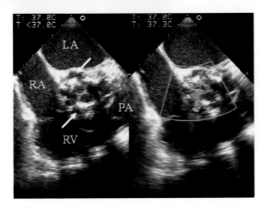

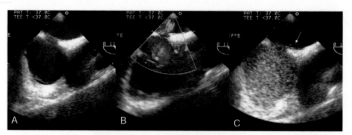

Plate 20 Transoesophageal echocardiogram images. (See Fig. 42.1 p 326)

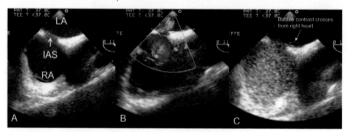

Plate 21 Transoesophageal echocardiogram demonstrating patent foramen ovale. The RA and LA are separated by the inter-atrial septum (IAS; A). There is no flow visible across the IAS when colour Doppler is applied (B), excluding an ASD. However, bubble contrast can be seen to cross the IAS (C; arrowed). This demonstrates the presence of a patent foramen ovale (PFO). (See Fig. 42.2 p 328)

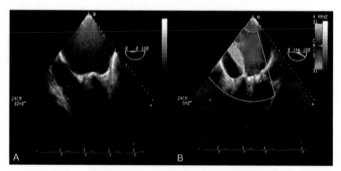

Plate 22 Transoesophageal echocardiogram. A, The mid-oesophageal four-chamber view. B, The mid-oesophageal long-axis view with colour Doppler overlay. (See Fig. 49.1 p 390)

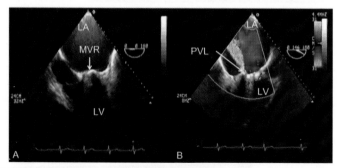

Plate 23 Transoesophageal echocardiogram demonstrating PVL. A, The mid-oesophageal four-chamber view demonstrates a giant left atrium (LA; 12 × 14 cm). B, The colour Doppler overlay on the mid-oesophageal long-axis view demonstrates severe mitral regurgitation due to PVL. (See Fig. 49.2 p 392)

Table 27.2 Haemodynamic classification of PH

Haemodynamic class of pulmonary hypertension	Characteristics				Causes (group; Table 27.1)
	Mean PA pressure (mmHg)	PA wedge pressure (mmHg)	Pulmonary blood flow	Pulmonary vascular resistance (Wood units, mmHg/L/min; dynes/cm^5)	
Pre-capillary	>25	≤15	Normal or reduced	> 3 Wood units > 240 dynes/cm^5	PAH, hypoxia, CTEPH, miscellaneous (1, 3, 4, 5)
Pre-capillary hyperkinetic	>25	≤15	Increased	Usually <2 Wood units Can be high if vasculature damaged <160 dyne s/cm^5	Systemic-to-pulmonary shunts and porto-pulmonary hypertension
Post-capillary	>25	>15	Normal or reduced	Passive < 2 Wood units < 160 dyne s/cm^5 Reactive >2 Wood units >160 dyne s/cm^5	Pulmonary venous hypertension (2)
Post-capillary hyperkinetic	>25	>15	Increased	< 2 Wood units < 160 dyne s/cm^5	Pulmonary venous hypertension (2)

3) **What symptoms and signs are associated with PH?**

Progressive shortness of breath is the most common presenting symptom of PH, followed by ankle swelling, dry cough, fatigue, syncope or pre-syncope, and chest pain. The signs of PH are listed in Table 27.3. The last three signs are late findings suggestive of right-heart failure. These symptoms and signs are non-specific and frequently lead to misdiagnosis.

Table 27.3 Signs of pulmonary hypertension

Loud pulmonary component of the second heart sound (equal to or louder than aortic component)

Right-ventricular heave (suggesting right-ventricular hypertrophy)

Tricuspid regurgitation

Peripheral oedema and ascites

Right-sided third and fourth heart sounds

4) How would you investigate the patient?

Interpretation of the investigations of PH requires knowledge of the anatomical location of potential causes (Fig. 27.1) and the effects on pulmonary haemodynamics (Table 27.2). A suggested approach is shown in Fig. 27.2.

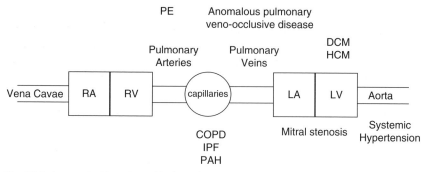

Fig. 27.1 Anatomical location of lesions that cause PH.

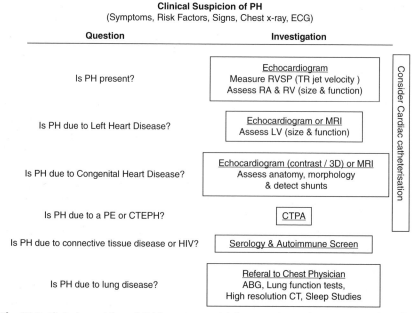

Fig. 27.2 Clinical suspicion of PH (symptoms, risk factors, signs, chest X-ray, and ECG).

5) **What causes of secondary PAH should be specifically considered in this case?**

PAH may be primary or secondary (associated). Secondary causes possible in this case include HIV and drugs (fenfluramine–phentermine, methamphetamines, cocaine).

The incidence of primary PAH is highest in younger women of childbearing age. The average reported female-to-male ratio is around 4:1.

As a group the incidence and prevalence of secondary (associated) PAH is higher than for primary PAH. It is important to ask about use of appetite suppressants as the incidence of dieting and anorexia is increased in homosexual men. In all, 1 in 20 000 people who took fenfluramine–phentermine for over 6 months develop PAH.

In this case, the patient denied use of appetite suppressants and urine toxicology was negative for cocaine and amphetamines.

The prevalence of PAH in patients infected with HIV is much higher (1/200) than in the general population and PAH may develop before AIDS. It is associated with high viral loads and delayed diagnosis and treatment. The prognosis is poor despite antiretroviral therapy and the median survival after diagnosis of PAH is 6 months.

The pathogenesis of PAH in patients with HIV remains unclear. Both viral and host factors are likely to be important. However, the relative contributions of each are difficult to determine because many patients with HIV have coexisting diseases that are independently associated with PAH (e.g. intravenous drug use, hepatitis B or C infection).

Plexiform lesions are the characteristic histopathological feature in patients with severe PAH of any cause. Plexogenic arteriopathy is characterized by abnormal vascular endothelium, disruption of the vessel intima, hypertrophy of the media, thrombosis, and obliteration of the lumen with subsequent recanalization. This occlusive vasculopathy results in increased pulmonary vascular resistance and PH. Plexogenic arteriopathy develops in patients infected with HIV, even in the absence of AIDS. The plexiform lesions of HIV-associated PAH are indistinguishable from those caused by idiopathic PAH (IPAH). HIV does not infect endothelial cells and so probably does not cause these lesions directly. However, the pathogenesis of HIV-induced PH may involve the same pathways that cause plexiform lesions in other types of PAH.

6) **How should the patient's previous HIV test results be interpreted?**

Despite the patient's claim of celibacy since last being tested, a single HIV negative test is not conclusive, particularly if further exposure may have occurred during the window period of screening tests.

Enzyme-linked immunosorbent assay is the first-line investigation for HIV. If positive (i.e. antibodies to HIV are present), the test is usually repeated to confirm the diagnosis. If ELISA is negative, other tests are not usually needed. However, seroconversion may occur 3 months (window period) after the original infection.

During this period, serological investigations for HIV infection may be negative but carriers can still spread the disease.

The current fourth-generation screening assays permit the simultaneous detection of HIV p24 antigen and antibody, and have reduced the diagnostic window between the time of HIV infection and laboratory diagnosis significantly (27.4 days). Genomic testing in the form of HIV quantitative assays (viral load tests) should be considered only in suspected primary HIV infection. The fourth-generation assay is as effective as genomic testing (viral load assays) in identifying acute HIV infection. Viral load tests have high false-positive results, which are potentially devastating for patients. Although UK guidelines for HIV testing recommend fourth-generation assays as first-line screening, these are not provided by all laboratories. Patients with suspected primary HIV infection should either be referred to specialist services urgently or retested 7 days later.

In this case, the patient was offered another HIV test as it was suspected that the previous result could have been a false negative.

7) **What is the prognosis if the PH is left untreated?**

There is no cure for idiopathic or primary PAH. The overall survival rate is 30% at 3 years if primary PAH is left untreated. The survival rate in untreated HIV-associated PAH is similar (see below) if antiretroviral treatment is given, but worse if not.

The main causes of death are right-heart failure and thromboembolism. Prostacyclin analogues and endothelin receptor antagonists may improve the prognosis.

8) **How is this condition staged?**

The NYHA functional class is a simple but subjective description of severity. More objective methods include signs of heart failure on examination, exercise capacity (e.g. 6-minute walk, maximal oxygen uptake (VO_2 max), and haemodynamic data (right-heart catheterization). Raised serum cardiac troponin and the presence of a pericardial effusion suggest a worse prognosis.

9) **What treatment is available for PAH?**

Idiopathic (primary) PAH is rare and patients should be referred to specialist centres for medical and surgical management.

The standard medical treatment for primary PAH includes oxygen for hypoxia at rest or on exertion, anticoagulation, diuretics for oedema, and digoxin for right-heart failure. Although several studies have suggested that these treatments are beneficial in PAH, there are no RCT data.

Calcium channel blockade (CCB) reduces pulmonary vascular resistance through vasodilatation, which may increase the cardiac output and decrease pulmonary artery pressure. CCB has greatest utility before the onset of right-heart failure. CCB may worsen heart failure but improve quality of life and survival rate in responders. Responders (<20% of primary PAH and <10% of secondary PAH) have an acute vasodilator response to intravenous or inhaled pulmonary vasodilator challenge (e.g. adenosine). The prognosis of non-responders treated with CCB is less good than responders.

Intravenous vasodilator therapy should be considered for non-responders and responders intolerant of CCB with NYHA class III or IV right-heart failure. The mechanisms of action of prostanoids and endothelin receptor agonists are unclear and may include inhibition of pathologic intimal fibrosis and smooth muscle proliferation as well as the obvious reduction in PA pressure.

Surgical care

Lung transplantation (single or double) may be considered for patients with who do not respond to medical therapy. Simultaneous cardiac transplantation may be required if right-heart failure has developed.

Atrial septostomy is palliative. This allows atrial right-to-left shunting, increasing cardiac output, and oxygen delivery despite the potential for a lower overall arterial saturation.

Management of HIV-associated PH

Treatment for patients with HIV-associated PH is more limited than for other forms of PAH. Lung transplantation is contraindicated, calcium channel blockers are rarely effective, and there are no RCTs in HIV-associated PAH. At present, antiretroviral therapy is not indicated for the sole purpose of improving PAH in patients with HIV, although there is some suggestion of potential benefit. However, specific treatment for PAH may improve outcome.

Open label, uncontrolled studies and case reports suggest potential benefit from prostacylins (e.g. epoprostenol), endothelin receptor antagonists (e.g. bosentan), and phosphodiesterase inhibitors (e.g. sildenafil). A review of over 500 published cases of HIV-associated PAH found that the survival of patients who received specific therapy for PAH (76%) was greater than those who did not (32%; Cicalini *et al.*, 2009). Screening for PAH should be considered in patients with HIV who report breathlessness. Specific therapy for PAH should be considered for patients with HIV-associated PAH.

In this case an HIV test was positive, the CD4 cell count was 150 cells/μL and the viral load was 2 00 000 copies/mL. There was no evidence of any AIDS-defining conditions. The patient was prescribed antiretroviral therapy and oral anticoagulation therapy and then discharged home with cardiology and infectious diseases follow-up. The patient subsequently had a trial of nifedipine. This did not improve his symptoms or reduce the PA pressure as measured by PA catheter and serial echocardiography. Six months later the viral load was 'undetectable' (i.e. suppressed to <40 copies/mL) and the CD4 count was 200 cells/mL. However, the PH did not improve and the patient developed cor pulmonale despite trials of sildenafil and epoprostenol. He passed away 12 months after presentation.

Reference

Cicalini S, Chinello P, Grilli E, Petrosillo N. (2009). Treatment and outcome of pulmonary arterial hypertension in HIV-infected patients: a review of the literature. *Curr HIV Res*; 7: 589–596.

Further reading

Simonneau G, Galiè N, Rubin LJ, Langleben D, Seeger W, Domenighetti G, Gibbs S, Lebrec D, Speich R, Beghetti M, Rich S, Fishman A. (2004). Clinical classification of pulmonary hypertension. *J Am Coll Cardiol*; **43**Suppl S::5S–12S.

Barst R, McGoon M, Torbicki A, Sitbon O, Krowka MJ, Olschewski H, Gaine S. (2004). Diagnosis and differential assessment of pulmonary arterial hypertension. *J Am Coll Cardiol*; **43**: S40–47.

British HIV Association, British Association of Sexual Health and HIV, British Infection Society (2008). UK national guidelines for HIV testing 2008. London: BHIVA. www.bhiva.org/files/file1031097.pdf.

Degano B, Guillaume M, Savale L, Montani D, Jaïs X, Yaici A, Le Pavec J, Humbert M, Simonneau G, Sitbon O. (2010). HIV-associated pulmonary arterial hypertension: survival and prognostic factors in the modern therapeutic era. *AIDS*; **24**: 67–75.

Case 28

A 70-year-old woman with type 2 diabetes mellitus was referred to a respiratory clinic with a 2-year history of increasing dyspnoea. Although her symptoms had improved with furosemide 40 mg once daily, she remained short of breath on climbing one flight of stairs or walking 50 m on level ground. She had 5 pillow orthopnoea, but denied paroxysmal nocturnal dyspnoea. Examination revealed raised venous pressure, AF with controlled ventricular rate, a right-sided pleural effusion, a palpable liver edge, and pitting oedema of the ankles.

Routine blood tests, including full blood count, renal, bone, and liver profiles, were normal. Dipstick examination of the urine was normal. Chest radiography (Fig. 28.1) confirmed the right-sided pleural effusion, which was aspirated. Biochemical analysis of the pleural fluid found 42 g/L protein, LDH 212 iu/L, glucose 6.2 mmol/L, and pH 7.4. Routine microscopy and culture of pleural fluid were negative. Ziehl Nielsen staining and culture for tuberculosis were also negative. Cytological analysis revealed large numbers of lymphocytes but no malignant cells.

The ECG is shown in Fig. 28.2. The report of the echocardiogram is shown in Table 28.1. In summary there is biatrial dilation, marked symmetrical LVH, and mildly impaired LV systolic function.

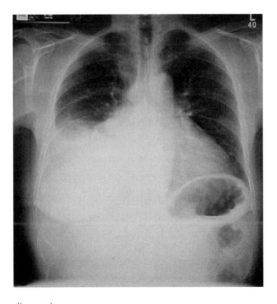

Fig. 28.1 Chest radiograph.

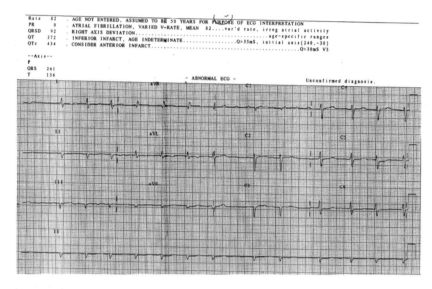

```
Rate   82    AGE NOT ENTERED, ASSUMED TO BE 50 YEARS FOR PURPOSE OF ECG INTERPRETATION
PR      0    ATRIAL FIBRILLATION, VARIED V-RATE, MEAN  82....var'd rate, irreg atrial activity
QRSD   92    RIGHT AXIS DEVIATION..........................................age-specific ranges
QT    372    INFERIOR INFARCT, AGE INDETERMINATE.................Q>35mS, initial axis(240,-30)
QTc   434    CONSIDER ANTERIOR INFARCT.................................................Q>30mS V3

--Axis--
P
QRS   261
T     156                                 - ABNORMAL ECG -              Unconfirmed diagnosis.
```

Fig. 28.2 Electrocardiograph.

Table 28.1 Report of initial echocardiogram

Interventricular spectum (IVS)	2.0 cm
Posterior wall (PW)	1.9 cm
LV end diastolic diameter (LV EDD)	3.6 cm
LV end sustolic diameter(LV ESD)	2.8 cm

Mitral valve (MV) normal–mild mitral regurgitation (MR), dilated left atrium (LA) 4.9 cm
Aortic valve(AV) tricuspid–no aortic stenosis (AS)/aortic regurgitation (AR); aortic root 3.1 cm
No LVOT flow acceleration
Mild TR; pulmonary artery pressure (PAP) 18 mmHg + JVP

The patient was treated for AF and heart failure. She was started on digoxin 125 µg od and warfarin for the AF. Her furosemide was increased to 80 mg od and she was started on ramipril 1.25 mg od, which was titrated up to 10 mg od. The pleural effusion was drained for symptomatic relief. However, the effusion recurred and required five further aspirations for symptomatic relief over the next 4 months. On each occasion the biochemical and cytological analysis was as described above.

Malignancy was suspected so CT of the chest, abdomen, and pelvis was performed. This confirmed the presence of the pleural effusion and also revealed ascites, mesenteric lymphadenopathy and a cyst on the right ovary. The serum tumour marker CA 125 was raised (276 u/mL; normal <38 u/mL) but carcino embryonic antigen (CEA) was normal. Thoracoscopy, pleural biopsy, and talc pleurodesis were performed. Thoracoscopic examination of the pleura was unremarkable. However, the pleural biopsy was reported to show lymphocytic infiltration, which was 'reactive' in nature. Ziehl Nielsen stain and culture for tuberculosis were again negative.

The patient was admitted to hospital from clinic 3 weeks post thoracoscopy. She was short of breath on minimal exertion and unable to walk more than 25 m. Clinically and radiologically there was only a small residual right pleural reaction. Examination also revealed AF, tricuspid regurgitation with high venous pressure, a palpable pulsatile liver edge, marked ascites, and severe pitting oedema to the abdomen.

The ECG on admission from clinic is shown in Fig. 28.3. Echocardiography was repeated (Fig. 28.4).

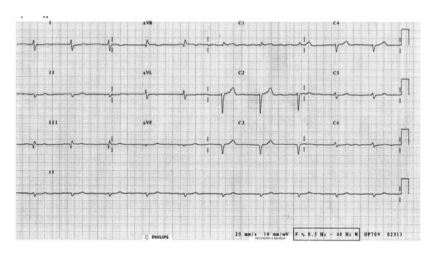

Fig. 28.3 Electrocardiograph.

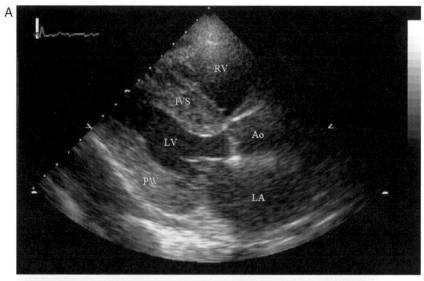

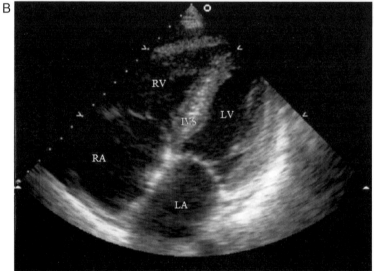

Fig. 28.4 A, Parasternal long-axis two-dimensional TTE. B, Apical four-chamber two-dimensional TTE. IVS, interventricular septum.

Questions

1. What does the pleural fluid analysis suggest? What are the possible causes of this?
2. Why is the CA 125 raised?
3. What abnormalities are present on the ECG in Fig. 28.1? What are the differences between the ECGs in Figs 28.1 and 28.3? What do these suggest?
4. What abnormalities does the echocardiogram (Fig. 28.4) show?
5. What is the differential diagnosis in view of the clinical features and echocardiogram results? What is the most likely diagnosis?
6. How would you investigate the patient?

Answers

1) **What does the pleural fluid analysis suggest? What are the possible causes of this?**

Exudates must meet one or more of the following criteria, whereas transudates meet none:

Pleural fluid/serum protein ratio >0.5 or absolute value > 3g/dL.

Pleural fluid/serum LDH ratio >0.6 or absolute value >0.45 upper normal serum limit

Pleural fluid specific gravity >1.018

In this case, the pleural fluid total protein was greater than 30 g/L, suggesting that the effusion was exudative. The causes of exudative pleural effusions are listed in Table 28.2.

Table 28.2 Aetiology of exudative effusions*

Parapneumonic
Simple
Complicated
Empyema
Tuberculosis
Other infections
Fungal
Parasitic
Malignant
Primary lung cancer
Metastatic disease
Mesothelioma
Pulmonary embolism
Collagen vascular disease
Rheumatoid arthritis
Systemic lupus erythematosus
Wegener's granulomatosis
Churg–Strauss syndrome
Familial Mediterranean fever
Abdominal disease
Pancreatitis
Subphrenic abscess
Oesophageal rupture

Table 28.2 (continued) Aetiology of exudative effusions*

Postoperative
Atelectasis
Acute respiratory distress syndrome
Amyloid
Asbestos exposure
Hemothorax
Chylothorax
Cholesterol effusions
Drug reactions
Dressler's syndrome
Meigs' syndrome
Uraemia
Sarcoidosis
Yellow nail syndrome
Radiation therapy
Ovarian hyperstimulation syndrome

2) **Why is the CA 125 raised?**

Although the abdominal CT scan revealed ascites and mesenteric lymphadenopathy, which suggested malignancy, cytological analysis of the ascites was negative. A pelvic ultrasound revealed only a cyst on the right ovary, which appeared benign. In view of the negative cytology and the absence of an adnexal mass, the raised CA 125 in this case was attributed to the congestive cardiac failure and ascites. The CA 125 fell (100 u/mL) after drainage of the ascites.

Malignant adnexal tumours are usually associated with levels of serum CA 125 > 38 u/mL and generally in the range 100–10000 u/mL. Although the level of serum CA 125 associated with benign disease is generally much lower (<38 u/mL), the ranges overlap. Ascites can significantly increase levels of CA 125. In a small series 10 patients with benign ascites were associated with CA 125 levels of 396 ± 287 u/mL (Xiao & Liu, 2003). The mechanism is unclear but peritoneal stretch may be important as CA 125 levels fall after paracentesis. Inappropriate measurement of serum CA 125 in women with congestive cardiac failure and ascites can lead to unnecessary investigations or even surgery.

3) **What abnormalities are present on the ECG in Fig. 28.1? What are the differences between the ECGs in Figs 28.1 and 28.3? What do these suggest?**

The initial ECG (Fig. 28.1) revealed AF with poor R-wave progression across the anterior leads. Importantly, there is no evidence of LVH as suggested by the report of the TTE. The ECG after the thoracoscopy (Fig. 28.3) revealed a regular junctional rhythm with no P waves, suggesting either AF or sinus node arrest. Ventricular voltages are further reduced.

4) **What abnormalities does the echocardiogram (Fig. 28.4) show?**

The echocardiogram demonstrates biatrial dilatation with marked thickening of both ventricles. Taken in conjunction with the ECG, these findings suggest the possibility of an infiltrative restrictive cardiomyopathy. The septum appears speckled, an echocardiographic feature suggestive of amyloid infiltration.

Restrictive cardiomyopathy is characterized by non-dilated ventricles with impaired ventricular filling (diastolic dysfunction). Although infiltrative and storage diseases may increase LV wall thickness, hypertrophy is typically absent. Systolic function usually remains normal, at least early in the disease. The elevated left atrial and pulmonary venous pressures and/or impaired stroke volume, which result from diastolic dysfunction, can cause dyspnoea and reduce exercise tolerance. In this case, these symptoms were exacerbated by tense ascites and marked peripheral oedema, and improved with paracentesis and cautious diuresis.

In contrast, dilated cardiomyopathy (see Cases 10 and 11) is characterized by ventricular dilatation and reduced contractility. This commonly causes systolic dysfunction but diastolic dysfunction may also occur.

In this case, the patient remained breathlessness despite drainage of the pleural effusions. There was no evidence of pulmonary oedema or cardiomegaly on the chest X-ray (Fig. 28.1). However, the venous pressure was elevated and there was severe peripheral oedema and ascites. The differential diagnosis for these clinical features includes restrictive cardiomyopathy, constrictive pericarditis (see Case 43), tricuspid regurgitation with an enlarged compliant right atrium, right heart failure (e.g. due to right ventricular infarction or pulmonary hypertension), or circulatory overload with systemic congestion. The discrepancies between the ECG (Figs 28.1 and 28.3; pseudoinfarction pattern and low-voltage QRS complexes) and the report of the first TTE (Table 28.1; preserved LV systolic function and LVH) raised the suspicion of an infiltrative process. Further evidence of an infiltrative process was obtained from the second TTE (Fig. 28.4).

5) **What is the differential diagnosis in view of the clinical features and echocardiogram results? What is the most likely diagnosis?**

The causes of infiltrative restrictive cardiomyopathy include amyloidosis (primary or secondary to a chronic inflammatory disease), sarcoidosis, hypereosinophilia (Loffeler syndrome), malignancy, and the storage diseases (e.g. glycogen storage disease, haemochromatosis, Gauchers disease, and Fabry disease). In the absence of specific features of any other disease, but normal full blood count (excluding eosinophilia) and absence of radiographic evidence of pulmonary sarcoidosis the most likely diagnosis is primary cardiac amyloidosis.

Primary amyloidosis is a monoclonal plasma cell dyscrasia, with an annual incidence of 8 per million. The diagnosis is frequently delayed because of its non-specific clinical presentation. Amyloidosis should be considered in patients with congestive heart failure in the absence of valvular disease, hypertension, or ischaemia.

The most common ECG abnormalities in patients with cardiac amyloidosis are low voltage and a pseudoinfarction pattern (Figs 28.2 and 28.3), occurring in approximately 50% of patients. The pseudoinfarction pattern can lead to the erroneous view that the patient sustained a silent infarction and subsequently developed ischemic cardiomyopathy. Other changes that can occur include conduction abnormalities (such as second- and third-degree atrioventricular block) and AF. Other ECG abnormalities include first-degree AV block in 21%, nonspecific intraventricular conduction delay in 16%, and second- or third-degree AV block in 3%. These ECG abnormalities are non-specific.

Arrhythmias are also common in patients with AL cardiac amyloidosis. In one study of 24 patients with amyloid light chain (AL) cardiac amyloidosis who had telemetry monitoring whilst receiving stem cell transplantation over 500 recorded episodes of arrhythmia were detected (Goldsmith et al., 2009). Of these episodes 36% were supraventricular and 64% were ventricular. The most common arrhythmias in order of decreasing frequency were non-sustained VT, sinus tachycardia, premature ventricular contractions/couplets, supraventricular tachycardia, AF, sinus bradycardia, and atrial ectopics. In this study three patients developed life-threatening arrhythmias (Goldsmith et al., 2009). These were fast AF with hypotension probably secondary to sepsis, asymptomatic sustained VT, and a bradycardia with a junctional escape rhythm at 40 bpm.

As demonstrated in this case echocardiography can also be deceptive in patients with cardiac amyloid. Myocardial thickening may be attributed to LVH rather than infiltration.

Pleural effusions are a rare complication of amyloidosis and the mechanism of effusion formation is poorly understood. Transudative pleural effusions may occur as a consequence of amyloid-induced cardiomyopathy or, more rarely, nephrotic syndrome. Cardiac failure that has been partially treated with diuretics may result in a transudative effusion being erroneously misclassified as an exudate. True exudative effusions may occur as a result of amyloid infiltration of the pleural tissue, which is likely in this case.

6) **How would you investigate the patient?**

The most important investigations are serum and urine protein electrophoresis and a biopsy to screen for amyloid deposition. Possible sites for a screening biopsy include the rectum, subcutaneous fat, and bone marrow. If a screening biopsy is negative, transvenous ventricular biopsy should be considered.

Serum amyloid P-component (SAP) is a normal plasma protein and a universal constituent of amyloid deposits. Radiolabelled SAP scintigraphy is a non-invasive method for detecting amyloid. It is diagnostic in most patients with systemic amyloidosis, but the intracardiac blood pool and heart movement prevent detection of cardiac amyloid. However, SAP scintigraphy can be used to demonstrate extracardiac amyloid infiltration.

In this case, serum electrophoresis showed polyclonal hypogammaglobulinaemia but urine protein electrophoresis revealed urinary-free monoclonal lambda light chains. A slight excess of plasma cells was noted on bone marrow aspirate and trephine. However, only 6% of B lymphocytes were lambda light-chain specific, and congo red staining was negative.

As there was no evidence of amyloid infiltration of the bone marrow, the screening biopsy was negative. A myocardial biopsy was then performed. This confirmed the presence of primary cardiac amyloidosis (Fig. 28.5). Immunostaining confirmed the presence of lambda light chains within the amyloid deposits and excluded secondary amyloid. Retrospective staining of the pleural biopsy also found amyloid infiltration.

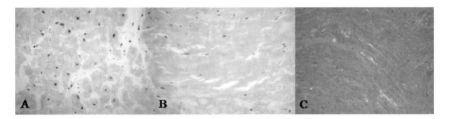

Fig. 28.5 Cardiac biopsy. A, Haematoxylin and eosin (H&E) stained section of normal cardiac muscle. B, H&E stained section of cardiac biopsy showing eosinophilic infiltrate. C, Congo red stained section of cardiac biopsy photographed under polarized light showing apple-green biorefringence. (See colour plate 9)

The diagnosis was primary (AL) lambda amyloidosis with pleural and cardiac involvement. Melphalan was started, but the response was poor and the patient was readmitted on several occasions for drainage of ascites. Unfortunately the patient died 14 months after presentation.

Primary amyloid deposits include immunoglobulin light chains or fragments. Thus, the screening tests of choice are serum and urine immunoelectrophoresis and immunofixation. These detect monoclonal light chains in about 90% of patients with primary amyloid. If a monoclonal protein is found, a biopsy is required to confirm amyloidosis.

Although amyloidosis is a multisystem disease, the prognosis is determined principally by cardiac involvement. Cardiac amyloid deposition causes four overlapping clinical presentations: restrictive cardiomyopathy, systolic heart failure, orthostatic hypotension, and conducting system disease.

Patients without cardiac or renal involvement have a median survival of 40 months. Patients with congestive heart failure have a median survival of 8 months. Echocardiography is helpful in determining the extent of cardiac involvement.

This case describes the classical presentation of primary amyloidosis. As there are no specific signs or symptoms, diagnosis can be difficult and often follows a protracted, fruitless search for malignancy. This case also highlights the importance of reviewing the result of each investigation in the context of what is already known from the history, examination, and previous investigations.

References

Goldsmith YB, Liu J, Chou J *et al.* (2009). Frequencies and types of arrhythmias in patients with systemic light-chain amyloidosis with cardiac involvement undergoing stem cell transplantation on telemetry monitoring. *Am J Cardiol*; **104**: 990–994.

Xiao W-B, Liu Y-L (2003). Elevation of serum and ascites cancer antigen 125 levels in patients with liver cirrhosis. *J Gastroenterol Hepatol*; **18**: 1315–1316.

Further reading

John L, Berk JL, Keane J, Seldin DC, Sanchorawala V, Koyama J, Dember LM, Falk RH (2003). Persistent pleural effusions in primary systemic amyloidosis: etiology and prognosis. *Chest*; 124: 969–977.

Gertz MA, Kyle RA (1989). Primary systemic amyloidosis—a diagnostic primer. *Mayo Clin Proc*; **64**: 1505–1509.

Kyle RA, Gertz MA (1995). Primary systemic amyloidosis: clinical and laboratory features in 474 cases. *Semin Hematol*; **32**: 45–59.

Murtagh B, Hammill SC, Gertz MA, Kyle RA, Tajik AJ, Grogan M (2005). Electrocardiographic findings in primary systemic amyloidosis and biopsy-proven cardiac involvement. *Am J Cardiol*; **95**: 535.

Goldsmith YB, Liu J, Chou J, Hoffman J, Comenzo RL, Steingart RM (2009). Frequencies and types of arrhythmias in patients with systemic light-chain amyloidosis with cardiac involvement undergoing stem cell transplantation on telemetry monitoring. *Am J Cardiol*; **104**: 990–994.

Xiao WB, Liu Y-L (2003). Elevation of serum and ascites cancer antigen 125 levels in patients with liver cirrhosis. *J Gastroenterol Hepatol*; **18**: 1315–1316.

Case 29

A 44-year-old school teacher with no previous medical history was training to climb Mount Kilimanjaro. She had recently increased the intensity of her exercise programme. Whilst running she felt 'funny' and so returned home. She visited a friend before going home, explained that she was 'not feeling right', collapsed, and lost consciousness at the front door. Her friend could not feel a pulse and so called for an ambulance and began cardiopulmonary resuscitation. The paramedics confirmed cardiac arrest and on connecting a monitor obtained the ECG rhythm strip in Fig. 29.1.

Resuscitation was successful. Cardiac output and spontaneous respiratory effort were restored. However, she remained unconscious (GCS 3), hypotensive (80/40 mmHg), and peripherally cyanosed with clinical signs of pulmonary oedema. She was intubated by the paramedics, ventilated, and brought to hospital. On arrival she was immediately admitted to the intensive therapy unit (ITU), where inotropes were started.

A 12 lead ECG was performed on admission to ITU (Fig. 29.2). The 12-hour cTnI was raised (3.7 ng/dL), but TTE was unremarkable. Systolic function was preserved, there were no regional wall motion abnormalities, and valve structure and function were normal. Right-ventricular systolic pressure was estimated to be 12 mmHg by Doppler. Within 24 hours of admission the patient was weaned off inotropic support and extubated, fully alert, and orientated.

The patient did not experience any symptoms during a Bruce protocol ETT (Fig. 29.3) performed 3 days after admission. This was stopped by the cardiac technician at 11 minutes. A myocardial perfusion scan and a coronary angiogram were subsequently performed (Figs. 29.4 and 29.5).

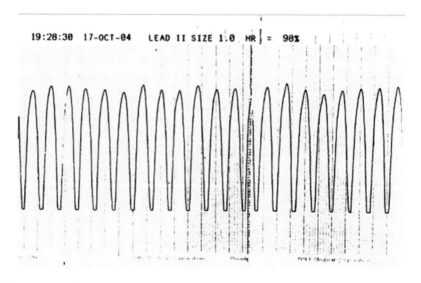

19:28:30 17-OCT-04   LEAD II SIZE 1.0 HR = 98%

Fig. 29.1 ECG rhythm strip performed at the scene of out-of-hospital cardiac arrest.

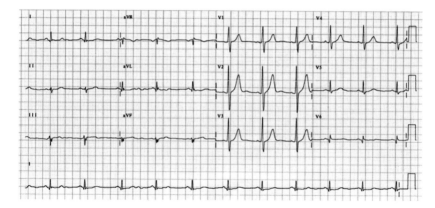

Fig. 29.2 12 lead ECG on admission to the ITU.

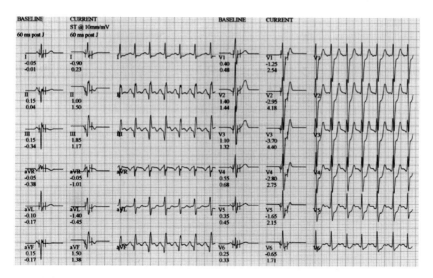

Fig. 29.3 12 lead ECG at 11 minutes of Bruce protocol ETT. The patient had no symptoms.

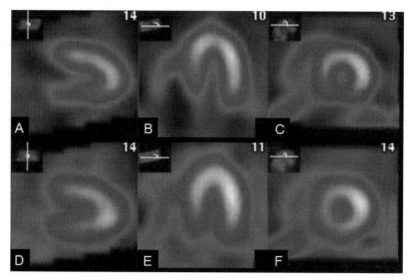

Fig. 29.4 Myocardial perfusion scan. (See colour plate 10)

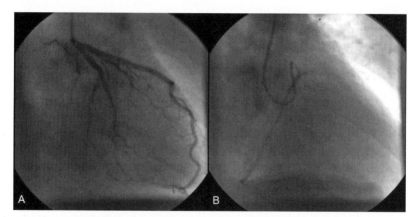

Fig. 29.5 Coronary angiogram RAO view showing the left (A) and right (B) coronary arteries.

Questions

1. What does the rhythm strip (Fig. 29.1) show? What is the appropriate management?
2. Report the 12 lead ECG performed on admission to ITU (Fig. 29.2).
3. Why was the ETT stopped?
4. Report the myocardial perfusion scan (Fig. 29.4).
5. What is the most likely cause for her aborted sudden cardiac death?
6. What investigation, if any, is required?
7. What do the coronary angiogram images (Fig. 29.5) show?
8. What are the management options?

Answers

1) **What does the rhythm strip (Fig 29.1) show? What is the appropriate management?**

   The ECG rhythm strip (lead II) demonstrates a regular broad complex tachycardia. There is no cardiac output. This is pulseless VT. Cardiopulmonary resuscitation should be initiated and defibrillation performed as soon as possible. CPR should resume immediately after a single shock. CPR should continue for at least 1 minute before the patient is reassessed for signs of life. In this case, sinus rhythm was restored after a single shock and the patient regained a cardiac output.

2) **Report the 12 lead ECG performed on admission to ITU (Fig. 29.2).**

   The ECG in Fig. 29.2 shows sinus rhythm at a rate of 70 bpm. The QRS axis is within normal limits. The R wave in V1 is dominant. A Q wave and a biphasic T wave are seen in V6. See Case 4 for a discussion of the causes of a dominant R wave in V1.

3) **Why was the ETT stopped?**

   Fig. 29.3 shows an ECG taken at 11 minutes of a Bruce protocol ETT and demonstrates ST depression in V1–V6 (>2 mm V1–V4). Although the patient did not experience symptoms, the ETT was clearly positive and was therefore stopped.

4) **Report the myocardial perfusion scan (Fig. 29.4).**

   The selected images from the myocardial perfusion scan in Fig. 29.4 show a moderate-to-large perfusion defect in the inferior and inferoseptal walls (A–C) in the distribution of the RCA (Fig. 29.6). The defect is completely reversible (D–F), indicating inferior inducible ischaemia and myocardial viability.

5) **What is the most likely cause for her aborted sudden cardiac death?**

   Sudden cardiac death results from either VF or hypotensive sustained VT. The incidence is estimated to be 1/1000/year. The most common cause, by far, is atheromatous coronary artery disease (75–80%). Idiopathic DCM is the second most common cause (10–15%). Other causes (Table 29.1) are much less common.

   In this case, the ETT and myocardial perfusion scan demonstrated inducible myocardial ischaemia. The small troponin rise probably reflects indirect myocardial damage from either hypoperfusion or defibrillation. The echocardiogram excluded cardiomyopathy and valvular heart disease. In this case, the most likely cause of aborted sudden cardiac death is coronary atherosclerosis.

6) **What investigation, if any, is required?**

   As a coronary arterial atherosclerosis is likely, a coronary angiogram is required to guide further management.

7) **What do the coronary angiogram images (Fig. 29.5) show?**

   The RAO image shown in Fig. 29.5A reveals a normal left coronary artery (Fig. 29.7A). A wisp of contrast seen in the left coronary artery during the angiogram of the RCA shown in the left-anterior-oblique (LAO) image in Fig. 29.7B, demonstrates that both the left and the right coronary arteries arise from the left coronary cusp. The distal RCA is under filled. The proximal segment of the RCA winds anteriorly between the pulmonary trunk and ascending aorta (Fig. 29.7B). The ostium of the RCA is narrowed and slit like (ostial stenosis; Fig. 29.7B). The stenosis is smooth and confined to the segment of the artery that runs between the pulmonary trunk and aorta. This stenosis could be due to atheroma; however, intravascular ultrasound (IVUS) demonstrated that the stenosis was anatomical as no plaque was seen.

Anomalous coronary artery anatomy has a reported incidence of 0.3% based on necropsy studies, and 1% in coronary angiography based studies. It is generally associated with normal myocardial development and function. Most anomalies, such as the circumflex artery arising from the R coronary ostium, do not affect daily activity. However, anomalies such as the left or right coronary artery arising from the opposite aortic sinus and coursing between the great vessels with a slit-like origin can lead to compressive vessel occlusion during exercise, when the great vessels expand. Presentation on vigorous exertion is common and sudden death in young athletes recognized. Other presentations include symptoms of volume over-loading (coronary fistulas) or ischaemia (probably due to spasm and anatomical narrowing), such as chest pain, syncope, dyspnoea, arrhythmias, and MI.

The most common anomaly is a split RCA (approximate 20%), where the poste-rior descending branch of the RCA is duplicated. An ectopic circumflex artery arising from the right aortic sinus accounts for a further 20% of anomalies, where-as an ectopic RCA from the left aortic sinus (as in the present case) is less prevalent (≅15%). Coronary artery fistulas account for around 10% of anomalies.

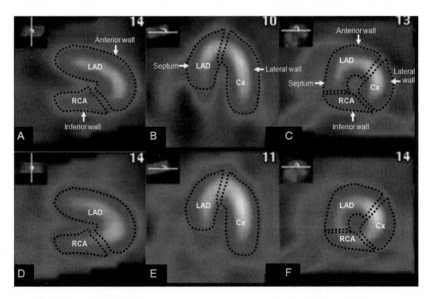

Fig. 29.6 Myocardial perfusion scan demonstrating reversible perfusion defect in the distribution of the RCA. These images from the myocardial perfusion scan show a moderate-to-large perfusion defect in the inferior and inferoseptal walls (A–C) in the distribution of the RCA. The defect is completely reversible (D–F), indicating inferior inducible ischaemia and myocardial viability. (See colour plate 11)

Table 29.1 Causes of sudden cardiac death

Cause		Frequency
1. Coronary artery disease		>90%
2. Dilated cardiomyopathy		
3. Other cardiomyopathies	a. Hypertrophic cardiomyopathy	
	b. Arrhythmogenic right ventricular cardiomyopathy	
4. Primary electrical disorders	a. Long QT syndrome	
	b. Brugada's syndrome	
	c. Catecholaminergic polymorphic VT	
	d. WPW syndrome	<10%
	e. Sinus or AV node disease	
5. Mechanical disease	a. Aortic stenosis	
	b. Anomolous origin of coronary arteries	
6. Myocarditis		
7. Chest trauma		
8. Drug-induced polymorphic VT		

Origin of left coronary artery from the right aortic sinus accounts for only 2% of anomalies, but is associated with sudden death in around half of cases, with 80% of the events occurring in association with exercise. Some anomalies are syndromic, notably a left coronary artery originating from the pulmonary artery (Bland–White–Garland syndrome or the anomalous left coronary artery arising from the pulmonary artery (ALCAPA) syndrome), which has an 80% mortality at 4 months of age, with survival being determined mainly by the extent of septal collaterals from the RCA. In adulthood, this syndrome is characterized by angina, congestive heart failure, mitral regurgitation, and sudden death.

8) **What are the management options?**

Documented sustained syncopal VT is a significant risk factor for sudden cardiac death, and any precipitating factors should be eliminated. In this case the RCA ostium was successfully stented, improving RCA flow significantly. Beta-blockers were started and an ICD was implanted. She remained well without recurrence of syncope or VT at 2 years.

Several RCTs have confirmed the role of ICD implantation in secondary prevention after aborted arrhythmic sudden cardiac death.

The antiarrhythmics versus implantable defibrillators (AVID) trial ($n = 1016$) demonstrated a mortality benefit (relative risk reduction 30%) with ICD therapy compared to medical treatment (amiodarone) in symptomatic VT and VF with LV impairment (EF <40%, mean 32%) mainly in the context of ischaemic heart disease. There was a trend towards benefit if EF was >35% and the Canadian implantable defibrillator study (CIDS) trial ($n = 659$) hoped to confirm this in a

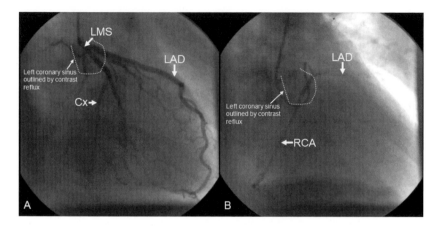

Fig. 29.7 Coronary angiogram demonstrating an ostial stenosis in anomalous RCA.

similar cohort (mean EF 34%). However, although total death rate was reduced this was not statistically significant. The cardiac arrest study hamburg (CASH) trial (*n* = 346) randomized to medical treatment (propafenone, amiodarone, metoprolol) or ICD with a 37% relative survival benefit in those receiving an ICD. The mortality benefit (mean 4.4 months) was from a reduction in death due to arrhythmia. The mortality benefit was confirmed in a meta-analysis of all available trial data. The greatest benefit seen in patients with ejection fraction was <35% and NYHA class III or IV heart failure. There was also a mortality benefit in the small cohort with idiopathic DCM (20–40%). See Case 10 for discussion of the role of ICD in primary prevention.

Primary and secondary prevention strategies also include specific antiarrhythmic and non-antiarrhythmic medical therapy. For example, use of ACE inhibitors in heart failure or after myocardial infarction reduces rates of sudden death significantly. Aldosterone receptor blockers reduce the relative risk of sudden death (30%; randomised adactone evaluation study (RALES) trial). Beta-blockers also reduce risk of sudden death and are used for primary and secondary prevention.

Although predominantly a class III agent (potassium channel blocker), amiodarone has antiarrhythmic properties characteristic of all Vaughan Williams classes. Amiodarone inhibits fast sodium channels (class I), adrenoceptors (α and β; class II), and L-type calcium channels (class IV). Although amiodarone reduces arrhythmia burden it has no mortality benefit sudden cardiac death in heart failure trial (SCD-HeFT) and should not be used as primary prevention.

Further reading

Zipes DP, Camm AJ, Borggrefe M, Buxton AE, Chaitman B, Fromer M, Gregoratos G, Klein G, Moss AJ, Myerburg RJ, Priori SG, Quinones MA, Roden DM, Silka MJ, Tracy C, Priori SG, Blanc JJ, Budaj A, Camm AJ, Dean V, Deckers JW, Despres C, Dickstein K, Lekakis J, McGregor K, Metra M, Morais J, Osterspey A, Tamargo JL, Zamorano JL, Smith SC Jr, Jacobs AK, Adams CD, Antman EM, Anderson JL, Hunt SA, Halperin JL, Nishimura R, Ornato JP, Page RL, Riegel B; American College of Cardiology; American Heart Association Task Force; European Society of Cardiology Committee for Practice Guidelines; European Heart Rhythm Association; Heart Rhythm Society. (2006). ACC/AHA/ESC 2006 guidelines for management of patients with ventricular arrhythmias and the prevention of sudden cardiac death: a report of the American College of Cardiology/American Heart Association Task Force and the European Society of Cardiology Committee for Practice Guidelines (Writing Committee to Develop guidelines for management of patients with ventricular arrhythmias and the prevention of sudden cardiac death) developed in collaboration with the European Heart Rhythm Association and the Heart Rhythm Society. *Europace*; **8**: 746–837.

Angelini P, Velasco JA, Flamm S. (2002). Coronary anomalies: incidence, pathophysiology, and clinical relevance. *Circulation*; **105**: 2449–2454.

Case 30

The wife of a 78-year-old man had noticed that he would occasionally wake from sleep, sit up, gesture whilst mumbling a few confused words, collapse back then 'return to sleep'. The frequency of the episodes was increasing and for the past week had occurred almost every night. On each occasion he was pale, cold, and unresponsive for several minutes after returning to sleep. On waking he would be distressed by short periods of retrograde amnesia lasting up to 4 hours from before he went to bed. He was otherwise completely unaware of these episodes. Neurological and cardiovascular examinations were normal in the clinic.

Questions

1. Is the syncope due to a cardiac cause or a neurological cause?
2. What investigations are required?
3. What is seen on the combined ECG and electroencephalography (EEG) (Fig. 30.1)?
4. What is the diagnosis?
5. How should the patient be managed?
6. What advice should be given regarding driving?

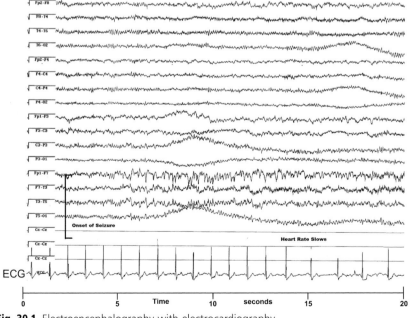

Fig. 30.1 Electroencephalography with electrocardiography.

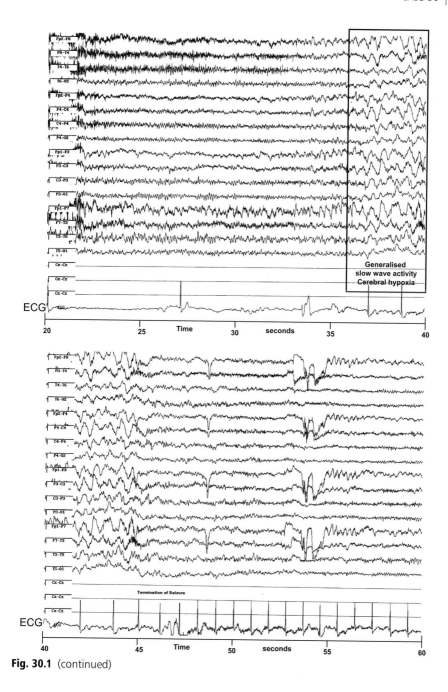

Fig. 30.1 (continued)

Answers

1) **Is the syncope due to a cardiac cause or a neurological cause?**

   The differential is broad. Pallor and cold peripheries suggest a cardiac cause of syncope. However, the preceding confusion, unusual and stereotyped behaviour, and retrograde amnesia suggest a neurological cause.

2) **What investigations are required?**

   In this case ECG, carotid sinus massage, echocardiography, and 24-hour Holter monitoring were unremarkable. Computed tomography and MRI of the brain showed only atrophic changes consistent with age. Overnight combined EEG and ECG monitoring (Fig. 30.1) was requested on review by a neurologist.

3) **What is seen on the combined ECG and EEG (Fig. 30.1)?**

   The EEG revealed a left temporal lobe focus. Contemporary ECG monitoring revealed that the seizure was followed 10 seconds after onset by bradycardia and episodes of asystole lasting up to 10 seconds, which abruptly ended with termination of the seizure (Fig. 30.1).

4) **What is the diagnosis?**

   The diagnosis is ictal bradycardia (seizure induced bradycardia).

   Seizures can affect any aspect of automonic function in the peri-ictal (pre-ictal, ictal, or post ictal) periods. Although palpitations, sinus tachycardia, and hypertension commonly occur as a result of sympathetic activation by seizure activity, fits rarely provoke clinically significant arrhythmias. Peri-ictal bradyarrythmias are particularly uncommon, occurring in 3.3% of focal seizures in one study. However, this is probably an underestimate and the incidence may be increased in those with pre-existing cardiac disease.

   ECG abnormalities may occur during 35% of generalized seizures. Although most are benign, potentially significant ECG changes (ST-segment or T-wave abnormalities) occur during up to 13% of seizures. Seizures may be prolonged in those patients with such changes in comparison to those without ECG abnormalities. In all, 40% of patients with refractory epilepsy have peri-ictal cardiac rhythm or repolarization abnormalities.

   Peri-ictal bradycardia and asystole may be life threatening and contribute to the syndrome of sudden unexplained death in epileptic patients. Ictal bradycardia should be excluded in patients with a history suggestive of both cardiac syncope and epileptic seizures. Differentiation between cerebral and cardiac bradyarrhythmia is only possible with simultaneous EEG and ECG recording. Identification of ictal bradycardia and asystole is vital as management requires both anti-epileptic therapy and cardiac pacemaker implantation.

5) **How should the patient be managed?**

   Treatment includes control of seizures and management of bradyarrythmias. In this case, sodium valproate was started and a permanent dual-chamber cardiac pacemaker was sited.

In this case, the frequency of the nocturnal seizures was significantly reduced by antiepileptic treatment but still occurred approximately once every 6 months. However, when the seizures recurred the pacemaker would maintain the heart rate. The seizures did not cause facial pallor but the duration of the seizures was prolonged up to 5 minutes and the patient still remained unresponsive for several minutes after termination of the seizure.

6) **What advice should be given regarding driving?**

Epileptic seizures are the most common medical cause of loss of consciousness whilst driving. The DVLA guidance for group 1 vehicles (cars and motorcycles) prohibits people who have had an epileptic seizure whether awake or asleep from driving for at least 1 year. In this case, although the patient has only had seizures whilst asleep he is still prohibited from driving for at least 1 year. However, if he continues to have seizures whilst asleep he may regain his licence 3 years after his first seizure so long as he does not have any seizures whilst awake. He must also comply with advised treatment and follow-up for epilepsy. In contrast, a person who has an epileptic seizure whilst awake can not regain their license if they continue to have seizures whilst awake. They may regain their driving license once free of seizures for 5 years.

This must be clearly explained to the patient and documented in the medical notes and correspondence with the patient's GP. However, it is the responsibility of the patient to inform the DVLA.

Although superseded by the DVLA guidance for epilepsy in this case, patients who experience arrhythmias are barred from driving if the arrhythmia has caused or is likely to cause incapacity. However, driving may be resumed 4 weeks after the cause has been identified and controlled. Patients who undergo pacemaker implantation or box change should not drive for 1 week after the procedure.

Further reading

Keilson MJ, Hauser A, Magrill JP, Goldman M (1987). ECG abnormalities in patients with epilepsy. *Neurology*; **37**:1624–1626.

Blumhardt LD, Smith PEM, Lynne O (1986). Electrocardiographic accompaniments of temporal lobe epileptic seizures. *Lancet*; **ii**: 1051–1055.

Reeves AL, Nollet KE, Klass DW, Sharbrough FW, So. EI *et al.* (1996). The ictal bradycardia syndrome. *Epilepsia*; **37**: 983–987.

Schernthaner C, Lindinger G, Poetzelberger K, Zeiler K, Baumgartner C (1999). Autonomic epilepsy: the influence of epileptic discharges on heart rate and rhythm. *Wien Klin Wochenschr*; **111**: 392–401.

Devinsky O (2004). Effects of seizures on autonomic and cardiovascular function. *Epilepsy Currents*; **4**: 43–46.

Jay G, Leetsma J (1981). Sudden death in epilepsy: a comprehensive review of the literature and proposed mechanisms. *Acta Neurol Scand*; **63**(suppl 82): 1–66.

Drivers Medical Group, DVLA (2010). Neurological disorders. In 'At a Glance Guide to the Current Medical Standards of Fitness to Drive' – A Guide for Medical Practitioners. http://www.dvla.gov.uk/medical/ataglance.aspx, pp 6–18.

Case 31

A 75-year-old retired policeman consulted his GP after his wife noticed him to be breathless on exertion. His symptoms had started after a severe respiratory infection 3 months previously. He had been a heavy smoker but had stopped 15 years ago. He had a history of hypertension and raised cholesterol, but was not diabetic.

He admitted to one previous episode of breathlessness on exertion, which occurred when walking in the hot weather whilst on holiday in Spain 3 years earlier. On that occasion he also felt faint and needed to sit down, but denied any loss of conciousness. He had been seen by the hotel doctor, who diagnosed dehydration and heat stroke. The patient was advised to seek medical attention when he got home if his symptoms persisted, but as he felt significantly better when he returned home he did not do so.

In the surgery, physical examination revealed a BP of 120/80 mmHg, regular pulse of 72 bpm, temperature of 36.7°C, and O_2 saturations of 99% on breathing air. The JVP was not raised and the apex beat was not displaced. The first heart sound was normal, but the second was quiet. A loud systolic murmur was heard by his GP across the precordium, which radiated to the carotids. There were no stigmata of endocarditis and no signs of cardiac failure.

He was urgently referred to the cardiology clinic where a 12 lead ECG (Fig. 31.1) and a TTE (Fig. 31.2) were performed.

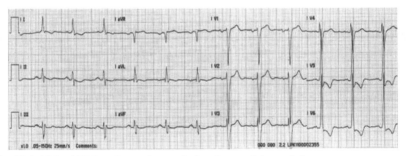

Fig. 31.1 12 lead ECG performed on arrival at the cardiology clinic.

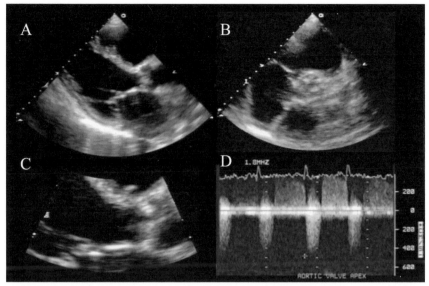

Fig. 31.2 Selected images from the echocardiogram performed in the cardiology clinic. A, Parasternal long-axis view. B, Zoomed parasternal short-axis view. C, Basal parasternal long-axis view. D, Continuous wave Doppler trace through aortic valve.

Questions

1. Report the ECG in Fig. 31.1.
2. Report the TTE images in Fig. 31.2. What is the diagnosis?
3. What is the likely aetiology?
4. Why did the symptoms develop in Spain?
5. Could the process have been slowed or prevented?
6. What is the prognosis?
7. How should this condition be managed?

Answers

1) **Report the ECG in Fig. 31.1.**

The ECG in Fig. 31.1 shows sinus rhythm at a rate of 72 bpm with a leftward QRS axis. There is evidence of LVH by voltage criteria (depth of S wave in V1 or 2 + height of R wave in V5 or V6 > 35 mm) and the repolarization abnormalities are consistent with a 'strain' pattern. Atrioventricular conduction is maintained.

2) **Report the TTE images in Fig. 31.2. What is the diagnosis?**

The parasternal long axis (Figs. 31.2A and 31.2C) and parasternal short axis view at the level of the aortic valve (AV; Fig. 31.2B) demonstrate a heavily calcified AV (Fig. 31.3B). The continuous wave Doppler measured a peak velocity >4.5 m/s (Fig. 31.3D). The modified Bernoulli equation ($\Delta P = 4 \times \Delta V^2$) suggests an instantaneous peak pressure gradient >90 mmHg across the AV. Aortic regurgitation is present on the Doppler signal, but the shape of the velocity envelope suggests this is only mild.

The valve area was calculated as 0.7 cm^2 using the continuity equation (Equation 1). This allows the calculation of the area of AV orifice using simple ratios and assumes that the flow into the valve has to equal the flow across the stenosed valve, i.e.:

Equation 1 The continuity equation

$$\text{If flow (F)} = \text{velocity (V)} \times \text{orifice area (A)}$$
$$\text{then } F_{LVOT} = F_{across\ AV}$$
$$\text{and so } A_{AV} = (V_{LVOT} \times A_{LVOT})/V_{AV}$$

The normal AV area is 2–4 cm^2. There is resistance to blood flow through the valve when the valve area is <1.5 cm^2. Severe aortic stenosis (AS) is associated with areas <1 cm^2 [0.6 cm^2/m^2 body surface area (BSA)]. Estimations of AV area make some allowance for changes in forward flow as a result of LV dysfunction but with severe impairment may underestimate severity. LV function can potentially be improved with a low-dose dobutamine infusion. The valve area calculated under these conditions will approximate more closely to the actual valve area.

The primary diagnosis is therefore calcific AS. Aortic stenosis is usually suspected on auscultation of a crescendo-decrescendo systolic ejection murmur radiating to the neck. In mild disease the thickened valve causes no appreciable obstruction to LV outflow; hence the murmur peaks early in systole and the second heart sound and carotid upstrokes are normal. Although this level of valve abnormality, sometimes referred to as aortic sclerosis, is benign, its pathophysiology is similar to that of atherosclerosis. Hence it is associated with coronary disease. As the stenosis progresses, the murmur becomes louder, peaks progressively later in systole, and may be associated with a thrill. With more severe stenosis, the murmur intensity decreases as stroke volume reduces. Carotid upstrokes are reduced in volume and the rate of rise is slowed. Conversely, the LV apical impulse increases, reflecting the obstruction between the ventricle and the aorta.

Although AS often presents with an incidental systolic murmur, the most common symptoms are exertional dyspnoea, fatigue, and angina. Altered consciousness during effort reflects either arrhythmias or cerebral hypoperfusion when systemic vascular resistance falls in the context of a fixed cardiac output. Angina is an unreliable predictor of CAD, which is present in 25% of patients without angina and absent in 40–80% of those with angina. Sub-endocardial ischaemia can occur in AS because of reduced diastolic perfusion time and increased LV diastolic pressures. Ventricular hypertrophy occurs in around 80% with severe AS and this is reflected in an abnormal ECG. Other ECG abnormalities that commonly occur in patients with AS include left atrial enlargement, left-axis deviation, and LBBB. The presence of atrioventricular block reflects encroachment of calcium from the valve annulus into the conduction system; atrial fibrillation reflects the higher filling pressures.

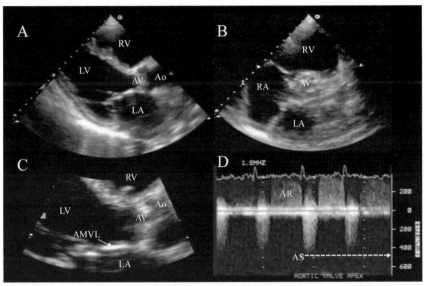

Fig. 31.3 Transthoracic echocardiogram demonstrating severe AS. A, Parasternal long-axis view showing a calcified AV. B, Zoomed parasternal short-axis view showing calcified AV. C, Basal parasternal long-axis view showing calcified AV. D, Continuous wave Doppler trace showing severe AS with a peak velocity >4.5 m/s through the valve and mild aortic regurgitation. Ao, aorta; AMVL, anterior mitral valve leaflet; AR, aortic regurgitation.

3) **What is the likely aetiology?**

Up to 10% of the population over the age of 85 years has significant calcific AS. Most cases (80%) of AS in an adult are due to degeneration of tri-leaflet valves through mechanisms similar to those involved in atherosclerosis (see answer to question 5 below). Calcification initially develops at the base of the cusps but progresses towards the edges without commissural fusion. Rheumatic AS was previously the most common cause in the West and remains a major public health problem in developing countries (5.7 per 1000). Rheumatic fever causes commissural fusion and fibrosis, with retraction and stiffening of the cusps.

Congenital bicuspid valves are of unequal size and progressively thicken and calcify, requiring replacement by the age of 60–70 years in about a third of cases. Other rarer associations with aortic stenosis are shown in Table 31.1.

The appearance of symptoms differs between these various aetiologies, with rheumatic AS becoming symptomatic earlier in adulthood, bicuspid AS in middle or late middle age, and degenerative disease presenting with symptoms in later life. When the valve is heavily calcified and deformed the aetiology is often uncertain. In view of the age at presentation degenerative AS is the most likely cause in this case.

Table 31.1 Rare causes of aortic stenosis

Familial hypercholesterolaemia
Hyperuricaemia
Hyperparathyroidism
Paget disease
Ochronosis
Fabry disease
Systemic lupus erythematosus

4) **Why did the symptoms develop in Spain?**

Aortic stenosis results in a fixed cardiac output that is dependent on preload, heart rate, and systemic vascular resistance. Vasodilatation reduces peripheral vascular resistance, which impairs venous return, increases the pressure gradient across the AV, and reduces coronary perfusion. Tachycardia reduces the time available for diastole, which impairs LV filling and coronary artery perfusion. Hypovolaemia, tachycardia, and vasodilatation result in severe hypotension, myocardial ischaemia, and a downward spiral of reduced contractility, causing further falls in blood pressure and coronary perfusion. Whilst in Spain the patient became dehydrated and increased his level of activity. He developed symptoms when his fixed cardiac output was not able to cope with the increased demand for oxygen delivery.

5) **Could the process have been slowed or prevented?**

The pathophysiology of degenerative AS was thought to be 'wear and tear' as a result of ageing. However, recently an active inflammatory process similar to atherosclerosis has been suggested. Epidemiological studies have demonstrated similar risk factors for coronary disease and degenerative AS. Histological studies show the presence of lipid particles and inflammatory infiltrates in the valves. Theoretically, risk factor modification in the early stages of the degenerative process could slow progression. Whether prevention would be possible if individuals at risk of degenerative AS could be identified is unclear. However, it is unlikely that risk factor modification would be beneficial after valve destruction and calcification have occurred. Current published trial data on slowing of AV disease progression by statin therapy are controversial.

6) **What is the prognosis?**

The prognosis from AS depends on the consequences of valve narrowing. On average, valve area decreases in a linear fashion by approximately 0.1 cm^2 per year. This increases the pressure gradient by 7 mmHg per year and the peak aortic jet velocity 0.25 m/s per year. However, there is considerable individual variability in the occurrence of symptoms.

Faster progression is associated with advanced age, smoking, and the presence of coronary disease, hypertension, or dyslipidaemia. The peak aortic jet velocity, the documentation of a rapid increase in peak velocity, and moderate-to-severe valve calcification also carry a less good prognosis.

The gradual pressure overload on the LV triggers reactive concentric hypertrophy. The rate of hypertrophy varies between individuals, but when present increases myocardial oxygen demand. Extracellular changes increase total collagen volume alongside the increased muscle mass, contributing to a stiffening of the ventricle and delaying relaxation of the myocardium (diastolic dysfunction). Eventually, systolic dysfunction develops, with further progression of the valve stenosis. This results in a decline in cardiac output, a paradoxical fall in the transvalvular gradient, and a progressive rise in ventricular end diastolic pressures.

Prognosis depends on the patient's position on this continuum. The presence of symptoms of AS is associated with a 50% increase in risk of major adverse cardiovascular events and 5-year survival rates of 15–50%. Asymptomatic patients have a better prognosis (incidence of sudden death being <1% per annum) if there is no evidence of LV strain on the ECG. An abnormal exercise capacity is a strong predictor of poor outcome. A positive stress test, in those who are fit and mobile enough to perform one, predicts an event-free survival at 2 years of only 19% compared to 85% event-free survival if exercise capacity is normal. In addition, exercise-induced hypotension or inadequate rises in blood pressure are both predictors of poorer outcomes.

7) **How should this condition be managed?**

Surgical aortic valve replacement is the definitive treatment for severe AS. The operative mortality is 2–5% in patients under 70 years and 3–15% in older patients, depending on comorbidities such as CAD. Factors that increase operative mortality are shown in Table 31.2. The need for concomitant bypass surgery approximately doubles the operative mortality. However, the long-term survival rates are excellent, with marked improvement in symptoms and quality of life. Indeed, several studies suggest that prognosis with successful surgery is close to that of age-matched controls.

The timing of AV surgery is critical to minimize risk and maximize benefit. Current recommendations are to operate soon after symptom onset in patients with severe AS. Surgery can be offered to asymptomatic patients with severe AS if the response to exercise is abnormal, peak aortic jet velocity is >4 m/s, the rate of progression of peak aortic velocity is >0.3 m/s per year, AV calcification is severe, LV systolic dysfunction (EF <50%) is present, or there is severe LV hypertrophy (>15-mm wall thickness) or significant ventricular arrhythmias.

Table 31.2 Factors that increase the operative mortality risk for aortic valve surgery

Older age
Associated comorbidities
Female gender
Higher functional class
Emergency operation
LV dysfunction
Pulmonary hypertension
Coexisting coronary disease
Previous bypass or valve surgery

Patients not fulfilling these criteria require regular surveillance. Patients with moderate-to-severe calcification and peak jet velocity ≥4 m/s require reassessment every 6 months to detect symptoms or changes in exercise tolerance/echo parameters. Annual clinical and echocardiographic follow-up is sufficient for patients who do not meet these criteria. However, follow-up of patients with borderline values should be more frequent.

Percutaneous retrograde arterial or transapical AV replacement is increasingly available but currently lacks systematic assessment of long-term durability or prognostic improvement. Currently, this procedure is advocated to palliate the symptoms of those patients felt unsuitable for cardiac surgery.

Further reading

Yetkin E, Waltenberger J. (2009). Molecular and cellular mechanisms of aortic stenosis. *Int J Cardiol*; **135**: 4–13.

Carabello BA, Paulus WJ. (2009). Aortic stenosis. *Lancet*; **373**: 956–966.

Rafique AM, Biner S, Ray I, Forrester JS, Tolstrup K, Siegel RJ. (2009). Meta-analysis of prognostic value of stress testing in patients with asymptomatic severe aortic stenosis. *Am J Cardiol*; **104**: 972–977.

Bonow RO, Carabello BA, Chatterjee K, de Leon AC Jr, Faxon DP, Freed MD, Gaasch WH, Lytle BW, Nishimura RA, O'Gara PT, O'Rourke RA, Otto CM, Shah PM, Shanewise JS; American College of Cardiology/American Heart Association Task Force on Practice Guidelines (2008). 2008 focused update incorporated into the ACC/AHA 2006 guidelines for the management of patients with valvular heart disease: a report of the American College of Cardiology/American Heart Association Task Force on Practice Guidelines (Writing Committee to revise the 1998 guidelines for the management of patients with valvular heart disease). Endorsed by the Society of Cardiovascular Anesthesiologists, Society for Cardiovascular Angiography and Interventions, and Society of Thoracic Surgeons. *Circulation*; **118**: e523–661.

Vahanian A, Baumgartner H, Bax J, Butchart E, Dion R, Filippatos G, Flachskampf F, Hall R, Iung B, Kasprzak J, Nataf P, Tornos P, Torracca L, Wenink A; Task Force on the Management of Valvular Hearth Disease of the European Society of Cardiology; ESC Committee for Practice Guidelines. (2007). Guidelines on the management of valvular heart disease: The Task Force on the Management of Valvular Heart Disease of the European Society of Cardiology. *Eur Heart J*: **28**; 230–268.

Case 32

A 30-year-old primigravida Gudjurati woman presented with increasing shortness of breath and swollen ankles. She was 14 weeks pregnant and spoke little English but denied previous medical or obstetric history. Examination revealed sinus rhythm, a loud first heart sound, an opening snap, and a mid diastolic murmur. Echocardiography confirmed moderate mitral valve (MV) stenosis (MS; valve area 1.2 cm^2). She was started on frusemide, anticoagulated, and discharged home with cardiology outpatient follow-up.

She did not attend follow up and 4 months later she presented to the ED, 26 weeks pregnant, in acute left ventricular failure and AF with a fast ventricular response.

Questions

1. What cardiovascular changes occur during pregnancy?
2. What is the differential diagnosis for causes of MS and which is most likely in this case?
3. Why did the patient develop symptoms when only 14 weeks pregnant?
4. What is the likely cause of the acute deterioration at 26 weeks?
5. How would you manage the MS?
6. The patient wishes to give birth at her local midwife-led unit. What do you recommend?
7. How would you anticoagulate the patient?
8. The patient's dentist writes to you requesting guidance on antibiotic prophylaxis against endocarditis. How would you respond?

Answers

1) **What cardiovascular changes occur during pregnancy and why?**

Blood volume and cardiac output

The most significant cardiovascular change is the increase in blood volume, which almost doubles by the end of pregnancy. Blood volume increases from the sixth week, rising rapidly in the second trimester but stabilizes in the last 8 weeks. Red cell mass increases later and by a smaller amount. This results in haemodilution and the physiological 'anaemia' of pregnancy. These changes are more marked in twin or multiple pregnancies. In the last trimester, arterial vasodilatation causes a relative reduction in intravascular volume. This induces sodium and water retention via the renin–angiotensin–aldosterone axis. Total body water increases by 6–8 L during pregnancy.

CO increases by about 40% as a result of increases in stroke volume and HR. Most of this change occurs early in pregnancy and peaks at 20–24 weeks. In late pregnancy, the increase in venous return is affected by posture: when the mother is supine, a sharp drop in preload due to uterine compression of the IVC may cause hypotension, with weakness and light headedness or syncope and secondary foetal distress. This resolves rapidly if the patient is turned into a lateral position.

Heart rate

Heart rate increases in the first weeks of pregnancy and peaks by the first-half of the third trimester. The average increase in resting HR is 10–20 bpm. Atrial tachyarrhythmias can occur even in women with normal hearts due to increases in plasma catecholamines and/or adrenoreceptor sensitivity, as well as the stretching of the atria by increased heart volumes.

Vascular tone

Maternal systemic systemic vascular resistance (SVR) and pulmonary vascular resistance fall as a result of the low-resistance uteroplacental circulation and direct effects of pregnancy-associated hormonal changes. Venous return increases and LV end-diastolic volume rises. The LV end-diastolic pressure does not rise because structural changes increase ventricular compliance. In the first two trimesters, the fall in SVR, which exceeds the increase in CO, leads to a drop in both systolic and, especially, diastolic BP, widening the pulse pressure.

The aim of the haemodynamic changes induced by pregnancy is to provide the developing foetus with an adequate supply of nutrients and remove its waste products. However, these changes can induce heart failure.

2) **What is the differential diagnosis for causes of mitral stenosis and which is most likely in this case?**

Mitral stenosis, nearly always rheumatic, is one of the most common (90%) and important cardiac valvular problems during pregnancy. Rare causes of mitral stenosis include: congenital mitral stenosis, radiotherapy to the chest, non rheumatic mitral annular calcification, systemic lupus erythematosus rheumatoid arthritis, carcinoid and methysergide therapy. Worldwide, rheumatic heart disease is still responsible for most of the cardiac complications during pregnancy. Mortality among pregnant women with mild symptoms is less than 1% but can reach 5% if MS is severe. Women are most at risk during labour, delivery, and immediately postpartum.

Heart disease is present in 0.5–1% of all pregnant women and accounts for 10–15% of maternal mortality. Although the incidence of acquired disease has fallen (to below 0.2%) in Western countries due to the decreased incidence of rheumatic fever, rheumatic heart disease is still the most common cause. Congenital heart disease is becoming an increasing problem during pregnancy as a result of the success of neonatal corrective or palliative cardiac surgery. Symptomatic coronary disease, although currently rare, can occur and is likely to increase with increasing maternal age and smoking.

3) **Why did the patient develop symptoms when only 14 weeks pregnant?**

The haemodynamic changes begin early in pregnancy and are usually well tolerated. However, women with previously silent heart disease can decompensate.

In MS the pressure gradient across the diseased MV increases significantly during pregnancy. This occurs as a result of the physiological increase in heart rate (HR; reduced LV diastolic filling time) and cardiac output (CO). This increases LA and PA wedge pressures and may result in a relatively fixed CO state (i.e. limited increase in CO during exercise). Symptoms (excessive fatigue, breathlessness, orthopnoea, and paroxysmal nocturnal dyspnoea) may occur even in women with mild–moderate MS who were previously asymptomatic. Symptoms usually develop or increase by the second trimester.

4) **What is the likely cause of the acute deterioration at 26 weeks?**

The onset of AF probably triggered acute pulmonary oedema. The shortened diastolic filling time associated with faster ventricular rates during atrial fibrillation is especially prone to cause sudden rises in LA pressure and pulmonary oedema. DC cardioversion was performed under general anaesthesia. The patient reported that she had been anticoagulated with treatment dose LMWH for 4 months prior to this presentation. However, as the patient had not attended follow-up, TOE was performed to exclude LA thrombus prior to cardioversion.

5) **How would you manage the MS?**

Tachyarrhythmias with haemodynamic compromise require consideration of immediate cardioversion. Anticoagulation is required for AF. Thereafter, the management of moderate MS (valve area 1.1–1.5 cm^2), depends on the severity of symptoms before and during pregnancy, and the rise in PA pressure. Women with NYHA I–II symptoms should be followed closely with regular clinical evaluation and echocardiographic assessment (measurement of mean transmitral gradient and PA pressure). If symptoms persist despite optimal medical therapy, percutaneous balloon valvuloplasty or repair/replacement should be considered during pregnancy.

In the present case, percutaneous balloon valvuloplasty was performed after treatment of the LVF when the patient was 27 weeks pregnant. Percutaneous balloon valvuloplasty is successful and safe (low maternal and foetal mortality). It is the first-line intervention for anatomically suitable valves in young patients with pliable, non-calcified valves, without significant subvalvular thickening or significant mitral regurgitation.

Patients with mild MS (valve area >1.5 cm^2) should be cautious with salt intake and may limit physical activity. They benefit from drug therapy, including diuretics and beta-blockade (to reduce HR and increase diastolic filling time) unless symptoms are severe. If MS is severe (valve area <1 cm^2), valvuloplasty or valve repair/replacement should be considered.

6) **The patient wishes to give birth at her local midwife-led unit. What do you recommend?**

Delivery should occur in a specialist centre with facilities for emergency Caesarean section and expertise in maternal medicine. Bedside ECG monitoring is required as arrhythmias are common. PA catheters are often used to monitor fluid balance in patients with moderate or severe MS. In this case elective Caesarean section was performed under combined spinal and epidural anaesthesia to avoid the cardio-vascular stress of labour. There were no complications during the Caesarean section. The patient had a healthy baby boy. Following delivery of the baby the patient's symptoms rapidly improved and she was discharged home 3 days postpartum. Cardiology outpatient follow-up was arranged.

Labour and delivery require careful planning. Significant haemodynamic shifts occur during labour, delivery, and immediately postpartum. During uterine con-tractions venous return increases and CO may rise by a further 25%. Pain and anxiety increase sympathetic tone, which also increases CO and BP. These changes are affected by analgesia and the mode of delivery.

About 500 mL of blood is lost during vaginal delivery and at least 750 mL of blood loss is expected during uncomplicated Caesarean section. However, CO increases abruptly postpartum as the contracted uterus returns blood to the systemic circulation and the IVC is decompressed (autotransfusion). The cardiovascular system returns to normal by 6 weeks postpartum. There are no haemodynamic differences between breastfeeding and non-breastfeeding women, but some medications should be avoided by breastfeeding mothers.

If vaginal delivery is considered, an epidural catheter should be sited for analgesia to reduce anxiety. Management involves cardiologists, obstetricians, anaesthetists, neonatologists, and cardiac surgeons.

7) **How would you anticoagulate the patient?**

There are no RCTs to guide management of anticoagulation during pregnancy and unfortunately there is no consensus of opinion. The options include the following.

LMWH and warfarin combination

The teratogenic effect of warfarin occurs mainly after the sixth week of gestation so warfarin may be continued until the pregnancy test is positive. Administer LMWH for the first trimester, switch to warfarin in the second trimester, but change back to

LMWH at 36 weeks or 2 days prior to expected delivery. LMWH should be given sub-cutaneously twice daily, and the dose adjusted to body weight to maintain anti-Xa levels 0.5–1.0 U/mL 4–6 h after injection. LMWH does not cross the placenta. Care must be taken when shifting from warfarin to LMWH and vice versa because most complications occur at these times.

A recent retrospective analysis of pregnancies in patients with mechanical heart valves suggested that resumption of warfarin after the first trimester increased foetal loss. However, mechanical heart valves require high levels of anticoagulation. Thus, whether warfarin should not be reinitiated after the first trimester in patients anticoagulated for other reasons is unclear.

Warfarin for the whole pregnancy

This may be appropriate after careful discussion of the potential risks and benefits with the patient if low doses are needed to maintain appropriate INR or the patient is at very high risk of thromboembolism (e.g. older generation mechanical MV or previous thromboembolism).

LMWH for the whole pregnancy

LMWH is administered subcutaneously twice daily with dose adjusted to body weight as above. This regime was used in this case.

LMWH is much less likely to cause thrombocytopenia than unfractionated heparin. However, platelet counts should be checked before and 7–10 days after starting therapeutic heparin. Thereafter, platelet counts are required at least monthly or if unexpected bruising or bleeding occurs.

To minimize the risk of epidural haematoma, epidural or spinal anaesthesia should not be performed until at least 12 hours after a prophylactic dose of LMWH or 24 hours after the last dose of LMWH if a twice-daily therapeutic regime is in use. If elective Caesarean section is planned prophylactic LMWH should be given the day before delivery. Omit the morning dose on the day of delivery, and operate in the morning. If Caesarean section is performed prophylactic LMWH should be given at 3 hours post-operatively and the therapeutic dose restarted that evening. LMWH should not be administered until 4 hours after an epidural catheter is removed.

8) **The patient's dentist writes to you requesting guidance on antibiotic prophy-laxis against endocarditis. How would you respond?**

Antibiotic prophylaxis against endocarditis has become a contentious issue in the UK. Until recently, patients at high risk of developing endocarditis (Table 32.1) undergoing various invasive procedures (Table 32.2) had been advised to take periprocedural antibiotics (Table 32.1). The aim of this practice was to abolish or reduce the bacteraemia caused by these procedures to reduce the risk of develop-ing endocarditis. A class 1C status in guidelines (1 = general agreement that the intervention is beneficial, useful and effective; C = consensus opinion of experts based on clinical experience) was given.

However, there is little evidence that this strategy is effective and potential complications include anaphylaxis, diarrhoea, and increasing antibiotic resistance.

In 2008, the National Institute for Health and Clinical Excellence (NICE) in the UK produced guidance on antibiotic prophylaxis. This recommended that in most cases endocarditis prophylaxis should not be given in view of the potential complications associated with antibiotic administration.

The NICE guidance stated that there was no consistent association between undergoing an interventional procedure (dental or non-dental) and developing endocarditis. Furthermore, the clinical effectiveness of antibiotic prophylaxis is not proven, so prophylaxis may cause more deaths from fatal anaphylaxis than would occur if antibiotic prophylaxis were not given.

In the NICE guidelines, antibiotic prophylaxis against endocarditis was only recommended if a patient at risk of infective endocarditis required antibiotic therapy prior to a gastrointestinal or genitourinary procedure at a site where there is a suspected infection. In this situation, NICE recommended that the antibiotic administered should cover organisms that could cause infective endocarditis.

However, NICE stated that antibiotic prophylaxis against endocarditis for dental procedures was not cost-effective and recommended that it should not be given. Despite this the European and American guidelines remain unchanged and include the class 1C recommendation for periprocedural administration of antimicrobial prophylaxis for patients at high risk of endocarditis. Many UK cardiologists still follow these guidelines. This has caused confusion with the dental profession and amongst patients.

In this case, the patient and her dentist were advised that antibiotic prophylaxis was not required.

Table 32.1 Cardiac conditions in which antimicrobial prophylaxis is indicated (ESC Guidelines)

Prosthetic heart valves
Complex congenital cyanotic heart diseases
Previous infective endocarditis
Surgically constructed systemic or pulmonary conduits
Acquired valvular heart diseases
Mitral valve prolapse with valvular regurgitation or severe valve thickening
Non-cyanotic congenital heart diseases (except for secundum type ASD), including bicuspid AVs
Hypertrophic cardiomyopathy

Table 32.2 Risk procedures: diagnostic and therapeutic interventions likely to produce bacteraemia

Bronchoscopy (rigid instrument)
Cystoscopy during urinary tract infection
Biopsy of urinary tract/prostate
Dental procedures with the risk of gingival/mucosal trauma
Tonsillectomy and adenoidectomy

Further reading

Bates SM, Greer IA, Pabinger I, Sofaer S, Hirsh J (2008). Venous thromboembolism, thrombophilia, antithrombotic therapy, and pregnancy: American College of Chest Physicians Evidence-Based Clinical Practice Guidelines (8th edition). *Chest*; **133**: 844S–886S.

Kim BJ, An SJ, Shim SS, Jun JK, Yoon BH, Syn HC, Park JS (2006). Pregnancy outcomes in women with mechanical heart valves. *J Reprod Med*; **51**: 649–654.

Silversides CK, Colman JM, Sermer M, Siu SC (2003). Cardiac risk in pregnant women with rheumatic mitral stenosis. *Am J Cardiol*; **91**: 1382.

Carabello BA (2005). Modern management of mitral stenosis. *Circulation*; **112**: 432.

Bruce CJ, Nishimura RA (1998). Newer advances in the diagnosis and treatment of mitral stenosis. *Curr Probl Cardiol*; **23**: 125.

Bonow RO, Carabello BA, Chatterjee K *et al.* (2008). 2008 Focused update incorporated into the ACC/AHA 2006 guidelines for the management of patients with valvular heart disease: a report of the American College of Cardiology/American Heart Association Task Force on Practice Guidelines (Writing Committee to Revise the 1998 Guidelines for the Management of Patients With Valvular Heart Disease): endorsed by the Society of Cardiovascular Anesthesiologists, Society for Cardiovascular Angiography and Interventions, and Society of Thoracic Surgeons. *Circulation*; **118**: e523.

National Institute for Health and Clinical Excellence. NICE clinical guideline 64. *Prophylaxis against infective endocarditis*. www.nice.org.uk/CG064.

Jain D, Halushka MK (2009). Cardiac pathology of systemic lupus erythematosus. *J Clin Pathol*; **62**: 584–592.

Roldan CA (2008). Valvular and coronary heart disease in systemic inflammatory diseases: Systemic disorders in heart disease. *Heart*; **94**: 1089–1101.

Zipes DP, Camm AJ, Borggrefe M, Buxton AE, Chaitman B, Fromer M, Gregoratos G, Klein G, Moss AJ, Myerburg RJ, Priori SG, Quinones MA, Roden DM, Silka MJ, Tracy C, Smith SC Jr, Jacobs AK, Adams CD, Antman EM, Anderson JL, Hunt SA, Halperin JL, Nishimura R, Ornato JP, Page RL, Riegel B, Blanc JJ, Budaj A, Dean V, Deckers JW, Despres C, Dickstein K, Lekakis J, McGregor K, Metra M, Morais J, Osterspey A, Tamargo JL, Zamorano JL; American College of Cardiology/American Heart Association Task Force; European Society of Cardiology Committee for Practice Guidelines; European Heart Rhythm Association; Heart Rhythm Society (2006). ACC/AHA/ESC 2006 Guidelines for Management of Patients With Ventricular Arrhythmias and the Prevention of Sudden Cardiac Death: a report of the American College of Cardiology/American Heart Association Task Force and the European Society of Cardiology Committee for Practice Guidelines (writing committee to develop Guidelines for Management of Patients With Ventricular Arrhythmias and the Prevention of Sudden Cardiac Death): developed in collaboration with the European Heart Rhythm Association and the Heart Rhythm Society. *Circulation* **114**:e385–484.

Case 33

A 23-year-old Asian woman presented to the ED with a 2-hour history of palpitations that began whilst she was carrying washing up stairs. It was associated with chest tightness, 'heaviness' in the left arm, and presyncope. She was unable to give any more history. On examination she was drowsy, tachycardic (over 200 bpm), and had a BP of 100/60 mmHg. There were no signs of cardiac failure, but a symmetrical rash was noted on the face.

The admission ECG is shown in Fig. 33.1. Adenosine (6 mg followed by 12 mg intravenous bolus), amiodarone (300 mg), and magnesium (8 mmol) intravenously had no effect on the tachycardia, but her dizziness increased and systolic pressure fell to 80 mmHg. She was sedated and electrically cardioverted into sinus rhythm. The ECG recorded post cardioversion is shown in Fig. 33.2.

The chest pain subsided and she became more haemodynamically stable. As she improved, further history was revealed: a diagnosis of systemic lupus erythematosus (SLE) had been made aged 7 because of an episode of lupus nephritis. She was known to have the antiphospholipid antibody syndrome with a previous popliteal artery thrombus and was taking warfarin. She denied previous chest pain. Admission cardiac troponin I was raised at 6 ng/dL. Echocardiography demonstrated inferior hypokinesia and an EF of 45%. The subsequent coronary angiogram is shown in Fig. 33.3.

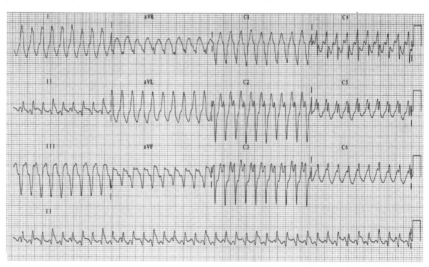

Fig. 33.1 Admission 12 lead ECG

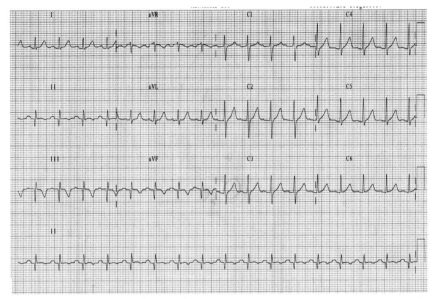

Fig. 33.2 Post cardioversion 12 lead ECG

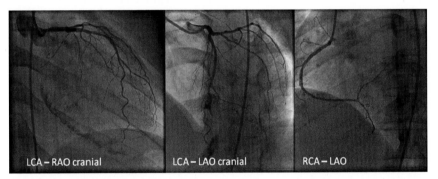

LCA – RAO cranial   LCA – LAO cranial   RCA – LAO

Fig. 33.3 Selected images from coronary angiogram

Questions

1. What was the admission heart rhythm? Is there a differential diagnosis and where is its origin?
2. Report the post-cardioversion ECG. Is her heart likely to be structurally normal?
3. What is the cause of the arrhythmia?
4. What does the angiogram show?
5. Is there an indication for implanting an ICD?
6. Is the background of SLE relevant?

Answers

1) **What was the admission heart rhythm? Is there a differential diagnosis and where is its origin?**

Figure 33.1 shows a regular monomorphic broad complex (QRS duration >120 ms) tachycardia (230 bpm). This is due to either VT (80%) or supraventricular tachycardia with aberrant ventricular conduction (20%). Various methods of differentiating SVT from VT have been described but if there is uncertainty, the patient should be treated for VT as it is more common and threatening. Importantly, haemodynamic stability does not discriminate SVT from VT.

   i. A history of myocardial infarction or heart failure suggests VT (positive predictive value 95%).

   ii. The interval from the start of the R wave to the nadir of the S wave in V1 ≥100 ms suggests VT (Fig. 33.4A).

   iii. Evidence of atrioventricular dissociation implies VT and fusion or capture beats can occur when a sinus beat is conducted. However, this is only obvious on the surface ECG in 20–50% of cases. Fusion beats are the complex resulting when an ectopic ventricular beat coincides with normal conduction to the ventricle that arrives outside of the myocardial refractory period, hence confirming atrioventricular dissociation. They appear on the surface ECG as QRS complexes of different morphology to the ectopic activity (see Fig. 33.4B).

   iv. If all precordial leads are predominantly positive or negative VT is the likely diagnosis (concordance).

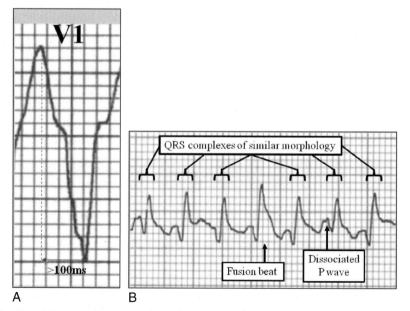

A   B

Fig. 33.4 (A) Zoomed image of QRS complex demonstrating prolonged time to nadir of S wave in V1. (B) Signs of AV dissociation on ECG.

v. QRS durations of >140 ms with RBBB or >160 ms with LBBB favours VT.

vi. If the QRS axis is between −90 and ±180 degrees VT is more likely.

vii. Termination with slowing of atrioventricular conduction (Valsalva manoeuvre, carotid sinus massage, or adenosine) suggests SVT, but can also occur with rare VT that originates within the conduction system in the ventricle (fascicular VT).

In this case the first, sixth, and eleventh complexes on the rhythm strip (Fig. 33.1) are fusion beats with some variation in QRS morphology in other complexes. There is an LBBB pattern with a QRS duration >120 but there is no concordance and the QRS axis is normal.

2) **Report the post-cardioversion ECG. Is her heart likely to be structurally normal?**

The post-cardioversion ECG shows sinus rhythm (100 bpm), with borderline left-axis deviation. Pathological Q waves are present in the inferior leads with an upright T wave in V1. This would be consistent with previous inferior MI.

3) **What is the cause of the arrhythmia?**

There are no flow-limiting stenoses in the left or right coronary arteries. However, the RAO cranial view shows extensive myocardial calcification, which probably represents post-infarct scarring on the inferior wall of the left ventricle and a substrate for slowed conduction and conduction block.

4) **What does the angiogram show?**

In this case, the absence of flow-limiting stenoses and the presence of post-infarct scarring suggests VT associated with a myocardial scar rather than acute ischaemia. Propagation of monomorphic VT requires a re-entry circuit. The development of a re-entry circuit requires retrograde conduction of the normal activation wavefront and re-excitation of the tissue where the activation wavefront originated, usually round an area of conduction block or markedly slowed conduction.

Chronically diseased (scarred) myocardium has multiple conducting pathways with different refractory periods. This increases the chance of re-entry. Similar circuits can occur in dilated or hypertrophic cardiomyopathy, where diffuse interstitial fibrosis and myofibrillar disarray provide multiple pathways and conduction block.

Although a re-entry mechanism is much the most likely mechanism in this case, a minority of automatic ventricular arrhythmias are due to altered myocyte electrical activity. This is associated with infarction (first 24–48 hours), ischaemia, and electrolyte abnormalities. The mechanism of polymorphic VT is discussed in Case 38.

5) **Is there an indication for implanting an ICD?**

In this case, the EF was >35% and there was no evidence of cardiomyopathy so ICD implantation was not indicated (see Cases 10 and 29). The patient was treated with bisoprolol and discharged with cardiology outpatient follow-up.

6) **Is the background of SLE relevant?**

Mortality in SLE is bimodal. Early deaths are due to active disease or sepsis; late deaths result from coronary and neurovascular disease. Atherosclerosis is both accelerated and premature. Autopsy series of women with SLE aged 16-37 dying of non-cardiac causes found that over 90% had more severe atherosclerosis than age-matched controls. The incidence of MI is five times higher than in the general population, with the overall prevalence of CAD around 7%. The mean age at first MI is 49 years, compared with that of the general population of 69 years. Conventional risk factors do not account for the increased risk; SLE is an independent risk factor. Other risk factors in patients with SLE include high cumulative corticosteroid dose, antiphospholipid antibodies, elevated homocysteine, renal insufficiency, and a 'lupus pattern' of hyperlipidaemia (raised very low density lipoprotein and triglycerides, low HDL). Inflammation is central to the pathogenesis of atherosclerosis. SLE is a chronic inflammatory autoimmune disease that drives accelerated atherosclerosis and immune complex mediated endothelial injury and dysfunction.

Further reading

Jain D, Halushka MK (2009). Cardiac pathology of systemic lupus erythematosus. *J Clin Pathol*; **62**: 584–592.

Roldan CA (2008). Valvular and coronary heart disease in systemic inflammatory diseases: Systemic disorders in heart disease. *Heart*; **94**: 1089–1101.

Zipes DP, Camm AJ, Borggrefe M, Buxton AE, Chaitman B, Fromer M, Gregoratos G, Klein G, Moss AJ, Myerburg RJ, Priori SG, Quinones MA, Roden DM, Silka MJ, Tracy C, Smith SC Jr, Jacobs AK, Adams CD, Antman EM, Anderson JL, Hunt SA, Halperin JL, Nishimura R, Ornato JP, Page RL, Riegel B, Blanc JJ, Budaj A, Dean V, Deckers JW, Despres C, Dickstein K, Lekakis J, McGregor K, Metra M, Morais J, Osterspey A, Tamargo JL, Zamorano JL; American College of Cardiology/American Heart Association Task Force; European Society of Cardiology Committee for Practice Guidelines; European Heart Rhythm Association; Heart Rhythm Society (2006). ACC/AHA/ESC 2006 Guidelines for Management of Patients With Ventricular Arrhythmias and the Prevention of Sudden Cardiac Death: a report of the American College of Cardiology/American Heart Association Task Force and the European Society of Cardiology Committee for Practice Guidelines (writing committee to develop Guidelines for Management of Patients With Ventricular Arrhythmias and the Prevention of Sudden Cardiac Death): developed in collaboration with the European Heart Rhythm Association and the Heart Rhythm Society. *Circulation* 114:e385–484.

Case 34

A 43-year-old civil servant presented with 30 minutes of central chest tightness that began at rest and radiated to his jaw. It was associated with anxiety, some sweating, and nausea. He was a non-smoker, treated hypertensive (lisinopril 5 mg), not diabetic, and had a total cholesterol of 3 mmol/L but had a strong family history of cardiac disease. His sister had had a heart attack aged 39 years, his father had collapsed at work with a heart attack aged 37 years, and his paternal grandfather had died suddenly at the age of 51 years.

Observations were BP 165/90 mmHg (equal in both arms) and HR 80 bpm. On examination he was in obvious discomfort. The JVP was not raised, heart sounds were normal and there were no clinical signs of cardiac failure. The admission ECG is shown in Fig. 34.1.

The patient was promptly thrombolysed with rtPA and admitted to the CCU. Transthoracic echocardiography demonstrated good systolic function with no regional wall motion abnormalities. The 12-hour troponin I was normal. However, despite almost complete resolution of the ECG changes (Fig. 34.2) the patient's chest pain persisted over the next 24 hours.

The patient was transferred to a tertiary centre for angiography. Only minor, non-flow-limiting, plaque disease in the LAD was seen and the LV angiogram was normal. Diagnoses suggested were either of an MI secondary to thrombosis on a ruptured atherosclerotic plaque that was aborted by prompt rtPA administration or coronary artery vasospasm. Aggressive risk factor modification was recommended. He was prescribed clopidogrel for 1 year and lifelong aspirin and discharged home.

He subsequently submitted a critical illness claim to his insurance company for the time spent in hospital. The insurance company organized a medical examination, which included an ECG (Fig. 34.3). This was reviewed by a medical officer, who referred the patient to a consultant cardiologist for a second opinion.

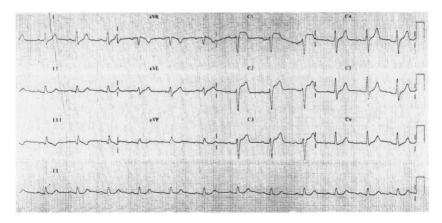

Fig. 34.1 ECG on admission during chest pain.

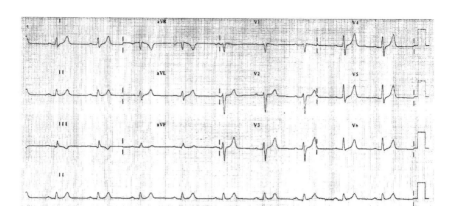

Fig. 34.2 ECG at 90 minutes post thrombolysis with rtPA.

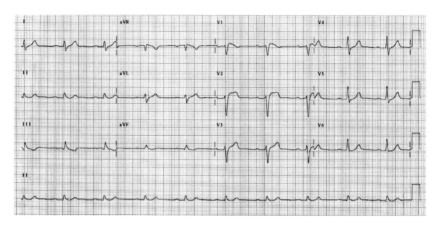

Fig. 34.3 ECG at rest and pain-free for medical examination 6 weeks later.

Questions

1. Report the ECG in Fig. 34.1.
2. Report the ECG in Fig. 34.2.
3. Report the ECG in Fig. 34.3.
4. What is the possible underlying diagnosis?
5. What may have caused the ECG changes noted in Figs 34.1 and 34.3?
6. How would you confirm and assess this further?
7. How would you manage this patient?

Answers

1) **Report the ECG in Fig. 34.1.**

    The admission ECG shows sinus rhythm at a rate of 70 bpm. The QRS axis is normal. The PR interval and QRS durations are normal. There is >2 mm ST elevation in V1–3. There are no associated Q waves or ST depression but T waves are inverted in III and flattened in aVF.

2) **Report the ECG in Fig. 34.2.**

    The anterior ST elevation has resolved post-thrombolysis. There is T-wave flattening in V1. This trace is within normal limits.

3) **Report the ECG in Fig. 34.3.**

    The ECG shows sinus rhythm at 66 bpm. There is coved ST elevation in V1 and 'saddle-back' ST elevation in V2. The inferior repolarization abnormalities are again present.

4) **What is the possible underlying diagnosis?**

    Two of the three ECGs shown demonstrate an RBBB pattern and ST elevation of differing degrees in the right precordial ECG leads (Figs 34.1 and 34.3), an ECG pattern that is consistent with a type 1 Brugada syndrome. The transitory nature of the ECG findings, with the ECG in Fig. 34.2 being essentially normal, is also characteristic.

    Brugada syndrome, a cause of idiopathic VF, was first described in 1992. It is a cardiac channelopathy. The inherited forms are linked to a loss of function mutation in the α-subunit of the cardiac sodium channel (SCN5A) in 20–30% of patients. In the more common sporadic disease (70–80%) *de novo* mutations are more rarely found.

    Patients have an abnormal resting ECG that classically shows an RBBB pattern and ST elevation in the right precordial ECG leads (Figs 34.1, 34.3, and 34.4). It presents during adulthood (mean age 40 years but the age range is wide). Brugada syndrome causes syncope or SCD from polymorphic VT or VF. Symptoms mainly occur at night and prior to 1992 patients with Brugada syndrome were probably diagnosed with sudden unexpected nocturnal death syndrome. Brugada syndrome occurs in structurally normal hearts and accounts for 4–12% of all sudden deaths and 20–40% of sudden deaths in people without structural heart disease. See Cases 29, 33, 35, and 38 for further discussion of ventricular arrhythmias. It has a male preponderance and has its highest prevalence in South-East Asia and Japan (estimated at 26–38 deaths per 100 000).

The diagnosis of Brugada syndrome is based on the presence of characteristic ECG abnormalities and the exclusion of any structural heart disease (e.g. arrrhythmogenic RV cardiomyopathy) or myocardial ischaemia. Three ECG repolarization patterns are described in Brugada syndrome (Fig. 34.4):

i. Type 1 has 'coved' ST-segment elevation (≥2 mm) that descends with an upward convexity into an inverted T wave.

ii. Type 2 and type 3 patterns are 'saddle back' ST elevation that descends toward the baseline before rising again into an upright or biphasic T wave, differing in the degree of ST elevation (type 2: ≥1 mm; type 3: <1 mm).

Moving the right precordial chest leads (V1–2) up to the second intercostal space may increase the sensitivity of ECG screening for these abnormalities.

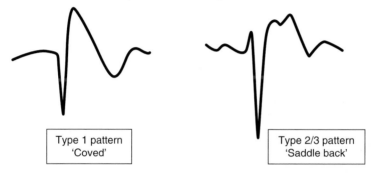

Type 1 pattern
'Coved'

Type 2/3 pattern
'Saddle back'

Fig. 34.4 The Brugada patterns of ST elevation.

5) **What may have caused the ECG changes noted in Figs 34.1 and 34.3?**

It is important to note that the ECG manifestations of Brugada syndrome may be transient or concealed (Fig. 34.2). The abnormalities can be unmasked by vagal stimulation or fever. Challenge with sodium channel blockers (e.g. ajmaline, flecainide) can also unmask the Brugada pattern ECG.

6) **How would you confirm and assess this further?**

The presence of a spontaneous type 1 pattern ECG is diagnostic of Brugada syndrome especially if clinical correlates are present. So in this case no further investigation is required to confirm the diagnosis.

A spontaneous 'saddle back' (type 2 or 3) pattern of ST elevation is suspicious and requires further investigation. Provocation testing with sodium channel blockers can be used to screen cases where ECG changes are suspicious or there is a family history of SCD or syncope but the resting ECG is normal. Ajmaline is commonly used and usually uncovers a clearer type 1 pattern in V1 and a type 2 pattern in V2 (Fig. 34.5).

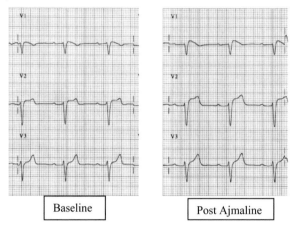

Baseline   Post Ajmaline

Fig. 34.5 ECG before and after administration of ajmaline to a patient with Brugada syndrome.

7) **How would you manage this patient?**

Management depends on the predicted risk of SCD or VF for each individual patient. High-risk features include history of syncope, spontaneously abnormal ECG, and susceptibility to sustained ventricular arrhythmia during programmed electrical stimulation (Table 34.1). However, the management of asymptomatic individuals with no family history and who are incidentally found to have an abnormal ECG is controversial. It is generally accepted that those presenting after aborted sudden death (i.e. successful resuscitation after cardiac arrest) have the highest risk of recurrence of arrhythmia.

There is as yet no proven pharmacological approach to risk reduction. Agents that shorten phase 0 (e.g. quinidine) or restore the balance of currents in phase 1 of the action potential (e.g. beta-adrenergic agonists or anticholinergic agents) may be helpful. Beta-blockers and amiodarone are not beneficial. The treatment of choice for primary and secondary prevention of sudden death is ICD implantation (see Cases 10 and 29).

In this case, the patient had a spontaneous type 1 Brugada pattern ECG that was intermittently concealed. There was no history of syncope and programmed stimulation could not induce a sustained ventricular arrhythmia. However, the cardiac disease in the family history could have actually been due to Brugada syndrome. His father's ECG also revealed a Brugada pattern, suggesting that his father's collapse and his grandfather's death were probably due to Brugada-related arrhythmias. In view of this an ICD was implanted. The chest pain settled with administration of Gaviscon, omeprazole, and metoclopramide, and gastroesophageal reflux was subsequently diagnosed at endoscopy.

Table 34.1 Risk of arrhythmia or sudden cardiac death in patients with Brugada syndrome

		Sustained ventricular arrhythmia	
		Non-inducible	**Inducible**
Prior syncope	Spontaneously abnormal ECG	Moderate risk (5% probability of SCD or VF at 24 months)	Very high risk (25% probability of SCD or VF at 24 months)
	ECG abnormal after drug challenge	Low risk (1–2% probability of SCD or VF at 24 months)	High risk (10–15% probability of SCD or VF at 24 months)
No prior syncope	Spontaneously abnormal ECG	Low risk (1–2% probability of SCD or VF at 24 months)	High risk (10–15% probability of SCD or VF at 24 months)
	ECG abnormal after drug challenge	Very low risk (<1% probability of SCD or VF at 24 months)	Moderate risk (5% probability of SCD or VF at 24 months)

Further reading

Fowler SJ, Priori SG.. (2009). Clinical spectrum of patients with a Brugada ECG. *Curr Opin Cardiol*; **24**: 74–81.

Junttila MJ, Gonzalez M, Lizotte E, Benito B, Vernooy K, Sarkozy A, Huikuri HV, Brugada P, Brugada J, Brugada R. (2008). Induced Brugada-type electrocardiogram, a sign for imminent malignant arrhythmias. *Circulation*; **117**: 1890–1893.

Case 35

A 48-year-old violinist presented to his GP after feeling faint whilst playing a solo piece in a concert. His wife also mentioned that his face would occasionally drain of colour but would return to normal a few seconds later. This symptom of intermittent facial pallor had developed over the preceding 2 months and had increased in frequency. It was particularly severe when he was under stress, when it could occur several times a minute. He denied palpitations, chest pain, breathlessness, or syncope. His exercise tolerance was unrestricted. There was no past medical or surgical history. He did not take any medications regularly. Examination revealed intermittent changes in facial appearance with episodes of pallor followed by flushing (Fig. 35.1), an irregularly irregular pulse, BP 140/75 mmHg, but otherwise unremarkable. His GP arranged blood tests and referred him for a 12 lead ECG (Fig. 35.2).

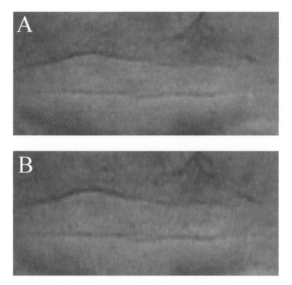

Fig. 35.1 Intermittent changes in facial appearance. Photograph of patient's forehead demonstrating pallor (A) and flushing (B). (See colour plate 12)

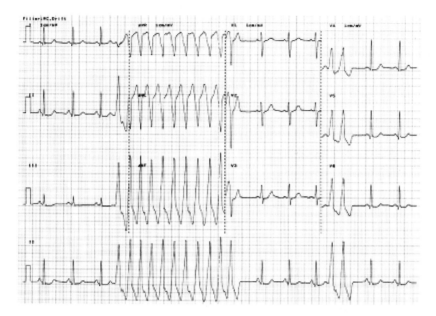

Fig. 35.2 12 lead ECG at rest.

Questions

1. The technician asks you to review the patient. What is the immediate management?

2. Report the ECG (Fig. 35.2).

3. Could the ECG explain the changes in facial appearance, dizziness, and irregular pulse?

4. Trans-thoracic echocardiography is normal. What are the potential causes of this arrhythmia?

5. What further investigation is required?

Answers

1) **The technician asks you to review the patient, what is the immediate management?**

   Venous access should be obtained and the patient should be admitted to the CCU for cardiac monitoring. Blood tests, including full blood count, serum creatinine and electrolytes, and magnesium and thyroid function tests are required. Echocardiography should also be performed.

2) **Report the ECG in Fig. 35.2.**

   At the start of the recording the patient was in sinus rhythm at a rate of 80 bpm. After three beats a non-sustained broad complex tachycardia at a rate of nearly 280 bpm is captured. This lasts for 3 seconds, after which sinus rhythm is restored spontaneously. The notching of the T waves of the 3rd, 5th, 7th and 10th complexes suggests atrioventricular dissociation. The tachycardia has an LBBB morphology with an inferior axis. This suggests that it is VT originating from the right ventricular outflow tract (RVOT) (see Table 35.1). Importantly, the ECG during sinus rhythm has a normal QT interval and there is no evidence of previous MI (although aVF is not seen in sinus rhythm). Septal Q waves are normal in sinus rhythm.

Table 35.1 12 lead ECG during ventricular tachycardia as a guide for site of origin

ECG feature		Site of origin of VT
Bundle branch block	LBBB	Exit in the RV or the septum
	RBBB	Exit in the LV
QRS axis	Superior	Exit in the inferior wall
	Inferior	Exit in the anterior (superior) wall
QRS duration	>140 ms	Free wall of the RVOT
	<140 ms	Septal side of the RVOT
Dominant R waves in V2–V4		Exit near the base of the ventricle

3) **Could the ECG explain the changes in facial appearance, dizziness, and irregular pulse?**

   The facial flushing was temporally associated with the intermittent VT, and was probably due to loss of cardiac output (pale episodes) followed by hyperaemia once the circulation was restored (flushing episodes) before his complexion returned to normal.

   The irregular pulse was due to intermittent loss of cardiac output, as shown in Fig. 35.3. The depression of the pulse oximeter trace during the tachycardia suggests reduction or loss of cardiac output. A prolonged run of VT or frequent bursts of VT could have caused the pre-syncopal episode.

   This case illustrates an unusual presentation of VT where the circulatory consequence of the tachycardia prompted the patient to present, and where the patient was asymptomatic from the VT itself.

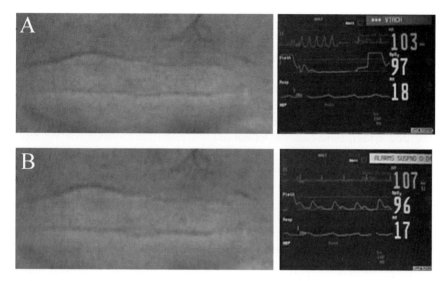

Fig. 35.3 Photographs demonstrating association of facial pallor with ventricular tachycardia. A, The facial pallor was associated with ventricular tachycardia. B, The facial flush was associated with spontaneous cardioversion to sinus rhythm. (See colour plate 13)

4) **Transthoracic echocardiography is normal. What are the potential causes of this arrhythmia?**

Ventricular tachycardia is most commonly associated with cardiac structural abnormalities (90%), such as scarring post infarction or cardiac surgery. Where no such macroscopic abnormalities are thought to exist, the VT is termed primary or idiopathic, and includes the 'channelopathy' subgroups. Idiopathic or primary VT begins either after re-entry of impulses into self-sustaining circuits: primary, triggered electrical activity; or secondary, catecholamine-mediated automatic electrical activity. Hence, in the present case, as the heart appeared to be structurally normal on echocardiography, the non-sustained VT was most likely to be an idiopathic VT. More detailed imaging with cardiac MRI is required to more definitively exclude structural cardiac disease.

Idiopathic VT has been variously classified by clinical presentation (sustained or non-sustained), precipitating factors (e.g. exercise), site of origin (LV or RV), response to antiarrhythmics (e.g. adenosine or verapamil), or underlying disease (primary electrical disorder or inherited myocardial disease).

One clinically useful classification is based on whether the resting ECG is abnormal and prognosis. Some types of VT cause SCD, particularly those associated with rapid polymorphic VT (torsade de pointes), whilst others can be cured by ablative therapy or have a good prognosis with medical treatment. In this system there are three subgroups:

   I. curable VT with a normal resting ECG

  II. malignant phenotypes with an abnormal resting ECG

 III. malignant phenotypes with a normal resting ECG.

I. Curable phenotypes with a normal resting ECG

The majority (70%) of patients with VT and structurally normal hearts are young, with a female preponderance, and have repetitive monomorphic VT originating from the RVOT due to a primary electrical abnormality. The spectrum of presentations range from recurrent extrasystoles to sustained VT brought on by exertion and stress. This spectrum includes bursts of non-sustained VT at rest that increased in frequency with exertion or sympathetic activity (repetitive monomorphic VT), as described in the present case. The VT has an LBBB pattern and inferior axis (Fig. 35.2; Table 35.2).

As ventricular function is usually preserved, the tachycardia is normally well tolerated and has a good long-term prognosis in comparison to VT associated with a structural abnormality. Beta-blockers, including sotalol, and calcium channel blockers can suppress the VT, but ablation of the RVOT focus is possible in those with breakthrough VT despite medical treatment.

A similar syndrome with a narrower complex VT of RBBB morphology and a superior axis is known as idiopathic LV tachycardia or fascicular VT (see Case 2). There is a young male preponderance and it is uncommonly associated with stress or exertion. It is not a primary electrical disorder. The most common mechanism is thought to be re-entry of delayed after depolarizations in the left posterior fascicle. Although it can be suppressed by therapy with beta-blockers and calcium channel blockers, catheter ablation is curative and should be considered early in the management of symptomatic patients.

II. Malignant phenotypes with an abnormal resting ECG

The long QT syndrome (LQTS) is the best characterized (see Case 38). A short QT syndrome (<300 ms) associated with familial sudden death, palpitations, syncope, and cardiac arrest has been described. Electrophysiological studies reveal short atrial and ventricular refractory periods and a low threshold for VF. Mutations in the cardiac potassium channel HERG (KCNH2) have been identified. Currently, ICD implantation is the treatment of choice, although beta-blockade and cardiac sympathectomy are possible alternatives.

III. Malignant phenotypes with a normal resting ECG

Catecholaminergic polymorphic ventricular tachycardia (CPVT) is a syndrome of syncope or SCD during physiological or emotional stress, associated with a strong family history of juvenile SCD and stress-induced syncope (30% of cases). Half die before the age of 30 years. Fifty per cent are linked to genetic mutations in either the *cardiac ryanodine receptor* gene or the *calsequestrin 2* gene.

Empirical use of beta-blockers, antiarrhythmic drugs, and ICD implantation has been described but there is no clear evidence of benefit. A significant minority (10%) of survivors of cardiac arrests have no identifiable structural or ECG abnormalities and do not have evidence of myocardial ischaemia, drug toxicity, or metabolic or electrolyte derangement.

This diagnosis is one of exclusion and as there is a 11% rate of sudden death within 1 year of presentation with VT or aborted SCD and a 30% recurrence rate at 5 years, ICD implantation is the treatment of choice.

For further discussion of VT see Cases 33 and 34.

Table 35.2 Causes of VT. The differentiation of RVOT VT and ARVC is clinically important

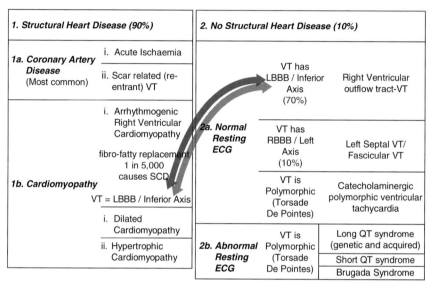

5) **What further investigation is required?**

Before diagnosing RVOT VT the RV and RVOT should be imaged to exclude arrhythmogenic right ventricular dysplasia/cardiomyopathy (ARVC). Although echocardiography can exclude major abnormalities, cardiac CT or MRI is required to detect more subtle abnormalities. As a primary myocardial disorder ARVC is characterized by structural changes with localized or diffuse atrophy of predominantly RV myocardium and replacement with fatty and fibrous tissue. However, clinically significant disease can be present, manifesting with VT or SCD before structural abnormalities become apparent, therefore other diagnostic criteria are important (Table 35.3).

Antiarrhythmic treatment of ARVC includes drug therapy, catheter ablation, and ICD implantation. Treatment is based on risk stratification using the features described in Table 35.4.

Table 35.3 Diagnosis of ARVC

Diagnosis of ARVC	Two major or one major and two minor or four minor criteria
	1) Extensive structural abnormalities in the RV
	2) Fibrofatty replacement of myocardium on biopsy
	3) Conduction abnormalities (QRS>110 ms in V1, epsilon wave)
	4) Family history of ARVC confirmed at necropsy or surgery
Major criteria	
	ε wave
Minor criteria	1) Mild-to-moderate structural abnormalities of the RV
	2) ECG abnormalities (T-wave inversion in V2–V3, late potentials)
	3) Ventricular arrhythmias (LBBB type VT, frequent ventricular ectopics)
	4) Family history of ARVC or SCD due to suspected ARVD

Table 35.4 Risk features of ARVD/C

High-risk features	Low-risk features
Severe RV dysfunction	Localized RV disease
LV involvement	
A history of syncope or cardiac arrest	
Family history of sudden cardiac death	Monomorphic VT suppressed by antiarrhythmic drugs
Inducible VT/VF	
ECG abnormalities (epsilon potential, late potential)	

Further reading

Wellens HJ (2001). Electrophysiology: Ventricular tachycardia: diagnosis of broad QRS complex tachycardia. *Heart*; **86**: 579–585.

Shah M, Akar FG, Tomaselli GF (2005). Molecular basis of arrhythmias. *Circulation*; **112**: 2517–2529.

ACC/AHA/ESC (2006). ACC/AHA/ESC 2006 Guidelines for Management of Patients with Ventricular Arrhythmias and the Prevention of Sudden Cardiac Death: ESC Clinical Practice Guidelines. *Europace*; **8**: 746–837.

Basso C, Corrado D, Marcus FI, Nava A, Thiene G. (2009). Arrhythmogenic right ventricular cardiomyopathy. *Lancet*; **373**: 1289–1300.

Case 36

A 61-year-old woman presented to the ED with a 1-day history of intermittent nausea, retching, and epigastric pain. Her past medical history included Nissen fundoplication for hiatus hernia 16 years previously. This was revised laparoscopically 1 year prior to this presentation when the hiatus hernia recurred. Her only regular medication was lansoprazole.

Examination revealed dehydration and mild epigastric tenderness but was otherwise normal. The patient was admitted for rehydration and endoscopy. Routine blood tests and ECG were unremarkable. Her chest X-ray is shown in Fig. 36.1. Abdominal X-ray was normal.

She was admitted under the surgical team on call, who prescribed analgesia (paracetamol and dihydrocodeine) and antiemetics (cyclizine), and requested an oesophagogastroduodensocopy (OGD).

Two days later, at 6 am, she developed intermittent dull retrosternal chest pain at rest and was referred to the resident medical officer. There were no risk factors for IHD. Her ECG is shown in Fig. 36.2. Treatment for acute coronary syndrome was started before the patient was transferred to the CCU. The ECG performed on admission to the CCU (whilst the patient was pain free) was normal.

Several attempts to pass a nasogastric tube were unsuccessful. The tube coiled in the mouth and would not pass into the oesophagus. The endoscopy was cancelled and a CT scan of the chest and abdomen was requested urgently.

However, shortly after admission to CCU the patient deteriorated and lost cardiac output. Monitoring still revealed sinus rhythm so CPR was started following the algorithm for an electromechanical dissociation (EMD) cardiac arrest. Cardiac output was restored after two cycles of CPR. No drugs were administered during CPR. The patient was intubated, ventilated, and started on inotropes.

On TTE it was difficult to visualize the left atrium, which appeared small and compressed by an extrinsic mass that moved asynchronously with the LA.

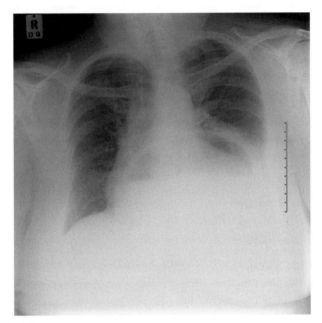

Fig. 36.1 Chest X-ray

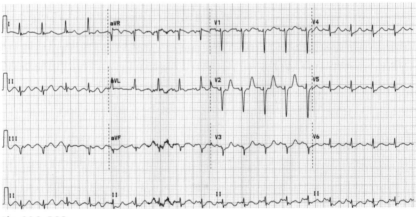

Fig. 36.2 ECG

Questions

1. What does the chest X-ray (Fig. 36.1) show?
2. What does the ECG (Fig. 36.2) show?
3. What are the most common causes of chest pain? What clinical features can guide further investigation?
4. What may cause extrinsic compression of the left atrium?
5. What does the failure to pass the nasogastric tube suggest?
6. What is the most likely cause of the chest pain, dynamic ECG changes, extrinsic left atrial compression and cardiac arrest in this case?
7. How would you investigate this patient?
8. What is the definitive management?

Answers

1) **What does the chest X-ray (Fig. 36.1) show?**

   The chest X-ray shows a large hiatus hernia with an air fluid level behind the heart.

2) **What does the ECG (Fig. 36.2) show?**

   The ECG shows sinus rhythm at a rate of 110 bpm. The QRS axis is normal. There is upsloping ST depression in leads V_3–V_6.

3) **What are the most common causes of chest pain? What clinical features can guide further investigation?**

   The common cardiac and non-cardiac sources of chest pain are listed in Table 36.1. The clinical features that can be used to guide further investigation include type of pain (visceral, somatic, neuropathic), associated tenderness, radiation, changes with posture, respiration or food/fluids, and response GTN or antacids.

Table 36.1 Common cardiac and non-cardiac sources of chest pain and the associated clinical features

Source				Affected by			
	Type	Radiate	Tender	Posture/ move	Breathing	Food/ fluid	GTN
ACS	Visceral	Yes Left arm/ neck/jaw	No	No	No	No	Yes
Dissecting aneurysm	Visceral	Yes Back/as ACS	No	No	No	No	Sometimes
Pericardium/ pleura/PE	Somatic	No	Sometimes	Yes	Yes	No	No
Lung tissue	Visceral/ somatic	No (usually)	No	No	Yes	No	No
Pneumo- thorax	Visceral/ somatic	No	No (usually)	No	No	No	No
Musculo- skeletal	Somatic	No	Yes	Yes	Yes	No	No
Nerve	Somatic/ neuro- pathic	Sometimes	Yes	Sometimes	No	No	No
GI	Visceral	Yes	Sometimes	No	No	Yes	Sometimes

4) **What may cause extrinsic compression of the left atrium?**

Extrinsic compression of the left atrium is a rare cause of haemodynamic compromise that can be caused by any abnormal adjacent structure. Examples reported in the literature include bronchogenic cysts, malignancy, thymoma, aneurysms of the aorta, diaphragmatic hernia, and intrathoracic gastric structures.

The investigation of choice for the diagnosis atrial compression is TTE. Extrinsic masses move asynchronously with the atria. In contrast, the movement of intrinsic atrial abnormalities (e.g. thrombus or myxoma) is synchronized with the movement of the atria. The stomach can be identified by ingestion of a carbonated drink, which produces air contrast. After identification of an LA mass, CT can provide more comprehensive assessment and determine the origin of the mass.

The electrical mechanical dissassociation (EMD) cardiac arrest in this case may have resulted from obstruction of inflow to the LA. This could directly reduce LV filling and cause functional tamponade.

5) **What does the failure to pass the nasogastric tube suggest?**

Consider oesophageal obstruction if it is not possible to pass a nasogastric tube in a patient with a hiatus hernia.

6) **What is the most likely cause of the chest pain, dynamic ECG changes, extrinsic left atrial compression, and cardiac arrest in this case?**

Acute intrathoracic gastric volvulus, a rare complication of hiatus hernia.

Gastric volvulus is defined as abnormal rotation of the stomach or part of the stomach through at least 180°, creating a closed-loop obstruction that can result in incarceration and strangulation. This torsion compromises the gastric blood supply and causes gastric outlet obstruction.

Acute volvulus and strangulation is a surgical emergency that often presents with Borchardt's triad (pain, retching, and inability to pass a nasogastric tube). Chronic gastric volvulus often present with chronic, non-specific symptoms of chest pain, abdominal pain, distension, and early satiety. However, the symptoms may fluctuate if the volvulus is intermittent, and abdominal symptoms and signs can be absent if the volvulus is intrathoracic.

If the volvulus is not reduced the stomach distends and eventually becomes necrotic. Intrathoracic gastric distension can cause cardiovascular compromise and may therefore masquerade as MI. If the stomach ruptures, the patient may die from sepsis and hypotensive shock. The mortality associated with gastric volvulus is high. Acute gastric volvulus is a surgical emergency.

Gastric volvulus is classified as either type 1 (idiopathic) or type 2 (congenital or acquired).

Type 1 (Idiopathic)

Two-thirds of cases are idiopathic. This type is more common in adults but has been reported in children. In these cases, gastric volvulus may be due to laxity of the gastro-splenic, gastroduodenal, gastrophrenic, and gastrohepatic ligaments. Laxity of these ligaments could predispose to volvulus by allowing approximation of the cardia and pylorus when the stomach is full.

Type 2 (congenital or acquired)

The remaining one-third of cases of gastric volvulus are associated with congenital or acquired abnormalities that result in abnormal mobility of the stomach.

The most common causes of gastric volvulus in adults are diaphragmatic defects. Other causes of secondary gastric volvulus in adults are listed in Table 36.2.

Table 36.2 Causes of secondary gastric volvulus in adults

Diaphragmatic defects	Hiatus hernia trauma
Surgery	Nissen fundoplication
	Total oesophagectomy
	Laparoscopic adjustable gastric band placement
	Hepatectomy (ligation of the hepatogastric ligament)
	Highly selective vagotomy
	Coronary artery bypass graft
Neuromuscular disease	Motor neuron disease
	Poliomyelitis
	Myotonic dystrophy
Raised intra-abdominal pressure	Abdominal masses
Causes of raised diaphragm	Phrenic nerve palsy
	Left-lung resection
	Intrapleural adhesions

7) **How would you investigate this patient?**

As the LA compression in this case was most likely to be due to a gastric volvulus OGD was performed on the CCU.

Whilst CT could characterize the nature of the mass in more detail, the patient would have to be transferred to the CT suite to perform this. Although the risk of oesophageal perforation during OGD is significant, it is probably lower than the risk involved in transferring a haemodynamically unstable patient to the radiology department. Furthermore, endoscopic reduction of a gastric volvulus may be considered in selected cases.

In this case, OGD confirmed that gastric volvulus had occurred and the intrathoracic hiatus hernia was strangulated with some areas of necrosis. In this case, endoscopic reduction was not attempted in view of the risk of gastric perforation.

Attempts at endoscopic reduction should be considered for patients with multiple comorbidities in whom surgery would not be appropriate. Endoscopic reduction may also be used as a temporizing measure to allow optimization before surgery.

8) **What is the definitive management?**

The definitive management of acute gastric volvulus requires decompression, reduction, and prevention of recurrence. This is best achieved by urgent surgery.

In this case, the patient was transferred to theatre immediately after the endoscopy. Laparotomy and reduction of the volvulus were performed. Necrotic areas were resected by segmental gastrectomy. A gastrostomy tube was sited to reduce the risk of recurrent gastric volvulus and allow postoperative decompression and enteral feeding. The fundoplication was also revised to reduce gastro-oesophageal reflux and recurrence of the hiatus hernia. The patient was then transferred to the ITU. There was no evidence of extrinsic atrial compression on postoperative TTE. The patient made a good recovery and was discharged from ITU 3 days later. She was discharged home with the gastrostomy *in situ* 7 days later.

On review in cardiology outpatients 3 months after discharge from hospital the patient denied any recurrence of the symptoms of chest pain. The patient completed stage 3 of the full Bruce protocol exercise tolerance test without difficulty and was discharged from follow-up.

Further reading

van Rooijen JM, van den Merkhof LFM (2008). Left atrial impression: a sign of extra-cardiac pathology. *Eur J Echocardiogr*; **9**: 661–664.

Gourgiotis S, Vougas V, Germanos S, Baratsis S (2006). Acute gastric volvulus: diagnosis and management over 10 years. *Dig Surg*; **23**: 169–172.

Teague WJ, Ackroyd RD, Watson DI, Devitt PG (2000). Changing patterns in the management of gastric volvulus over 14 years. *Br J Surg*; **87**: 358–361.

McElreath DP, Olden KW, Aduli F (2008). Hiccups: a subtle sign in the clinical diagnosis of gastric volvulus and a review of the literature. *Dig Dis Sci* **53**: 3033–3036.

Paut O, Mely L, Viard L, Silicani MA, Guys JM, Camboulives J (1996). Acute presentation of congenital diaphragmatic hernia past the neonatal period: a life threatening emergency. *Can J Anaesth*; **43**: 621–625.

Kalra PR, Frymann R, Allen DR (2000). Strangulated gastric volvulus: an unusual cause of cardiac compression resulting in electromechanical dissociation. *Heart*; **83**(5): 550.

Case 37

A 68-year-old retired school teacher was brought to the ED by ambulance with a 4-hour history of chest pain radiating to her jaw. For 4 weeks prior to this presentation she had noticed similar but less severe pain whilst gardening and had taken antacids to try to relieve the pain.

Her risk factors for IHD included type II diabetes (metformin 500 mg three times a day), treated hypertension (perindopril 4 mg daily), and hypercholestrolaemia (simvastatin 20 mg daily). She had been recently diagnosed with obstructive airways disease (COPD) from passive exposure to cigarette smoke at home. In addition, she had mild renal impairment (creatinine 140 μmol/L).

The observations recorded by the paramedics were BP 122/80 mmHg, HR 96 bpm (sinus), and O_2 saturations 99% on air. She was given sublingual GTN, which initially eased the pain, but her symptoms returned before arrival at the hospital.

On examination in the ED she was cold, clammy, and obviously distressed. The JVP was raised, the heart sounds were normal, but a pansystolic murmur was audible. Breath sounds were vesicular but fine inspiratory crepitations were audible in the bases of both lung fields.

An ECG was performed (Fig. 37.1) and the admission cTnI was 20 ng/mL (normal range <0.4 ng/mL). She was admitted to the CCU. She had ongoing pain and the cardiology registrar was therefore asked to review her.

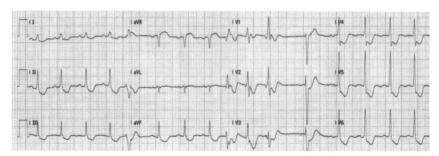

Fig. 37.1 ECG on admission to ED.

Questions

1. Report the ECG in Fig. 37.1.

2. What is the most likely diagnosis?

3. How should the patient be managed in the ED?

4. Which of the following would result in the largest reduction in risk of mortality: aspirin, clopidogrel, abciximab, metoprolol, or diltiazem?

5. Why are nitrates used?

6. Is heparin beneficial if patients have been given dual antiplatelet therapy?

7. What is her ongoing risk and how should this be managed?

8. What is the next investigation she requires and what may this show?

9. Are beta blockers contraindicated given her history of COPD?

10. How should her diabetes be managed on admission?

Answers

1) **Report the ECG in Fig. 37.1.**

The admission ECG shows sinus rhythm at a rate of 96 bpm with a normal QRS axis. There is widespread ST depression (V1–V6, I, II, aVL). There is ST elevation in aVR. During this recording there were frequent ventricular ectopic beats with a RBBB morphology, suggesting a left ventricular origin.

2) **What is the most likely diagnosis?**

The most likely diagnosis is an NSTEMI. The widespread ECG changes suggest left main stem disease. The frequent ectopic beats suggest significant LV ischaemia and electrical instability.

3) **How should the patient be managed in the ED?**

The patient should be given:

  i. oxygen

  ii. symptom control: analgesia (sublingual GTN, morphine iv); antiemetic (e.g. cyclizine iv)

  iii. antiplatelet therapy: aspirin (loading dose 300 mg po), clopidogrel (loading dose 300 mg po)

  iv. anticoagulation: low-molecular-weight heparin (ACS treatment dose)

  v. heart rate control (target 60 bpm): beta-blockers (oral and/or intravenous).

4) **Which of the following would result in the largest reduction in risk of mortality: aspirin, clopidogrel, abciximab, metoprolol, or diltiazem?**

Aspirin

Aspirin inhibits platelet function by irreversible modification of the enzyme cyclooxygenase to prevent conversion of arachidonic acid into thromboxane A_2. Administration of aspirin alone for NSTEMI causes a 53% relative risk (RR) reduction of death or MI (6.2% vs 12.2% events; OR 0.47, 95% CI 0.37–0.61). Hence guidelines recommend starting low-dose aspirin after the loading dose (>300 mg) and continuing medication during long-term follow-up.

Clopidogrel

This is a thienopyridine derivative that inhibits the platelet aggregation pathway that involves adenosine diphosphate (ADP). It is of proven benefit in the context of acute MI: the clopidogrel in unstable angina to prevent recurrent events (CURE) trial (12 562 patients) studied the acute use of clopidogrel in addition to aspirin, and continued for a median of 9 months, in NSTEMI. There was a 20% reduction in the incidence of cardiovascular death, MI, or stroke (9.3% versus 11.4% events with aspirin alone; hazard ratio 0.80, 95% CI 0.72–0.90) without any significant increase in life-threatening bleeding. These finding were confirmed by the NSTEMI subgroup in the clopidogrel for the reduction of events during observation trial (CREDO) trial. Current guidelines support the use of dual antiplatelet therapy in all patients.

Glycoprotein IIb/IIIa inhibitors (GP IIb/IIa, e.g. abciximab)

These act on the final common pathway of platelet aggregation: surface GP-IIb/IIIa receptor activation and prevent binding of fibrinogen to form platelet thrombi. They are highly effective in the treatment of NSTEMI: a meta-analysis of 10 RCTs (13 166 patients) demonstrated a 36% reduction in the incidence of death or MI at 30 days. Particular benefit was seen in the subgroups, who had early invasive evaluation and were troponin positive or diabetic.

Beta-blockers

These decrease cardiac work and oxygen demand, lengthen diastole, and improve coronary flow. Guidelines recommend them as a routine part of care in ACS. A meta-analysis of RCTs of acute intravenous beta-blockers followed by oral treatment for a week in NSTEMI demonstrated a 13% reduction in the risk of MI.

Calcium channel blockers

There are three subclasses of calcium channel blockers, differing in the degree of vasodilatation they cause:

 i. dihydropyridines (e.g. amlodipine and nifedipine) – most potent peripheral arterial vasodilators

 ii. benzothiazepines (e.g. diltiazem) – less potent peripheral arterial vasodilators

 iii. phenylalkylamines (e.g. verapamil) – least potent vasodilators but decrease contractility and delay atrioventricular conduction.

All subclasses cause similar coronary vasodilatation and are comparable to beta-blockers in symptom control but do not reduce mortality or morbidity. Hence, guidelines recommend CCBs for symptom relief in patients who do not respond to beta-blockers and nitrates.

5) **Why are nitrates used?**

The role of nitrates in the management of NSTEMI is based on extrapolation from pathophysiological principles and clinical observations. There are no RCTs of clinical efficacy.

Nitrates act on both the peripheral and the coronary circulations, predominantly causing venodilation. Nitrates reduce preload, LV end-diastolic volume, and therefore myocardial oxygen consumption. In addition, they dilate normal and atherosclerotic coronary arteries and increase coronary collateral flow, providing symptomatic relief of pain.

6) **Is heparin beneficial if patients have been given dual antiplatelet therapy?**

Although dual antiplatelet therapy inhibits the formation of platelet thrombi, the exposed tissue factor at the site of plaque rupture can still activate the clotting cascade and produce thrombin. Thrombin is a potent platelet activator and catalyses conversion of fibrinogen to fibrin, promoting thrombus propagation. Unfractionated heparin rapidly inhibits thrombin by binding antithrombin III, slowing thrombus formation, and facilitating endogenous fibrinolysis. However, the affinity of heparin for antithrombin III binding sites is variable so monitoring of APTT is required and anticoagulation with heparin is often subtherapeutic.

Low-molecular-weight heparins consist of fragments of heparin molecules that have increased antifactor Xa activity. LMWHs have a more predictable anticoagulant response and a longer plasma half-life. LMWHs are administered subcutaneously based on a weight-adjusted dose; laboratory monitoring is not necessary in routine practice.

Heparins are less active against thrombin that is already bound to fibrin. Thrombin bound to fibrin remains enzymatically active and propagates thrombus formation by continued clotting factor and platelet activation. In contrast, direct thrombin inhibitors (e.g. bivalirudin) bind to bound thrombin and block the enzyme's interaction with substrates.

NSTEMI RCTs evaluated the addition of heparin to aspirin for 2–7 days after admission, and also compared unfractionated heparin with LMWH. There was a 34% reduction in the incidence of death or MI with the addition of heparin (7.9% vs 10.4% events; OR 0.67 and 95% CI 0.44–0.99). LMWH produced a 61% event reduction compared with heparin (2.1% vs 5.2% events; OR 0.39 and 95% CI 0.22–0.86).

Direct thrombin inhibitors have also been evaluated in this setting. Overall there was a small additional reduction (8%) in the incidence of death or MI at 30 days compared with LMWH (9.7% vs 10.6% events; OR 0.92 and 95% CI 0.87–0.98), with a significantly lower major bleeding risk with bivalirudin. The recent organisation for the assessment of strategies for ischaemic syndromes 5 trial (OASIS 5 trial) reported that the factor Xa inhibitor fondaparinux was as effective as LMWH in terms of prevention of ischaemic complications, but there were fewer associated bleeding complications. This resulted in an overall mortality benefit from fondaparinux, which has therefore been included in the most recent NICE guidelines for ACS.

7) **What is her ongoing risk and how should this be managed?**

Risk stratification should address short-term risks of acute thrombotic events and long-term risks of disease progression. Recurrent episodes of ischaemic chest pain with dynamic ST-segment depression, ventricular arrhythmias (ventricular tachycardia, ventricular fibrillation), haemodynamic instability (symptoms of shock), and diabetes increase short-term risk.

An elevated cTn is an independent predictor. In a substudy of the fragmin during instability in coronary artery disease (FRISC) trial prognosis over a 5-month period correlated with absolute concentrations of cardiac tropins T, with the peak value during the first 24 hours being particularly useful in assessing risk (the TIMI IIIB trial demonstrated 7.5% mortality at 42 days in patients with the highest troponin I values). The negative predictive value is also useful, and in combination with a normal predischarge exercise test identifies a low-risk group (death and MI <1%).

Risk scores simplify assessment and triage. The TIMI risk score (Table 37.1) was derived from clinical trial data in STEMI populations and integrates historical (age, diabetes, hypertension, or previous ischaemic heart disease), physical (BP, HR, and Killip class) and other data (ST-segment deviation or LBBB) in determining risk. It has been validated against registry data [Correlation (C) index 0.74 overall]. The GRACE risk score (Fig. 37.2) was derived directly from registry data from all types of ACS with multivariate analysis identifying eight important components of risk for in-hospital and 6-month post-discharge death or MI. It was validated prospectively against the Global utilization of streptokinase and tissue plasminogen activator for occluded coronary arteries GUSTO-IIB data set [C index 0.84 (in-hospital) and 0.71 (post discharge)]. In addition, the Grace

Table 37.1 TIMI risk score for unstable anginas (UA)/ST elevation myocardial infarction (NSTEMI)

Age ≥ 65 years?	☑	Yes +1
≥ 3 risk factors for CAD?	☑	Yes +1
Known CAD (stenosis ≥ 50%)?	☐	Yes +1
ASA use in past 7d?	☑	Yes +1
Severe angina (≥ 2 episodes w/in 24 hrs)?	☑	Yes +1
ST changes ≥ 0.5mm?	☑	Yes +1
+ Cardiac marker?	☑	Yes +1
Score	6 points	

41% risk at 14 days of: all-cause mortality, new or recurrent MI, or severe recurrent ischemia requiring urgent revascularization.

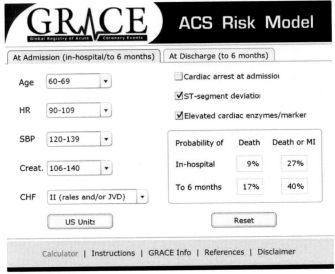

Fig. 37.2 GRACE risk score for UA/NSTEMI. Copyright (1998–2011) Center for Outcomes Research, University of Massachusettes Medical School.

6-month risk score, long-term risk of mortality is related to age, risk factor profile, ventricular function, and coronary anatomy, and biochemical markers of inflammation (CRP) are strongly associated with increased mortality.

One of the most important management considerations is whether early revascularization would be beneficial. The Grace and TIMI scores place her at high risk of ongoing or recurrent ischaemia that may lead to MI or death where the evidence for intervention is strongest.

8) **What is the next investigation she requires and what may this show?**

In patients with high-risk NSTEMI urgent coronary angiography is indicated. Given the ECG findings (Fig. 37.1), she is likely to have either critical three-vessel disease or a left main stem stenosis.

Figure 37.3 shows a selected image from the coronary angiogram. There is a distal left main stenosis. The evidence suggests that left main stem stenoses, particularly when they are distal and involving the bifurcation, are best treated surgically. The case was discussed with the on-call cardiothoracic team. However, in view of the history of airways disease the surgical risk in the setting of acute NSTEMI was deemed too high, and the patient was offered high-risk angioplasty and stenting. She agreed, and the left main bifurcation stenosis was treated successfully with drug-eluting stents.

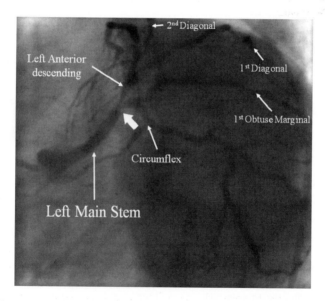

Fig. 37.3 Coronary angiogram 'spider view' demonstrating a long left main stem that has a critical distal stenosis (large arrow) involving the bifurcation into the LAD and circumflex coronary arteries.

The cornerstone of the management of non-ST elevation ACS (NSTE-ACS) is risk assessment for the presence of coronary disease that would benefit from revascularization and preventative risk-factor management strategies.

This case describes the assessment and management of a patient with 'high-risk' features. However, a large proportion patients with NSTE-ACS are stratified as being at 'low risk' of significant coronary disease on the basis of either calculated prediction scores (e.g. Grace or TIMI methods), or the presence of all the following clinical features:

I. No recurrence of chest pain (i.e. a single episode).

II. No signs of heart failure.

III. No abnormalities seen on the initial ECG or on a second ECG performed 6–12 hours later.

IV. No elevation of troponin either on arrival or after 6 hours and 12 hours from symptom onset.

There should be a low threshold for offering invasive angiography to 'low-risk' patients, particularly if there is concern that the predicted mortality risk is not insignificant. There is debate in the literature as to the optimal timing of this, but it is clear that angiography should occur within 72 hours.

9) **Are beta-blockers contraindicated because of her COPD?**

The benefits of beta-blockers that have been outlined above are often denied to those with or suspected to have COPD for fear of inducing bronchoconstriction. However, there is little evidence to support this, and selective beta-1-adrenergic blockers (e.g. metoprolol, bisoprolol, and atenolol) are well tolerated by patients with COPD who do not have reversible airway obstruction. Even in patients with mild-to-moderate reversible airway disease significant adverse respiratory effects have not been reported. In those with significant reversibility or who have active bronchospasm beta blockade is contraindicated. Hence, in this case the patient should be beta blocked. However, the beta-blocker should be discontinued if it causes a deterioration in symptoms or lung function.

10) **How should her diabetes be managed on admission?**

Hyperglycaemia in the context of an ACS predicts poor short- and long-term outcomes with RCTs trials of an insulin glucose infusion the diabetes mellitus insulin-glucose infusion in acute myocardial infarction trial (DIGAMI) being associated with an 11% reduction in mortality at 24 hours (number needed to treat of 9 to save one life) and if tight control was maintained with subcutaneous insulin a 30% reduction in mortality at 3.4 years. DIGAMI 2 did not show any clinically relevant differences between different blood glucose-lowering regimens. In those already identified as diabetic, acute glycaemic control was able to reduce 24-hour mortality and in-hospital mortality to that of non-diabetics.

Further reading

Salpeter SR, Ormiston TM, Salpeter EE (2005). Cardioselective beta-blockers for chronic obstructive pulmonary disease. *Cochrane Database Syst Rev*; **Issue 4**.

ESC Clinical Practice Guidelines (2007). Universal definition of myocardial infarction. *Eur Heart J*; **28**: 2525–2538.

Report of Taskforce of European Society of Cardiology (2007). Management of acute coronary syndromes (ACS) in patients presenting without persistent ST-segment elevation. *Eur Heart J*; **28**: 1598–1660.

The Task Force on Diabetes and Cardiovascular Diseases of the European Society of Cardiology (ESC) and of the European Association for the Study of Diabetes (EASD) (2007). Guidelines on diabetes, pre-diabetes, and cardiovascular diseases: executive summary. *Eur Heart J*; **28**: 88–136.

Case 38

A 43-year-old woman underwent elective Caesarean section for placenta praevia 36 weeks into her second pregnancy. She was readmitted 10 days after delivery with pneumonia and oral moxifloxacin was started. Two days later, she developed diarrhoea and vomiting, and admission blood cultures grew *Streptococcus pneumoniae*. She was treated with cyclizine and domperidone, and moxifloxacin was continued.

Seven days after readmission, the patient had a fit in bed that terminated spontaneously after 1 minute. Blood glucose was 6.0 mmol/L. Several hours later, the patient had a second fit whilst awaiting brain MRI. This was followed by cardiorespiratory arrest and CPR was commenced. The initial cardiac rhythm is shown in Fig. 38.1. The treatment of this resulted in the cardiac rhythm shown in Fig. 38.2.

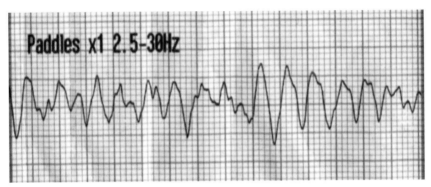

Fig. 38.1 Initial rhythm during cardiac arrest.

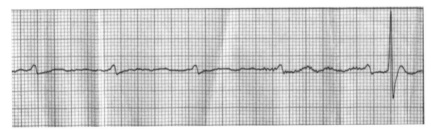

Fig. 38.2 Rhythm during cardiac arrest.

Blood taken during CPR revealed: Hb 12g/dL, WCC 16 × 10⁹ cells/L, platelets and CRP 200 mg/dL, glucose 7.8 mmol/L, Na+ 141 mmol/L, K+ 2.7 mmol/L, urea 1.7 mmol/L, and creatinine 85 μmol/L.

Cardiac output and spontaneous respiratory effort were restored within 3 minutes of cardiac arrest. The patient was extubated but remained drowsy with a GCS of 10 (E2, V3, M5) for nearly 1 hour. Examination was otherwise normal. Chest X-ray was unremarkable. Figure 38.3 is the 12 lead ECG performed on admission to hospital. Figure 38.4 shows the 12 lead ECG performed shortly after restoration of cardiac output after the cardiac arrest.

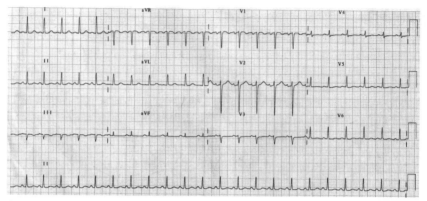

Fig. 38.3 ECG on admission.

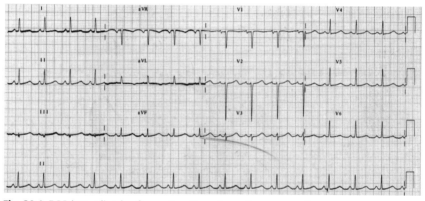

Fig. 38.4 ECG immediately after restoration of spontaneous cardiac output.

Questions

1. What is the cardiac rhythm shown in Fig 38.1? What is the treatment?
2. What is the cardiac rhythm shown in Fig. 38.2?
3. What is the difference between the pre-arrest (Fig. 38.3) and post-arrest (Fig. 38.4) ECGs? What is the most likely cause and is the pregnancy relevant?
4. What are the other causes of the abnormality noted in question 3?
5. What is likely to have caused the seizures in this case?
6. How would you manage this patient?

Answers

1) **What is the cardiac rhythm shown in Fig. 38.1? What is the treatment?**

Figure 38.2A shows ventricular fibrillation. The treatment is defibrillation and cardiopulmonary resuscitation.

2) **What is the cardiac rhythm shown in Fig. 38.2?**

The ECG rhythm strip in Fig. 38.2 initially shows regular P waves but no QRS complexes, that is, ventricular standstill. Defibrillation had restored atrial activity but as a result of transient AV block there was initially no ventricular activity. The last P wave on the rhythm strip is followed by a QRS complex. In this case, this was also associated with restoration of cardiac output and sinus rhythm.

If the AV block persists, percussion pacing or external pacing should be started. Transvenous pacing should then be considered.

3) **What is the difference between the pre-arrest (Fig. 38.3) and post-arrest (Fig. 38.4) ECGs? What is the most likely cause and is the pregnancy relevant?**

The 12 lead ECG performed on admission (Fig. 38.3) is normal. However, the post-arrest ECG (Fig 38.4) shows prolongation of the QT-interval at 0.44 seconds. Bazett's square root correction for rate suggests a QT_c of 0.55 seconds.

However, Bazett's correction over-reads the QT_c at faster heart rates, as in this case. If the cube root correction of Fridericia is used then QT_c is more modest (0.49 seconds) but clearly still prolonged. This observation is less relevant in this case, but is very important when considering the potential cardiotoxicity of drugs such as antibiotics and antipsychotic/antidepressants in clinical trials, when heart rate may vary significantly. The best method of analysis to detect drug-induced QT change within a clinical trial is to determine the relationship between QT and HR in the placebo population and apply the relevant correction to the treatment group.

In this case, the cause of the prolonged QT-interval is most likely to be the low serum potassium and moxifloxacin. However, congenital LQTS exacerbated by hypokalaemia and the co-prescription of QT prolonging drugs should be considered in the differential diagnosis.

Pregnancy is not associated with an increased incidence of cardiac events in LQTS. However, the incidence of cardiac events in women with congenital LQTS is increased postpartum. Treatment with beta-blockers during and following pregnancy is recommended for all affected women and relatives with prolonged QTc, even in the absence of previous symptoms.

4) **What are the other causes of the abnormality noted in question 3?**

Prolongation of the QT-interval may be congenital or acquired.

Congenital LQTS results from mutations in genes encoding for the sodium and potassium channels in cardiac cells. Delayed closure of the sodium channel results in prolongation of inward current while potassium channel mutations result in delayed repolarization. Both mechanisms result in prolongation of the QT-interval and increased disposition to early after-depolarizations and polymorphic VT (torsade de pointes), often preceded by an increase in sinus rate. Individual paroxysms of torsade de pointes are usually self-limiting but if persistent cardiac arrest will occur and emergency defibrillation is necessary.

A variety of congenital syndromes have been described, including Jervell–Lange–Nielsen, an autosomal recessive condition associated with neural deafness, and Romano Ward, an autosomal condition without deafness. To date, more than 250 different mutations in seven genes have been identified as potential causes of the LQTS. Episodes of torsade de pointes may be associated with sympathetic stimulation, including exercise and fear, and cause syncope and sometimes convulsion. As a result, patients may be misdiagnosed as epileptic. Congenital LQTS is probably under diagnosed, particularly as 10–15% of gene carriers may have normal QT_c. The prevalence of LQTS mutation carriers is therefore difficult to determine but estimates of up to 1 in 1000 have been suggested. Criteria used to assist the diagnosis of congenital LQTS are listed in Table 38.1.

Table 38.1 Diagnostic criteria for LQTS

Criteria	Points	
ECG[1]		
QTc	>480 ms	3
	460–469 ms	2
	450–459 ms (male)	1
Torsade de pointes		2
T-wave alternans		1
Notched T wave in 3 leads		1
Low heart rate for age		0.5
Clinical history		
Syncope	With stress	2
	Without stress	1
Congenital deafness		0.5
Family history		
A. Family members with definite LQTS		1
B. Unexplained sudden cardiac death <30 years in a first-degree relative		0.5

[1]In the absence of medications or disorders known to affect these electrocardiographic features. Definite LQTS is defined by an LQTS score ≥4.

In acquired LQTS, in contrast to the congenital syndromes, a slowing of the HR and postextrasystolic pause often initiates the arrhythmia. Patients with acquired LQTS may also be misdiagnosed with epilepsy or the patient may be thought to have self-terminating VT or VF unless the characteristic morphology of torsades de pointes and the QT prolongation is recognized. Accurate diagnosis is essential as empirical antiarrhythmic therapy may worsen the arrhythmia through further lengthening of the QT interval. Drugs that may cause acquired LQTS are listed in Table 38.2. It is interesting in this case that the initial ECG when tachycardic did not reveal clearcut QT prolongation, although the interval is difficult to measure with early P-wave onset.

Table 38.2 Some drugs known to cause prolongation of the QT interval

Adrenaline
Antihistamines
Antibiotics—erythromycin, septrin, fluoroquinolones (particularly moxifloxacin)
Antiarrhythmics—sotalol, amiodarone
Antifungal drugs—ketoconazole, fluconazole, cisapride
Psychotropic drugs
– tricyclics (amitriptyline)
– haloperidol, risperidone

Important risk factors for drug-induced QT prolongation are female sex, electrolyte disturbances (hypokalaemia and hypomagnesaemia), hypothermia, thyroid dysfunction, structural heart disease, bradycardia, and, of course, drugs.

Patients who have a drug-induced long QT-interval may be genetically predisposed because of the presence of an underlying mild or attenuated form of congenital LQTS. The principal ion channel affected by the QT-interval prolonging drugs is IKr (HERG), the same ion channel that causes congenital LQTS. However, data are insufficient to claim that all patients with drug-induced QT prolongation have a genetic LQTS-related mechanism.

5) **What is likely to have caused the seizures in this case?**

After the cardiac arrest, the seizures were thought to be secondary to global cerebral ischaemia resulting from polymorphic ventricular tachycardia (torsades de pointes).

In this patient, polymorphic VT degenerating into pulseless VT was captured by cardiac monitoring in association with a third seizure on the ITU. Defibrillation restored sinus rhythm and cardiac output.

Prior to the cardiac arrest, the differential diagnosis included neurological causes of syncope:

- Drug-induced reduction of seizure threshold
  - moxifloxacin
- Intracranial venous thrombosis
  - postpartum high-risk period
- Eclampsia
  - 25% of seizures occur postpartum
- Epilepsy

6) **How would you manage this patient?**

Management of this patient with acquired LQTS should include:

- cardiac monitor
- intravenous serum potassium replacement
- intravenous magnesium sulphate
- cessation of drugs that prolong the QT interval
- beta blockade
- echocardiography and a 24-hour tape.

In acquired LQTS, any predisposing drugs should be discontinued and electrolyte disturbance, particularly hypokalaemia, should be corrected. Intravenous magnesium is safe and may be effective. Since the arrhythmia is associated with brady-cardia and pauses, the heart rate should be increased, if necessary through overdrive pacing or isoprenaline infusion, although this should be done with caution in case acute ischaemia is triggered. High-dose beta blockade is effective in the congenital LQTS, although pacemaker or defibrillator implantation may be required in resistant cases. A thorough drug history should be taken in cases of unexplained prolonged QT interval and the patient should be asked about any previous episodes of syncope or seizures or family history of such events.

In this patient, administration of metoprolol and correction of the potassium to 4.5 mmol/L over the next 24 hours reduced the QT_c to 0.45 seconds (Fig. 38.5B). Echocardiogram was normal. There were no further convulsions or arrhythmias and within 1 week the QT_c had returned to the pre-arrest duration of 0.38 seconds. The patient was discharged on atenolol with outpatient follow-up arranged with a cardiac electrophysiologist. At this appointment a diagnosis of acquired LQTS was thought to be most likely as there had been no recurrence of symptoms and no previous or family history of syncope. The atenolol was stopped. The patient was advised which drugs she should avoid.

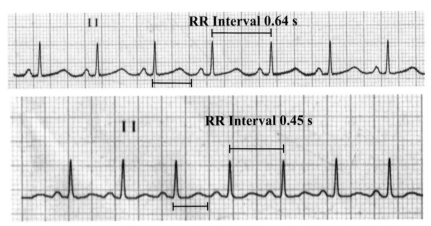

Fig. 38.5 A, Rhythm strip from ECG in Fig. 38.3. QT interval 0.44 seconds. QT_C interval 0.55 seconds ($0.44/\sqrt{0.64}$). B, Rhythm strip from ECG after correction of potassium and administration of atenolol and magnesium. QT interval 0.3 seconds. QT_C interval 0.45 seconds ($0.3/\sqrt{0.45}$).

Further reading

Priori SG, Napolitano C, Schwartz PJ (1999). Low penetrance in the LQTS: clinical impact. *Circulation*; **99**: 529–533.

Rashba EJ, Zareba W, Moss AJ, Hall WJ, Robinson J, Locati EH, Schwartz PJ, Andrews M. (1998). Influence of pregnancy on the risk for cardiac events in patients with hereditary long QT syndrome. LQTS Investigators. *Circulation*; **97**: 451–456.

Roden DM (2008). Long QT syndrome. *New Engl J Med*; **358**(2): 169–176.

Zipes DP, Camm AJ, Borggrefe M, Buxton AE, Chaitman B, Fromer M, Gregoratos G, Klein G, Moss AJ, Myerburg RJ, Priori SG, Quinones MA, Roden DM, Silka MJ, Tracy C, Smith SC Jr, Jacobs AK, Adams CD, Antman EM, Anderson JL, Hunt SA, Halperin JL, Nishimura R, Ornato JP, Page RL, Riegel B, Blanc JJ, Budaj A, Dean V, Deckers JW, Despres C, Dickstein K, Lekakis J, McGregor K, Metra M, Morais J, Osterspey A, Tamargo JL, Zamorano JL; American College of Cardiology/American Heart Association Task Force; European Society of Cardiology Committee for Practice Guidelines; European Heart Rhythm Association; Heart Rhythm Society. (2006). ACC/AHA/ESC 2006 Guidelines for Management of Patients with Ventricular Arrhythmias and the Prevention of Sudden Cardiac Death: a report of the American College of Cardiology/American Heart Association Task Force and the European Society of Cardiology Committee for Practice Guidelines (writing committee to develop Guidelines for Management of Patients With Ventricular Arrhythmias and the Prevention of Sudden Cardiac Death): developed in collaboration with the European Heart Rhythm Association and the Heart Rhythm Society. *Circulation*; 114(10): e385–484.

Morissette P, Hreiche R, Turgeon J (2005). Drug-induced long QT syndrome and torsade de pointes. *Can J Cardiol*; **21**: 857–864.

Hreiche R, Morissette P, Turgeon J (2008). Drug-induced long QT syndrome in women: review of current evidence and remaining gaps. *Gender Med*; **5**: 124–135.

www.QTdrugs.org–an updated list of drugs which cause prolongation of the QT interval.

Case 39

A 65-year-old man awaiting a laparoscopic right nephrectomy for renal cell carcinoma was referred for a preoperative cardiology opinion.

He had type 2 diabetes treated with metformin, hypertension, and was an ex-smoker. Three months prior to this referral, whilst on holiday in Greece, he had an anterior STEMI that was initially treated with thrombolysis. He was subsequently commenced on aspirin 75 mg daily, clopidogrel 75 mg daily, simvastatin 20 mg nocte, and ramipril 5 mg daily. He was not given a beta-blocker because 'his heart rate was too low'. Two days later an isolated mid LAD stenosis was found on angiography. Follow-on angioplasty and stenting with a tacrolimus drug-eluting stent was performed.

No other information about the admission or treatment in Greece was available. He had been advised to see a cardiologist on return to the UK but had forgotten to do so.

He denied having any further episodes of chest pain since returning from Greece. He walked 3 miles every day without difficulty and he could climb three flights of stairs before becoming breathless. However, he had an episode of painless haematuria 2 weeks prior to this referral. Urine cytology demonstrated renal cell carcinoma and CT confirmed the presence of T1N0M0 (stage 1) renal cancer in the right kidney. The patient continued to experience intermittent macroscopic haematuria. His Hb was stable at 14 g/dL.

The consultant anaesthetist reviewing him in the preoperative assessment clinic (PAC) requested an ECG (Fig. 39.1) and an outpatient cardiology opinion.

On examination in the cardiology outpatient clinic he was comfortable at rest, with a regular pulse of 50 bpm and BP of 160/50 mmHg. There were no physical signs of heart failure. Surgery was planned for 2 weeks after the cardiology outpatient appointment and the patient was very keen to proceed in view of the 'ticking time bomb' in his abdomen.

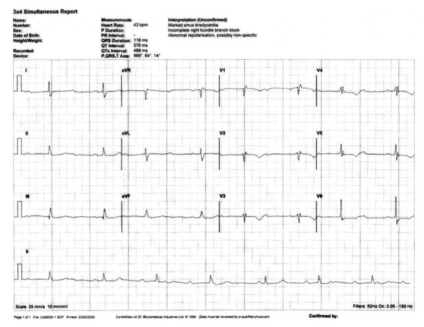

3x4 Simultaneous Report

Name:	Measurements	Interpretation (Unconfirmed)
Number:	Heart Rate: 43 bpm	Marked sinus bradycardia
Sex:	P Duration:	Incomplete right bundle branch block
Date of Birth:	PR Interval: -	Abnormal repolarisation, possibly non-specific
Height/Weight:	QRS Duration: 116 ms	
	QT Interval: 576 ms	
Recorded:	QTc Interval: 488 ms	
Device:	P,QRS,T Axis: 999°, 64°, 14°	

Scale 25 mm/s 10 mm/mV

Filters: 50Hz On; 0.05 - 150 Hz

Page 1 of 1 File LVAEE9–1 SCP Printed 23/02/2009   CardioView v4 25, Micromedical Industries Ltd. © 1999 (Data must be reviewed by a qualified physician)   Confirmed by:

Fig. 39.1 12 lead ECG recorded at preassessment clinic.

Questions

1. Is the automated report of the ECG (Fig. 39.1) correct? If not, what is your interpretation?

2. What clinical signs would confirm your interpretation of the ECG?

3. What is the most likely aetiology of the bradycardia?

4. Is the heart rate likely to respond to atropine?

5. Was any other treatment indicated after the anterior MI in Greece?

6. Is the patient medically optimized for surgery? If not, what should be done prior to surgery?

7. How would you manage the patient's heart rate if emergency surgery was required?

Answers

1) **Is the automated report of the ECG (Fig. 39.1) correct? If not, what is your interpretation?**

   The automated report of the ECG in Fig. 39.1 is not correct.

   The ECG demonstrates third-degree atrioventricular conduction block or complete heart block (CHB), with a narrow complex junctional escape rhythm at 43 bpm. The partial RBBB pattern is due to intraventricular conduction delay. The sinus rate is approximately 100 bpm. Although there is poor R-wave progression consistent with previous anterior MI, there are no pathological Q waves.

   Complete heart block is characterized by the dissociation of atrial and ventricular activity. Symptoms of reduced cardiac output, such as reduced exercise tolerance, breathlessness, fatigue, or syncope, usually occur. Atrioventricular conduction disturbance may occur at any point from the atrioventricular junction to the bundle branch Purkinje system. Varying degrees of block in the AVN, bundle of His, right or left bundle branches, or anterior or posterior divisions of the left bundle branch (left anterior or left posterior fascicular blocks) can occur. Block usually occurs at a single site but can affect two or more components of the conduction system. The AV node and the bundle of His, which form a narrow preferential conduction pathway between the atria and the ventricles, are particularly sensitive to ischaemia and trauma.

2) **What clinical signs would confirm your interpretation of the ECG?**

   Intermittent 'cannon a waves' in the waveform of the jugular venous pulsation indicate atrioventricular dissociation and are a feature of CHB. The intensity of the first heart sound may also vary due to variable positioning of the atrioventricular valves at the onset of ventricular activation. Intermittent atrial filling sounds can also occur.

3) **What is the most likely aetiology of the bradycardia?**

   As there are no reversible causes (i.e. drugs like beta-blockers and calcium channel blockers) in this case the most likely cause of CHB is ischaemic injury to the conduction system after the MI that occurred in Greece. Antecedent atrioventricular conduction delay cannot be excluded in this case. This possibility was considered because of the lack of symptoms; CHB after anterior MI is usually related to extensive myocardial damage.

   Myocardial ischaemia and autonomic derangement in the context of acute MI promote atrioventricular and intraventricular conduction abnormalities. Prompt reperfusion can limit myocardial damage and has reduced the incidence of atrioventricular block after acute MI to about 7%. However, the prevalence of intraventricular conduction disturbances after MI has not changed (18% and persist in 5%).

4) **Is the heart rate likely to respond to atropine?**

   In this case, the good exercise tolerance and the junctional escape rhythm suggest that the patient's heart rate increases in response to exercise and should also respond to atropine. Currently, atropine therapy is not indicated.

The heart rate and the duration of the escape QRS complex depend on the site of the escape rhythm pacemaker and reflect the site of the atrioventricular block. A sustained rhythm between 40 and 60 bpm with narrow QRS complexes suggests a junctional rhythm associated with supra-Hisian block. Patients with a junctional rhythm are often haemodynamically stable. The heart rate usually increases in response to exercise and atropine. Wide QRS complexes at a slower heart rate suggest a block lower in the His–Purkinje system, which is unresponsive to exercise and atropine, so therapeutic intervention is more urgently required.

5) **Was any other treatment indicated after the anterior MI in Greece?**

In patients with anterior MI and conduction disturbance below the bundle of His, first-degree block may progress to complete infra-Hisian block and ventricular stand still. Complete heart block after anterior MI is a sign of extensive myocardial necrosis and usually results in a wide QRS escape rhythm and high mortality (up to 80%).

Resolution of conduction block is uncommon after anterior MI so the threshold for permanent pacing should be lower than after inferior MI. Complete heart block and Mobitz type II second-degree heart block associated with bundle branch block after anterior MI are indications for permanent pacemaker implantation. In this case of the CHB may have been misdiagnosed as a sinus bradycardia in Greece.

Inferior MI is associated with more benign intranodal and atropine-sensitive conduction blocks with narrow QRS escape rhythms above 40 bpm. Heart block is often well tolerated and transient; resolving within 7 days in most cases. The associated mortality is low but permanent pacing is indicated if conduction abnormalities persist beyond 8–14 days.

6) **Is the patient medically optimized for surgery? If not, what should be done prior to surgery?**

The patient is not medically optimized for several reasons:

+ Perioperative cardiovascular morbidity and mortality is increased after a recent MI.
+ Dual-antiplatelet therapy with aspirin and clopidogrel significantly increases the risk of perioperative bleeding. However, clopidogrel should not be stopped within 6 months of implantation of a drug-eluting stent. The risk of acute stent thrombosis increases significantly when platelet function returns after 3–4 days. Furthermore, there is increasing evidence for the benefit of dual-antiplatelet treatment of all patients with stents for at least 12 months.
+ The patient also has CHB. Although the patient is asymptomatic and has an escape rate above 40 bpm, permanent pacemaker implantation is indicated.

The final decision on whether a patient is fit for surgery rests with the anaesthetist. However, in this case the risk of perioperative cardiovascular complications is higher than the risk of complications from the renal cancer. Cancer surgery is considered semielective but can be postponed briefly to allow medical optimization. In general, only life-saving emergency operations should be performed within 3 months of PCI and stenting. However, the patient and the surgeons will be concerned by the delay. Surgery should be performed as soon as possible.

In this case, after extensive discussion involving the surgeons, anaesthetists, cardiologists and the patient, a DDDR permanent pacemaker was implanted and surgery was postponed until 6 months after the anterior MI. Clopidogrel was then stopped and the patient underwent laparoscopic right nephrectomy. Aspirin was continued throughout the perioperative period. After the operation the patient was initially observed in the ITU but was transferred to the ward on the second postoperative day. There were no complications and the patient was discharged home 5 days later.

Urgent non-cardiac surgery after recent PCI is associated with a high risk of complications, particularly in view of the dual-antiplatelet therapy required after deployment of coronary stents.

Coronary balloon angioplasty

Restenosis after angioplasty may delay non-cardiac surgery and increase the risk of perioperative ischaemia. However, as the injury at the angioplasty site takes some time to heal, operating too soon could also be disadvantageous. The optimum timing is unclear but guidelines based on consensus of expert opinion recommend a delay of 2–4 weeks after balloon angioplasty. The benefit of aspirin should be balanced against the increased risk of bleeding complications from the planned surgery. However, aspirin should usually be continued in the perioperative period with neurosurgery an important exception.

Bare-metal coronary stents

If a stent is deployed, longer delays may be preferable. Instent thrombosis is most common within 2 weeks of stent placement but is rare (<0.3%) after 4 weeks. Stent thrombosis results in Q-wave MI or death in the majority of patients if it occurs. The risk of bare-metal stent thrombosis decreases after the stent has endothelialized (4–6 weeks). Delaying elective non-cardiac surgery by 4–6 weeks allows at least partial endothelialization of the stent. However, restenosis may also occur more than 12 weeks after bare-metal stent deployment and increase the risk of perioperative ischaemia.

Dual-antiplatelet therapy (clopidogrel and aspirin) is generally taken for 4 weeks after bare-metal stent placement to reduce stent thrombosis. However, the risk of bleeding is increased. Late stent thrombosis is rare because bare-metal stents endothelialize more quickly. However, the perioperative cardiac risk of early withdrawal of either or both antiplatelet agents (within 4 weeks) in the perioperative period of non-cardiac surgery is greater than the risk of major bleeding from most operations.

A course of dual-antiplatelet therapy can be completed if non-cardiac surgery is delayed 4–6 weeks after bare-metal stent placement. This reduces the risk of stent thrombosis. Non-cardiac surgery can proceed 1 week after stopping the clopidogrel but aspirin should continue.

The benefit of antiplatelet therapy should be balanced against the increased risk of bleeding complications from the planned surgery. However, aspirin is usually continued in the perioperative period.

Drug-eluting stents

Thrombosis of drug-eluting stents has occurred up to 18 months after deployment. Early withdrawal of antiplatelet therapy greatly increases the risks of stent thrombosis, MI, and death.

Elective operations with high risk of bleeding should be delayed until the required course of dual-antiplatelet therapy has been completed (12 months after drug-eluting stents and at least 1 month after bare-metal stents). Dual-antiplatelet therapy may need to continue after completion of a standard course if there is a high risk of stent thrombosis or the consequences of stent thrombosis could be catastrophic (Table 39.1). After clopidogrel has been stopped, patients with a drug-eluting stent should continue aspirin indefinitely.

Table 39.1 Risk factors for stent thrombosis or significant complications of stent thrombosis

Previous stent thrombosis
Left main stem stent
Multivessel stenting
Stent placement in the only patent coronary artery or graft conduit

If the operation cannot be delayed, the risk of stopping any antiplatelet therapy should be balanced against the benefit of reduction in bleeding complications from the planned surgery. If clopidogrel must be stopped prematurely, aspirin should be continued if possible. Clopidogrel should be restarted as soon as possible after the operation. If the risk of instent thrombosis is high the operation should be performed in an interventional centre where rescue PCI can be performed.

There is no evidence to suggest that warfarin, heparin, or glycoprotein IIb/IIIa agents reduce the risk of instent thrombosis if oral antiplatelet agents are stopped.

Percutaneous coronary intervention in patients requiring urgent non-cardiac surgery

The management of patients who require both PCI and non-cardiac surgery requires careful thought and review of the urgency and risk of bleeding of the non-cardiac surgery.

If the risk of bleeding is low or surgery can be delayed at least 12 months, PCI with drug-eluting stents could be considered. If non-cardiac surgery is required within 1–12 months, then bare-metal stenting and 4–6 weeks of dual-antiplatelet therapy with continuation of aspirin perioperatively should be considered. If the surgery is imminent (within 2–6 weeks) and the risk of bleeding is high, balloon angioplasty could be considered.

In each case aspirin monotherapy and vigilance for restenosis and stent thrombosis are required in the perioperative period. Repeat PCI may be necessary in the event of complications.

If the non-cardiac surgery is urgent or emergency, then cardiac risk, the risk of bleeding, and the benefits of coronary revascularization must be considered. In the rare cases when preoperative coronary revascularization is absolutely necessary, coronary artery bypass grafting and non-cardiac surgery can be performed simultaneously.

7) **How would you manage the patient's heart rate if emergency surgery was required?**

Severe bradycardia or asystole can occur under general anaesthesia in patients with dysfunction of the cardiac-conducting pathways. Anaesthetic agents can impair the function of the autonomic nervous system or directly depress the myocardium. If necessary, transvenous pacing can be performed in the operating theatre pre- or peroperatively, but should not delay surgical management. Balloon flotation pacing wires can be sited without X-ray guidance but X-ray screening is possible in the operating theatre.

In most cases, glycopyrrolate, atropine, isoprenaline, adrenaline, or external transthoracic pacing can be used to treat intraoperative bradyarrhythmias. However, a temporary transvenous pacing wire or permanent pacemaker should then be placed postoperatively.

Elective temporary pacing in the perioperative period is required if the patient has the inherent potential for bradycardia and asystole, or bradycardia and asystole are likely as a result of the operation (e.g. aortic valve surgery). Indications for temporary pacing in the perioperative period are listed in Table 39.2.

Table 39.2 Indications for temporary pacing in the perioperative period

Indications for perioperative temporary pacing
Third-degree AV block
Second-degree AV block
Intermittent AV block
Symptomatic first-degree AV block and bifasicular block
Symptomatic first-degree AV block and LBBB

Further reading

ESC (2009). Pre-operative Cardiac Risk Assessment and Perioperative Cardiac Management in Non-Cardiac Surgery: ESC guidelines. *Eur Heart J*; **30**: 2769–2812.

ACC/AHA (2007). ACC/AHA 2007 guidelines on perioperative cardiovascular evaluation and care for noncardiac surgery: a report of the American College of Cardiology/American Heart Association Task Force on Practice Guidelines. *J Am Coll Cardiol*; **50**: e159–241.

Elizari MV, Acunzo RS, Ferreiro M. (2007). Hemiblocks revisited. *Circulation*; **115**: 1154–1163.

Case 40

A 22-year-old nursery assistant was found collapsed at home by her partner. She was unrousable, had laboured breathing, and her left arm and leg were shaking. On arrival of the paramedics her GCS was 3/15, and she was in respiratory distress with coarse crepitations throughout her chest. Endotracheal (ET) intubation was performed and she was taken to hospital by ambulance. Her partner explained that she had been off work for the last 2 weeks with sinusitis. She had been taking antibiotics for 1 week with no improvement in the periodic fevers, night sweats, and arthralgia. For the preceding 24 hours she had complained of severe abdominal pain and worsening breathlessness. Her GP had attributed these symptoms to the antibiotics.

On arrival in the ED observations were BP 170/80 mmHg, HR 110 bpm (sinus rhythm), O_2 saturations 100% on 50% oxygen via the ET tube, and temperature 37.8°C. The GCS had improved to 9/15 but she appeared agitated. There was a left hemiparesis, nystagmus, and the left plantar response was up going. On auscultation of the heart sounds were normal but a quiet pansystolic murmur was heard over the apex and scattered basal crepitations were present. There was abdominal tenderness with guarding in the left upper quadrant.

Contrast-enhanced CT of the head and abdomen were performed (Figs 40.1 and 40.2). The CT was followed by MRI of the head (Fig. 40.3). She was admitted to the ITU and a cardiology opinion was sought. Both TTE and TOE (Figs. 40.4 and 40.5) were performed.

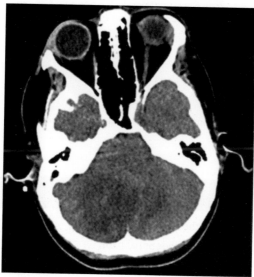

Fig. 40.1 CT head.

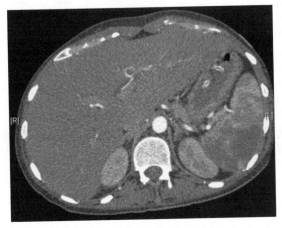

Fig. 40.2 CT abdomen.

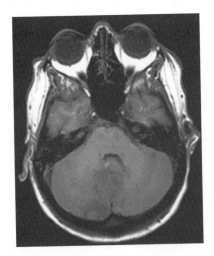

Fig. 40.3 MRI head.

Questions

1. What was the cause of the neurological signs?
2. What was the cause of the abdominal pain?
3. Report the echocardiograms. Is there a unifying diagnosis?
4. What is the next most important investigation?
5. How should this patient be managed?

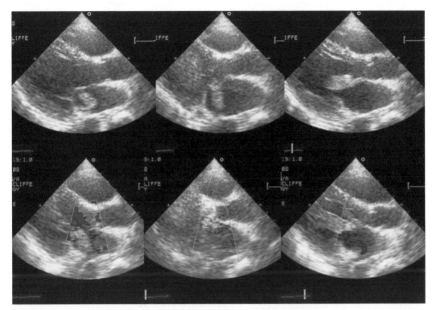

Fig. 40.4 TTE. Selected sequential images with corresponding colour flow beneath. (See colour plate 14)

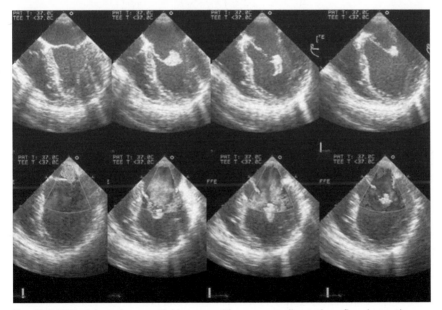

Fig. 40.5 TOE. Selected sequential images with corresponding colour flow beneath. (See colour plate 15)

Answers

1) **What was the cause of the neurological signs?**

The CT head (Fig. 40.1) demonstrates a hypodense area in the right cerebellar hemisphere suggestive of acute infarction (Fig. 40.6).

The image from the MRI head (Fig. 40.3) confirms the CT findings, but also reveals multiple areas of infarction (Fig. 40.6). These are consistent with the neurological signs and may also explain the agitation and the possible seizures.

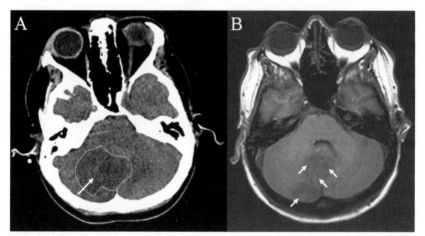

Fig. 40.6 The CT (A) and MRI (B) demonstrate multiple cerebellar lesions (arrowed) with surrounding oedema (dotted outline).

2) **What was the cause of the abdominal pain?**

The image from the CT abdomen (Fig. 40.2) demonstrates multiple hypodense areas in the spleen, which could represent infarction (Fig. 40.7). This could explain the abdominal pain that preceded the neurological event and the left upper quadrant tenderness and guarding. The spleen appeared only slightly enlarged.

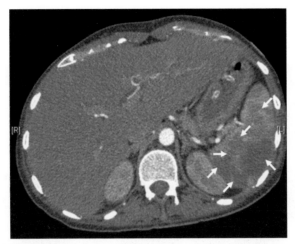

Fig. 40.7 CT of the abdomen demonstrating splenic infarction (arrowed).

3) **Report the echocardiograms. Is there a unifying diagnosis?**

The series of TTE images (Fig. 40.4) show a mass at the tip of the anterior mitral valve leaflet that prolapses into the ventricle during diastole (Fig. 40.8). At the base of the anterior leaflet there is a jet of mitral regurgitation (MR) seen on colour Doppler flow mapping (Fig. 40.8). This suggests a possible perforation.

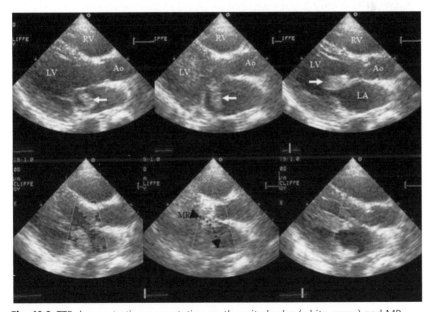

Fig. 40.8 TTE demonstrating a vegetation on the mitral valve (white arrow) and MR (black dotted arrow). (See colour plate 16)

The series of TOE images (Fig. 40.5) also shows valvular MR and evidence of transvalvular flow consistent with perforation (Fig. 40.9).

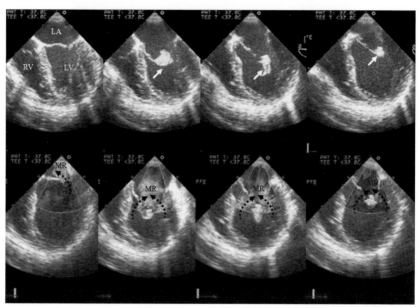

Fig. 40.9 TOE demonstrating vegetation (white arrow) on mitral valve and MR (black dotted arrows). A valvular and a para-valvular jet are visible. (See colour plate 17)

In this case, the mass is most likely to be a vegetation. Vegetations are often highly mobile structures with irregular borders attached to the low-pressure side of a valve leaflet. Vegetations can grow to several centimetres and prolapse through the valve orifice with each cardiac cycle, causing valvular regurgitation. This may be compounded by chordal rupture and leaflet perforation. Their echo-density is relatively low and similar to myocardium when of recent onset.

The unifying diagnosis is endocarditis. Infective endocarditis has an incidence of 1.7–6.2 per 100 000 person years, is believed to be uniformly fatal if not treated, and carries a mortality of 40% at 1 year. The echocardiographic signs of endocarditis are listed in Table 40.1.

Table 40.1 Echocardiographic signs of infective endocarditis

I. The presence of additional structures:
   a. vegetation
   b. abscess
   c. pseudoaneurysm

II. Defects within existing structures:
   a. regurgitant lesions
   b. perforations
   c. fistulae

The initial stages of endocarditis require microtrauma to the valvular endocardial surface either as a result of a high velocity and turbulent jet of blood (e.g. regurgitant, stenotic, or shunt flows) or from cardiac surgery or foreign bodies within the heart. Platelet adhesion then forms a sterile fibrin–platelet aggregate. This can become infected by circulating pathogens during bacteraemia. The bacteria multiply with the formation of macroscopic vegetations. These are often friable, seed infection, and are prone to embolization (30–50% of cases), particularly if large and mobile.

The constant, often low-grade, bacteraemia may seed infection to other organs in the absence of macroembolization. This can result in the formation of mycotic aneurysms (1–5% of endocarditis) within the vasculature. Screening for mycotic aneurysms with contrast CT or MRI is only required if neurological symptoms or signs develop. Mycotic aneurysms can heal with medical therapy, but may enlarge and rupture, which is fatal in many cases.

Embolization from left heart endocarditis results in infarction and/or metastatic abscesses in the brain, spleen, and kidneys. Lung abscess or pneumonia result from embolization from right heart infections. In many cases embolization is clinically silent but two-thirds involve the central nervous system.

Stroke complicates 10% of infective endocarditis and, as in this case, may be the mode of presentation. Ischaemic cerebral infarction occurs in most cases, usually within the first 2 weeks of appropriate antimicrobial therapy. These strokes result from embolic fragments from the vegetation, which tend to be multiple. Specific antimicrobial treatment can reduce the chances of further embolization. Chronic vegetations increase in density and can calcify. This actually reduces the risk of fragmentation and embolization.

Secondary intracranial bleeding can occur, both from haemorrhagic conversion of an ischaemic infarct or rupture of a cerebral artery mycotic aneurysm. This is associated with increased mortality. Use of anticoagulants after ischaemic stroke can cause haemorrhagic transformation and increase mortality. If prosthetic mechanical valve endocarditis is complicated by stroke the balance of risks is in favour of anticoagulants being stopped. If urgent valve replacement is necessary, stroke is not necessarily a contraindication. Cardiac bypass and cardiac surgery are possible within 72 hours of stroke if CT excludes haemorrhagic transformation.

4) **What is the next most important investigation?**

Diagnosis of acute endocarditis requires positive blood cultures and evidence of vegetations (see Duke criteria; Table 40.2).

Table 40.2 The Duke major and minor criteria for the diagnosis of endocarditis. For a definite diagnosis two major or one major and one minor, or three minor criteria are required. Endocarditis is rejected if a clear alternative source of bacteraemia exists and there is resolution of it with fewer than 4 days of antibiotic treatment

A. The two major criteria are:

   1. positive blood cultures (two or more sets) or serology for typical organisms

   2. visualization of endocardial involvement with echocardiography:

      i. vegetations

      ii. abscess formation

      iii. new dehiscence of prosthetic valves

      iv. new valvular regurgitation

B. The 10 minor criteria are:

   1. predisposing heart disease

   2. fever >38°C

   3. vascular phenomena

   4. a single positive blood culture for a typical organism or culture from a metastatic lesion

   5. elevated CRP or ESR

   6. splenomegaly

   7. haematuria

   8. clubbing

   9. splinter haemorrhages

   10. petechia and purpura

Multiple (≥3) separate aerobic and anaerobic blood cultures should be taken over a period of 24 hours. In endocarditis, bacteraemia is constant so cultures need not coincide with fevers. The skin at the site of sampling should be cleaned and prepared with antiseptic. At least 10 mL of blood should be added to the culture medium in each bottle.

In this case, blood cultures grew *Staphylococus aureus* after 3 days. This is a common cause of endocarditis (Table 40.3). The incidence of *Staphylococcal* infection and septicaemia has risen with the increased implantation of indwelling devices. However, a microbiological diagnosis is often hampered by the use of empirical antibiotics. In many cases no clear diagnosis is made before starting antibiotics. Worse, in up to 25% no blood cultures are taken at initial presentation. This misuse of antibiotics has increased bacterial resistance and contributed the phenomenon of culture-negative endocarditis.

Table 40.3 Common causes of endocarditis

I. **Gram-positive bacteria** *Most common cause*	**Streptococci** *Most frequent cause of endocarditis*	Originates in oropharynx
		Streptococcus bovis associated with colonic adenoma/adenocarcinoma
	Staphylococci *Second most common cause of native valve endocarditis*	*Staphylococcus aureus*	Aggressive and destructive 90% of staphylococcal endocarditis
		Staphylococcus Epidermidis	From skin, catheters and i.v. lines
			Early prosthetic valve endocarditis
II. **Zoonosis**	*Coxiella burnetii* (Q fever)	Intracellular rickettsia – 10% of cases affect the heart
		Frequent in France. From cattle, sheep, goats
		Diagnosis is by serology or polymerase chain reaction
		Doxycycline and rifampicin recommended
III. **Enterococcus**	*Enterococcus faecalis*	Most frequent enterococcus
		From gastrointestinal tract
		Antibiotic resistance frequent
IV. **Fungi**	Immunocompromised or long-term intravenous therapy
	Difficult to diagnose
	Usually requires surgery

Culture-negative endocarditis must be distinguished from endoarditis due to a fastidious organism (Table 40.4). If blood cultures remain negative at 5 days, but clinical suspicion remains high, subculture and prolonged incubation for atypical organisms is required. Samples should be sent for serology. Histological analysis of tissue obtained either at valve operation or from sites of septic embolization can also be useful.

Hence, negative cultures in the context of a clinical picture compatible with infective endocarditis suggest:

- the diagnosis is not endocarditis
- bacteraemia has been masked with antibiotics
- endocarditis is due to a fastidious organism requiring special diagnostic tests (Table 40.3).

Diagnosis then requires the presence of systemic inflammatory signs and clear evidence of intracardiac vegetations or an abscess.

Evidence of vegetations may be provided by TTE, but TOE is required if TTE is negative. A negative TOE in a patient with a low or medium pretest probability makes native valve endocarditis unlikely. Other sources of bacteraemia should be sought. However, if pretest probability is high, a clinical diagnosis of endocarditis can be made even if the TOE is negative. Imaging should be repeated at regular intervals to document any structural changes or detect the late appearance of vegetations.

Table 40.4 Pathogens associated with culture negative endocarditis

Coxiella	
Legionella	
The HACEK group	*Haemophilus* species
	Actinobacillus actinomycetemcomitans
	Cardiobacterium hominis
	Eikenella corrodens
	Kingella kingae
Chlamydia	
Bartonella	
Tropheryma whippelii	
Fungi	Candida
	Histoplasma
	Aspergillus
	Torulopsis glabrata

5) **How should this patient be managed?**

In general, once blood cultures have been taken and the diagnosis is clear or probable, intravenous antibiotics should be started empirically. The diagnosis must then be confirmed and the pathogen identified. At least 4 weeks of appropriate intravenous antibiotic therapy are required.

Daily 12 lead ECGs are useful to screen for the onset of heart block, which can result from involvement of the cardiac conduction system. Changes in clinical status, resolution of fevers, and falling CRP and leucocyte count are used to gauge response.

Echocardiography should be repeated to document resolution of vegetations and screen for complications. Echocardiographic features that suggest a need for surgery to prevent embolism include:

- ◆ persistent vegetation on the anterior mitral leaflet (particularly if >10 mm)
- ◆ one or more embolic events within first 2 weeks of antimicrobial treatment
- ◆ two or more embolic events later in treatment.

Outcomes are thought to be better when valve replacement is combined with antimicrobial therapy, particularly if a prosthetic valve is involved. However, there is no evidence from RCTs to support this. Close collaboration between cardiologists, microbiologists, and cardiac surgeons is required.

The initial clinical presentation in this case was the result of extensive systemic embolization. Embolization complicates 20–50% of endocarditis. Of these, 65% involve the central nervous system, causing ischaemic or haemorrhagic strokes, transient ischaemic attacks, or mycotic aneurysms. The embolic risk falls dramatically over the first weeks of successful antibiotic therapy. An argument for early surgery to reduce embolic events can be made on the basis of higher early embolic rates. This argument is stronger if valve-sparing conservative reconstructive surgical technique is appropriate and use of long-term anticoagulation can be avoided.

In patients with cerebral infarction as a result of embolization the risks of secondary haemorrhage during early valve surgery are not clearly defined. Surgery should not be excluded if indicated from a haemodynamic perspective. However, after cerebral haemorrhage valve surgery should be postponed for at least 4 weeks unless the rebleeding risk can be reduced by neurosurgical or endovascular intervention. Bioprosthetic valves reduce the need for long-term anticoagulation and are preferred to mechanical prostheses in these patients.

In this case, the patient was felt to be too unstable to undergo valve replacement. The risk of haemorrhagic transformation of the multiple cerebral and cerebellar infarcts during cardiac bypass was thought to be too high. Cure was attempted with medical therapy alone. This strategy was successful. There were no further embolic events after initiation of intravenous antibiotic therapy with benzylpenicillin and gentamicin. TOE performed 3 weeks after completion of the course of antibiotics demonstrated more complete resolution of the vegetations. Several sets of blood cultures over the following year were negative.

Further reading

Prendergast BD (2006). The changing face of infective endocarditis. *Heart*; **92**: 879–885.

Naber CK, Erbel R (2003). Diagnosis of culture negative endocarditis: novel strategies to prove the suspect guilty. *Heart*; **89**: 241–243.

Habib G, Hoen B, Tornos P, Thuny F, Prendergast B, Vilacosta I, Moreillon P, de Jesus Antunes M, Thilen U, Lekakis J, Lengyel M, Müller L, Naber CK, Nihoyannopoulos P, Moritz A, Zamorano JL; ESC Committee for Practice Guidelines. (2009). Guidelines on the prevention, diagnosis, and treatment of infective endocarditis (new version 2009): the Task Force on the Prevention, Diagnosis, and Treatment of Infective Endocarditis of the European Society of Cardiology (ESC). Endorsed by the European Society of Clinical Microbiology and Infectious Diseases (ESCMID) and the International Society of Chemotherapy (ISC) for Infection and Cancer. *Eur Heart J*; **30**: 2369–2413.

Wilson W, Taubert KA, Gewitz M, Lockhart PB, Baddour LM, Levison M, Bolger A, Cabell CH, Takahashi M, Baltimore RS, Newburger JW, Strom BL, Tani LY, Gerber M, Bonow RO, Pallasch T, Shulman ST, Rowley AH, Burns JC, Ferrieri P, Gardner T, Goff D, Durack DT; American Heart Association Rheumatic Fever, Endocarditis, and Kawasaki Disease Committee; American Heart Association Council on Cardiovascular Disease in the Young; American Heart Association Council on Clinical Cardiology; American Heart Association Council on Cardiovascular Surgery and Anesthesia; Quality of Care and Outcomes Research Interdisciplinary Working Group.

Mayo Clinic, USA. (2007). Prevention of infective endocarditis: guidelines from the American Heart Association: a guideline from the American Heart Association Rheumatic Fever, Endocarditis, and Kawasaki Disease Committee, Council on Cardiovascular Disease in the Young, and the Council on Clinical Cardiology, Council on Cardiovascular Surgery and Anesthesia, and the Quality of Care and Outcomes Research Interdisciplinary Working Group. *Circulation*; **116**: 1736–1754.

Baddour LM, Wilson WR, Bayer AS, Fowler VG Jr, Bolger AF, Levison ME, Ferrieri P, Gerber MA, Tani LY, Gewitz MH, Tong DC, Steckelberg JM, Baltimore RS, Shulman ST, Burns JC, Falace DA, Newburger JW, Pallasch TJ, Takahashi M, Taubert KA; Committee on Rheumatic Fever, Endocarditis, and Kawasaki Disease; Council on Cardiovascular Disease in the Young; Councils on Clinical Cardiology, Stroke, and Cardiovascular Surgery and Anesthesia; American Heart Association; Infectious Diseases Society of America. (2005). Infective endocarditis: diagnosis, antimicrobial therapy, and management of complications: a statement for healthcare professionals from the Committee on Rheumatic Fever, Endocarditis, and Kawasaki Disease, Council on Cardiovascular Disease in the Young, and the Councils on Clinical Cardiology, Stroke, and Cardiovascular Surgery and Anesthesia, American Heart Association: endorsed by the Infectious Diseases Society of America. *Circulation*; **111**: 3167–3184.

ESC (2009). ESC Clinical Practice Guidelines. Guidelines on Prevention, Diagnosis and Treatment of Infective Endocarditis. *Eur Heart J*; **30**: 2369–2413.

AHA (2007). Prevention of Infective Endocarditis: Guidelines from the American Heart Association. *Circulation*; **116**: 1736–1754.

AHA (2005). AHA Scientific Statement. Infective Endocarditis—Diagnosis, Antimicrobial Therapy, and Management of Complications: A Statement for Healthcare Professionals. *Circulation*; **111**: 3167–3184.

Case 41

A 72-year-old lady presented to the medical take with a 3-week history of a cough productive of green sputum and recent breathlessness. She had been treated with two courses of oral antibiotics by her GP but had not responded. Over the last 4 days she had suffered from night sweats and rigors. Over the last 24 hours she had become breathless at rest and had developed peripheral oedema. She had been sleeping in a chair for the last 3 nights. She had diabetes and hypertension treated with gliclazide (80 mg twice daily) and ramipril (5 mg daily), respectively. She had had a biological aortic valve replacement with coronary artery bypass grafts when she presented with breathlessness and syncope 5 years prior to this admission.

On admission she appeared to be in respiratory distress with a respiratory rate of 40 per minute and O_2 saturations 82% on high-flow oxygen administered via a non-rebreathe mask. She was jaundiced and febrile (38.2°C) but her extremeties were cold. Her BP was 110/50 mmHg and she was tachycardic at 140 bpm with an irregular pulse. The JVP was raised to her ears and there were sternotomy and vein harvest scars visible. There was a murmur audible but because of the tachycardia it was hard to characterize. Both lung bases were dull to percussion and there were coarse crepitations throughout the chest. There was ascites but no palpable organomegally. There was bilateral pitting oedema to her knees.

Blood gas analysis demonstrated PaO_2 9 kPa, $PaCO_2$ 5.5 kPa, pH 7.28, bicarbonate 21 mmol/L, base excess –6 mmol/L, and lactate 4 mmol/L. Admission blood tests were Na^+ 132 mmol/L, K^+ 4.3 mmol/L, urea 38 mmol/L, creatinine 450 µmol/L, Hb 7 g/dL, WCC 18×10^9 cells/L, MCV 96 fl, reticulocytes 8%, CRP 123 mg/dL, bilirubin 30 µmol/L, albumin 30 g/L, ALT 23 u/L, and alkaline phosphatase ALP 60 u/L. The ECG on admission is shown in Fig. 41.1. The admission chest X-ray demonstrated bilateral alveolar shadowing with pleural effusions and upper lobe blood diversion.

She was diagnosed as being in heart failure by the admitting doctor, who prescribed intravenous furosemide and commenced continuous positive airway pressure CPAP. Broad spectrum intravenous antibiotics were also commenced to treat the presumed community-acquired pneumonia. A urinary catheter was inserted. The residual volume was only 20 mL. Urine dipstick testing was positive for blood ++ and nitrites. The cardiology registrar was asked to review the patient and performed an echocardiogram (Fig. 41.2).

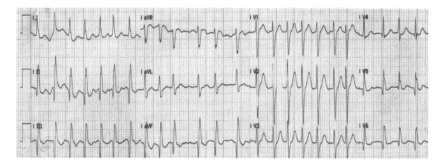

Fig. 41.1 Admission ECG.

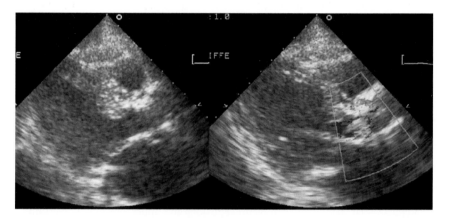

Fig. 41.2 Transthoracic echocardiogram: parasternal long-axis view with colour flow Doppler over the aortic valve prosthesis. (See colour plate 18)

Questions

1. Report the ECG.
2. What are the probable causes of the anaemia and how would you investigate it further?
3. Report the echocardiogram. What test would you like to do next to confirm the findings?
4. What is the underlying diagnosis?
5. How should this be managed?

Answers

1) **Report the ECG.**

The admission ECG showed atrial fibrillation with a ventricular response rate of about 140 bpm. The axis is normal and the QRS duration is not prolonged. There are T-wave inversion and Q waves inferiorly.

2) **What are the probable causes of the anaemia and how would you investigate it further?**

The patient has a normocytic anaemia. The mean cell volume is at the upper limit of normal. The differential diagnosis is broad. It would be useful to review the results of any previous laboratory investigations to determine the time course of the onset of the anaemia and the results of any other investigations.

The raised bilirubin and reticulocyte count suggest haemolysis. In order to confirm this it would be helpful to measure haptoglobins (usually absent), LDH (frequently raised), and examine a blood film for red blood cell fragments and spherocytosis.

Mild haemolysis is a common complication of normal prosthetic valves. It is more common with mechanical valve prostheses. This can cause anaemia if not counteracted by enhanced erythropoiesis. Other causes of anaemia can limit the capacity of the bone marrow to compensate for haemolysis and so measurement of iron indices, vitamin B12, and folate is still important. The raised creatinine suggests that renal failure could also be relevant. This would be more likely if the patient had chronic renal impairment and chronic anaemia.

Severe haemolysis is almost always associated with abnormal valve function such as paravalvular leaks or bioprothetic valve degeneration (see Case 49). Haemolytic anaemia secondary to prosthetic dysfunction is an indication for reoperation. Where reoperation is inappropriate the haemolytic anaemia can be palliated with iron supplementation, correction of any other deficiency, beta-blockers to reduce transvalvular flow velocities and shear stress, and in some cases erythropoietin therapy when other measures have failed.

3) **Report the echocardiogram. What test would you like to do next to confirm the findings?**

The TTE (Fig. 41.3) demonstrates a parasternal long axis view that shows the presence of a bioprosthetic AVR. Anterior to the valve there is a suggestion of an echo hypo-dense area. The colour flow Doppler has flow within it, suggesting antegrade diastolic flow. There is significant aortic regurgitation with a broad jet of colour flow Doppler seen in the outflow tract. These subtle findings, in conjunction with the clinical presentation, suggest prosthetic valve endocarditis until proven otherwise.

Prosthetic valve endocarditis tends to be more severe than native valve endocarditis. Early postoperative endocarditis (≤1-year postimplantation) is mainly due to perioperative colonization with *Staphylococcus epidermidis* and has a high mortality. The aetiology of late postoperative infection is similar to native endocarditis (risk ≤0.5% per year). Prosthetic mechanical and tissue valves are at risk of infection, particularly at the sewing ring. This may cause local invasion, necrosis, and the formation of para-prosthetic leaks and abscesses.

Bioprothetic valve leaflets themselves can be involved, just as pacemaker leads can develop adherent vegetations with infection spreading to contiguous cardiac structures. Abscess formation commonly predicts failure of conservative antibiotic treatment and the need for surgical reintervention. TOE can confirm this and assess the severity of any paravalvular leaks or abscesses. The TOE (Fig. 41.3) show a short axis of the aortic valve. The aortic valve cusps and pillars are clearly visible. There is an abscess cavity running from 9 o'clock to the anterior aspect of the valve. The colour flow Doppler suggests that the regurgitation is mainly paravalvular from the 7 to 12 o'clock positions.

4) **What is the underlying diagnosis?**

Prosthetic valve endocarditis. On the modified Duke's criteria (see discussion on case 40) she has one major criteria (evidence of valve dehiscence on echocardiography) and three minor criteria present on admission (predisposing heart disease, fever >38°C, and elevated CRP). If the prior treatment with antibiotics does not cause negative blood cultures then a second major criteria may also exist.

5) **How should this be managed?**

The focus of management should be to reverse the complications that have occurred as a result of endocarditis. The immediate priorities would be to support her ventilation and to treat the sepsis syndrome with appropriate doses of broad spectrum intravenous antibiotics once the appropriate cultures have been taken. Heart failure and pulmonary congestion can be treated with diuretics. When renal function is impaired large doses of loop diuretics may be required. Haemofiltration could be considered to achieve a euvolaemic state.

The anaemia should be corrected. This may improve ventricular function and reduce the tachycardia, but volume loading can exacerbate cardiac failure.

Digoxin may be used to slow the heart rate. However, renal clearance of digoxin will be reduced so the dosage of maintainance therapy should be reduced and digoxin levels should be closely monitored. Beta-blockers are contraindicated in all patients with pulmonary oedema until euvolaemic. However, if heart failure is primarily due to the severe acute regurgitation early surgery should be considered, particularly given the evidence for abscess formation. In *Staphylococcal* prosthetic valve endocarditis, mortality is around 75% with medical treatment and 25% with surgical treatment.

In this case, the patient could not be immediately stabilized with non-invasive ventilation and required sedation, intubation, and inotropic support. She required haemofiltration to achieve a negative fluid balance. The anaemia was treated with packed red cell transfusions to maintain Hb 10 g/dL. Blood cultures failed to identify the causative organism and broad spectrum antibiotics were continued (penicillin and gentamicin). Repeat TOE confirmed no further deterioration in valve function. Haemodynamic stability was eventually achieved and she was gradually weaned from the ventilator but remained dependent on CPAP because of frequent episodes of acute pulmonary oedema. Intermittent haemofiltration was required. However, given the patient's determination to get better, high-risk surgery was considered. After extensive discussion with the patient and her family she underwent extensive debridement of aortic root with implantation of an aortic homograft and a stentless bioprosthetic valve. Culture of the excised valve grew *Staphylococcus aureus*. Postoperative recovery was complicated by complete heart block, for which she received a single-chamber permanent pacemaker. She had a prolonged stay in the ITU, during which her renal function gradually improved. She received a total of 8 weeks of intravenous antibiotics and surveillance echocardiography demonstrated no evidence of recurrent abscess formation.

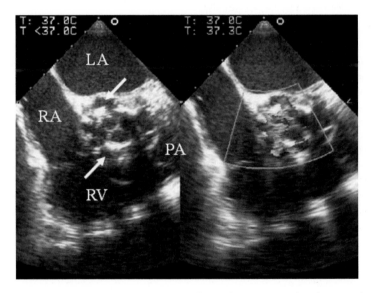

Fig. 41.3 TOE short axis AVR views. Arrows indicate the extent on the abcess cavity. (See colour plate 19)

She was returned home 3 months later after a period of convalescence and rehabilitation. She continues to be followed-up in the outpatient clinic and blood cultures remain negative to date.

Further reading

Habib G, Hoen B, Tornos P, Thuny F, Prendergast B, Vilacosta I, Moreillon P, de Jesus Antunes M, Thilen U, Lekakis J, Lengyel M, Müller L, Naber CK, Nihoyannopoulos P, Moritz A, Zamorano JL; ESC Committee for Practice Guidelines. (2009). Guidelines on the prevention, diagnosis, and treatment of infective endocarditis (new version 2009): the Task Force on the Prevention, Diagnosis, and Treatment of Infective Endocarditis of the European Society of Cardiology (ESC). Endorsed by the European Society of Clinical

Microbiology and Infectious Diseases (ESCMID) and the International Society of Chemotherapy (ISC) for Infection and Cancer. *Eur Heart J*; **30**: 2369–2413.

Wilson W, Taubert KA, Gewitz M, Lockhart PB, Baddour LM, Levison M, Bolger A, Cabell CH, Takahashi M, Baltimore RS, Newburger JW, Strom BL, Tani LY, Gerber M, Bonow RO, Pallasch T, Shulman ST, Rowley AH, Burns JC, Ferrieri P, Gardner T, Goff D, Durack DT; American Heart Association Rheumatic Fever, Endocarditis, and Kawasaki Disease Committee; American Heart Association Council on Cardiovascular Disease in the Young; American Heart Association Council on Clinical Cardiology; American Heart Association Council on Cardiovascular Surgery and Anesthesia; Quality of Care and Outcomes Research Interdisciplinary Working Group.

Mayo Clinic, USA. (2007). Prevention of infective endocarditis: guidelines from the American Heart Association: a guideline from the American Heart Association Rheumatic Fever, Endocarditis, and Kawasaki Disease Committee, Council on Cardiovascular Disease in the Young, and the Council on Clinical Cardiology, Council on Cardiovascular Surgery and Anesthesia, and the Quality of Care and Outcomes Research Interdisciplinary Working Group. *Circulation*; **116**: 1736–1754.

Baddour LM, Wilson WR, Bayer AS, Fowler VG Jr, Bolger AF, Levison ME, Ferrieri P, Gerber MA, Tani LY, Gewitz MH, Tong DC, Steckelberg JM, Baltimore RS, Shulman ST, Burns JC, Falace DA, Newburger JW, Pallasch TJ, Takahashi M, Taubert KA; Committee on Rheumatic Fever, Endocarditis, Kawasaki Disease; Council on Cardiovascular Disease in the Young; Councils on Clinical Cardiology, Stroke, and Cardiovascular Surgery and Anesthesia; American Heart Association; Infectious Diseases Society of America. (2005). Infective endocarditis: diagnosis, antimicrobial therapy, and management of complications: a statement for healthcare professionals from the Committee on Rheumatic Fever, Endocarditis, and Kawasaki Disease, Council on Cardiovascular Disease in the Young, and the Councils on Clinical Cardiology, Stroke, and Cardiovascular Surgery and Anesthesia, American Heart Association: endorsed by the Infectious Diseases Society of America. *Circulation*; **111**: 3167–3184.

Case 42

A 78-year-old lady with severe gastro-oesophageal reflux had an elective right total hip replacement (THR) under combined general anaesthesia and regional anaesthesia (femoral nerve block).

There were no intra-operative complications but she desaturated to 65% on being sat up shortly after extubation. Aspiration was suspected so she was reintubated and transferred to the ITU. There was no cardiovascular instability during or after the operation. The BP and HR were around 135/70 mmHg and 90 bpm, respectively, throughout the immediate perioperative period. Other than peripheral and central cyanosis there were no abnormal findings on examination of the cardiovascular or respiratory systems before or after the patient was reintubated.

She was a smoker and had recently been diagnosed with COPD by her GP, who started inhaled steroids. Four years prior to this admission, she had an elective left THR. Desaturation had also been noted in the perioperative period after the left THR, but was less profound (88%) and thought to be due to intraoperative cementing of the femoral shaft of the left THR. Her rehabilitation was complicated by an embolic stroke 4 days after the left THR. CT brain excluded haemorrhage and a TTE was reported to be normal. There was no residual neurological deficit prior to the right THR.

ECG and chest X-ray performed on admission to ITU were unremarkable and CTPA excluded pulmonary emboli.

She was ventilated with pressure support (PS) ventilation with positive end expiratory pressure (PEEP) 5 cm H_2O and PS 10 cm H_2O. These ventilator settings achieved PaO_2 8 kPa on FiO_2 0.6. However, increasing the PEEP resulted in a fall in O_2 saturations and PaO_2. Turning or sitting up also caused desaturation. When the patient lay flat O_2 saturations were 100%.

Questions – Part 1

1. What are the common causes of postoperative hypoxia?
2. What is the effect of supplemental oxygen on hypoxia due to shunt?
3. What are the adverse effects of PEEP on the cardiovascular system?
4. What is the most likely cause of hypoxia in this case?
5. What investigation is most likely to be diagnostic in this case?

Answers – Part 1

1) **What are the common causes of postoperative hypoxia?**

Postoperative hypoxia may be due to:

- reduced oxygen supply (ventilation perfusion mismatch, impaired alveolar diffusion)
- increased oxygen demand (stress response to surgery).

Common causes of hypoxia in the perioperative period are listed in Table 42.1.

Table 42.1 Common causes of perioperative ventilation perfusion mismatch and hypoxia

Alveolar hypoventilation *(increased shunt)*	Airway obstruction	Upper airway obstruction
		Bronchospasm
		Aspiration
		Collapse, atelectasis
		Pneumothorax
	Decreased ventilatory drive	Inhalational anaesthetics
		Benzodiazipines
		Opiates
		Central nervous system (stroke or trauma)
	Inadequate respiratory muscle function	Incomplete reversal of neuromuscular blockade
		Neuromuscular disease
		Diaphragmatic splinting (obesity, abdominal distension, pain)
		Thoracic or upper abdominal surgery
		Acute or chronic lung disease
Alveolar hypoperfusion *(increased dead space)*	Pulmonary embolism	
	Impaired cardiac output	
Impaired alveolar diffusion	Diffusion hypoxia (nitrous oxide)	
	Pneumonia	
	Aspiration pneumonitis	
	Pulmonary oedema	

2) **What is the effect of supplemental oxygen on hypoxia due to shunt?**

Right-to-left shunt causes severe ventilation/perfusion (V/Q) mismatch, increased arterial–alveolar oxygen (A-a pO_2) gradient, and hypoxia. Deoxygenated blood mixes with oxygenated blood returning to the systemic circulation. In a normal lung, less than 5% of blood is shunted, but if the shunt fraction is over 20–30% of cardiac output, the resulting hypoxia is resistant to correction with oxygen therapy.

Similar V/Q mismatches occur in atelectasis, severe pulmonary oedema, air-space consolidation (as may occur with pneumonia), arteriovenous malformation, and intracardiac shunts.

3) **What are the adverse effects of PEEP on the cardiovascular system?**

Excessive PEEP impairs cardiac output as LV compliance is reduced by the pressure transmitted through the lungs. Pulmonary capillary resistance is increased by alveolar distension as the alveolar transmural pressure gradient is reduced. The increased pulmonary vascular resistance increases right atrial and RV pressures. These changes can exacerbate any right-to-left intracardiac shunt.

4) **What is the most likely cause of hypoxia in this case?**

Platypnoea–orthodeoxia is an uncommon but striking syndrome characterized by dyspnoea and deoxygenation on sitting or standing from a recumbent position. Oxygenation is normal whilst flat. Causes include intracardiac and intrapulmonary shunting of different aetiology.

Platypnoea–orthodeoxia may be caused by interatrial communication (e.g. ASD, PFO, or a fenestrated atrial septal aneurysm) that allows right-to-left shunt when upright. A Chiari network and lipomatous atrial hypertrophy may also rarely route blood preferentially to the atrial septum when upright and cause right-to-left shunting in the presence of a PFO. When recumbent, the higher LA pressure effectively prevents the right-to-left shunt. Positional modification of intracardiac shunt has also been described in the presence of pericardial effusion and constrictive pericarditis. In these conditions, the septum may be stretched and deformed, altering the streaming of venous blood from the IVC through the defect. Positional changes in RA pressure may also modify shunt flow and direction. The syndrome is also described with liver cirrhosis associated with lower zone pulmonary arteriovenous shunting, which increases with the increase in lower zone perfusion in the upright position.

The most common cause of an intracardiac communication is a PFO. In the foetal circulation the foramen ovale enables oxygenated blood to bypass the uninflated lungs and enter the systemic circulation directly. The rapid drop in pulmonary vascular resistance at birth reverses the pressure gradient across the foramen ovale, closing the valve. Autopsy studies have shown that postnatal fusion of the septum primum and secundum fails in a quarter of people. The resultant PFO retains the potential to allow right-to-left shunting of blood if a driving pressure gradient or particular flow characteristics develop.

5) **What investigation is most likely to be diagnostic in this case?**

Trans-thoracic echocardiography with intravenous bubble contrast can be used to detect an intracardiac shunt. Contrast can be prepared by agitation of 8 mL of 0.9% saline with 1 mL of air and a few drops of aspirated blood to produce stabilized micro-bubbles of air within the saline. Macroscopic bubbles should be expelled before injection.

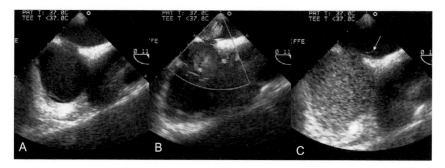

Fig. 42.1 Transoesophageal echocardiogram images. (See colour plate 20)

Questions – Part 2

6. Report Fig. 42.1. How is the image in Fig. 42.1C produced? What does Fig. 42.1C demonstrate?

7. What may have caused the stroke 4 years prior to this admission?

8. What are the management options in this case?

Answers – Part 2

6) **Report Fig. 42.1. How is the image in Fig. 42.1C produced? What does Fig. 42.1C demonstrate?**

The images from the TOE show the RA and LA separated by the interatrial septum (IAS; Fig. 42.2A). There is no flow visible across the IAS when colour Doppler is applied (Fig. 42.1B), excluding an ASD. However, bubble contrast can be seen to cross the IAS (Fig. 42.2C, arrowed). This demonstrates the presence of a PFO.

In this case, the echocardiogram performed after the initial injection of bubble contrast was normal, with bubble contrast only visible in the right heart. However, on repeating the study with increased PEEP, bubbles were seen in the LA after full right-sided cavity opacification, demonstrating the presence of a shunt. The interatrial and interventricular septae appeared intact. Interestingly, more bubbles crossed the septum when the patient sat upright.

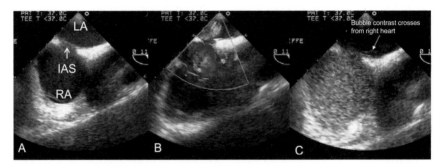

Fig. 42.2 Transoesophageal echocardiogram demonstrating patent foramen ovale. The RA and LA are separated by the inter-atrial septum (IAS; A). There is no flow visible across the IAS when colour Doppler is applied (B), excluding an ASD. However, bubble contrast can be seen to cross the IAS (C; arrowed). This demonstrates the presence of a patent foramen ovale (PFO). (See colour plate 21)

The echocardiogram performed 4 years prior to this presentation had been performed during spontaneous ventilation and without bubble contrast.

7) **What may have caused the stroke 4 years prior to this admission?**

The most common cause of thromboembolic stroke is atherosclerosis. However, paradoxical embolization of a venous thrombus across the PFO could also cause a stroke. Other cardiac causes of embolic stroke (Table 42.2) are unlikely as echocardiography was otherwise normal.

Patent foramen ovale has been associated with decompression sickness, migraine, platypnoea–orthodeoxia syndrome, and stroke. Most patients with an isolated PFO do not require specific treatment. However, there has been much recent debate and a lack of consensus about how PFOs should be managed in the context of stroke and transient ischaemic attacks (TIAs).

Table 42.2 Causes of embolic stroke

Atrial fibrillation	
Mitral stenosis	
Endocarditis	
Prosthetic valve	
Thrombus	
Left atrial myxoma	
Potential sources of cardioembolic events	Mitral valve prolapsed
	Annular calcification
	Septal aneurysm
	Patent foramen ovale

A definite cause is not found in around 40% of patients who have an ischaemic stroke. In these cases the stroke is described as cryptogenic. Up to half of cryptogenic stroke may be attributable to paradoxical venous thromboembolism through a PFO. However, whether the presence of a PFO in a patient who has had a cryptogenic stroke represents a causal relationship or a chance occurrence remains uncertain.

Case–control and registry data suggest that the incidence of PFO is higher patients who have had cryptogenic stroke than in the general population who have not had a stroke (OR 5). In addition, the odds of having a PFO in association with an atrial septal aneurysm are more than four times higher (OR 23.3) than controls who have not had a stroke. In those patients who have had a cryptogenic stroke and have a PFO, the risk of recurrent stroke or TIA within 1 year is higher (12%) than if the patient does not have a PFO (3.4%). At 4 years the risk of recurrent stroke or TIA is around 6% in those with a PFO and 19% if the PFO is associated with an atrial septal aneurysm.

However, these data have been criticized. They may simply represent the referral bias of cryptogenic stoke patients for further assessment with echocardiography. The prevalence of PFO in the non-cryptogenic stroke population may be similar if investigated to the same degree. Importantly, the risk of atrial arrhythmias, including AF is increased in the presence of a PFO. This suggests an alternative mechanism for the association of PFO with stroke.

Although medical treatment lacks the risks of an interventional closure procedure it does increase the risk of adverse drug effects, in particular bleeding complications. Furthermore, patients occasionally do not comply with treatment and medical treatment is contraindicated in certain circumstances, such as pregnancy.

Closure of a PFO is performed under local anaesthesia via a femoral venous puncture. The PFO is crossed with a wire under fluoroscopic guidance with adjunctive intracardiac echocardiography (TOE can be used but requires endotracheal intubation and general anaesthesia). A self-expanding device is deployed first to the left of the septum and then the right to hold the flap valve closed. Postprocedural antiplatelet therapy is recommended for 3–6 months whilst the device becomes endothelialized.

The risk of periprocedural complications with percutaneous PFO closure is small. Access site complications occur in 1.5%, TIA in 0.2%, tamponade in 0.3%, and device embolization in 1.1%. Later complications include a 7–15% risk of new onset AF, and new aortic regurgitation has been reported. Interestingly, in patients followed up after closure was performed, a residual right-to-left shunt was present in a fifth at 1 month and around 10% at 1 year.

Retrospective data and prospective non-randomized cohort data have suggested that PFO closure may be superior to medical therapy to prevent stroke. However, the major issue still remains that there are currently no RCT data available to support the use of PFO closure devices. The data from two trials are awaited with interest (a prospective, multicenter, randomized controlled trial to evaluate the safety and efficacy of the STARFLEX® septal closure system versus best medical therapy in patients with a stroke and/or transient ischemic attack due to presumed paradoxical embolisum through a patent foramen ovale (CLOSURE 1) and Randomized Evaluation of recurrent Stroke comparing PFO closure to Established Current standard of care Treatment (RESPECT)).

8) **What are the management options in this case?**

The management of right-to-left shunt through a PFO is to reduce or abolish the shunt. This can be achieved by reducing RA pressure, increasing LA pressure, or closing the PFO. Intermittent positive pressure ventilation and PEEP in particular increase RA pressure and should be discontinued. Inotropic agents can be used to support RV systolic function. Nitrate-induced venodilation can reduce RA and may be used as a bedside diagnostic test for the presence of right-to-left shunt, causing an immediate increase in systemic oxygen saturation. However, despite encouraging results, the clinical use of nitrates has limited acceptance. Arterial vasodilators can exacerbate the shunt by lowering LA pressure and so should not be used. Beta-blockers have been used with favourable results. Their mechanism of action is not well understood but they may improve RV function by reducing heart rate and oxygen consumption. Theoretically, in the setting of acute MI with RV involvement, early myocardial revascularization should improve RV function and thereby reduce the shunt fraction. Atrioventricular sequential pacing may also reduce RA pressure by maintaining atrial contraction.

Closure of PFO (surgical or percutaneous) has had varied clinical success in this particular situation. Under certain conditions, closure of a PFO could be detrimental, reducing LV filling and increasing filling of the non-compliant RV. In one series, five of eight patients who had a PFO closed died. Theoretically, in acute RV failure, creation of an atrial septal defect could improve RV function.

In this case, percutaneous occlusion of the PFO immediately improved the hypoxia, allowing extubation immediately and discharge from the ITU shortly afterwards. Fig. 42.3 is a fluoroscopic image taken after closing the PFO with an occlusion device in this patient.

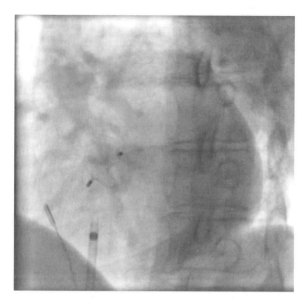

Fig. 42.3 Fluoroscopic image taken after closing the PFO with an occlusion device.

Further reading

Cujec B, Polasek P, Mayers I, Johnson D (1993). Positive end-expiratory pressure increases the right-to-left shunt in mechanically ventilated patients with patent foramen ovale. *Ann Intern Med*; **119**: 887–894.

Aslam F, Shirani J, Haque AA (2006). Patent foramen ovale: assessment, clinical significance and therapeutic options. *South Med J*; **99**: 1367–1372.

Kizer JR, Devereux RB (2005). Clinical practice. Patent foramen ovale in young adults with unexplained stroke. *New Engl J Med*; **353**: 2361–2372.

Somberg J (2007). Patent foramen ovale closure devices: thoughts from the circulatory device advisory panel. *Am J Cardiol*; **100**: 905–906.

Case 43

A 42-year-old steel worker initially presented to the ED with a 3-day history of intermittent, sharp, localized, left anterior chest pain at rest. His symptoms were worse on deep inspiration and bending forwards, and were increasing in frequency. He had been working more overtime at work to pay for a new car, and had attributed his symptoms to muscle strain.

He smoked but denied any other risk factors for IHD. There was no significant past medical history. He did not take any medications. On examination he was febrile (38°C), there was no evidence of raised JVP or cardiac failure, but a high-pitched, scratchy sound was audible at the left sternal edge that was not affected by breath holding.

On initial presentation to hospital blood tests were Hb 14 g/dL, WBC 13.3 × 10^9 cells/L, platelets 400 x 10^{12} cells/L, creatinine 120 μmol/L, urea 5 mmol/L, total cholesterol 3.8 mmol/L, cTn I 0.4 ng/mL, and CK 100 u/L. Electrolytes and liver function tests were normal. His ECG on admission is shown in Fig. 43.1. This ECG was recorded during an episode of pain. There was no progression of the ECG changes on serial recording.

Echocardiography demonstrated vigorous LV function, a normal-sized right heart and a small (<1 cm) rim of pericardial fluid. He completed 10 minutes (into stage IV) of a full Bruce protocol ETT without symptoms or new ECG abnormalities and was discharged home without follow-up. After the initial presentation his symptoms settled slowly over the next 2 months. Similar chest pains recurred every few months but usually settled within 1 week.

Two years after the initial presentation the patient was referred to a cardiologist by his GP with breathlessness on walking more than 100 m. His wife incidentally reported an increase in his collar size over the last 6 months. The ECG enclosed with the referral letter was normal, without repolarization changes. The chest X-ray is shown in Fig. 43.2. Physical examination revealed prominent and pulsating internal jugul veins, raised JVP, peripheral oedema and abdominal distension.

Questions

1. Report the ECG (Fig. 43.1).
2. What is the differential diagnosis for his initial clinical presentation and what is most likely?
3. Report the chest X-ray (Fig. 43.2).
4. Why is the patient breathless and what tests would confirm this?
5. How would you have managed the patient at the initial presentation?

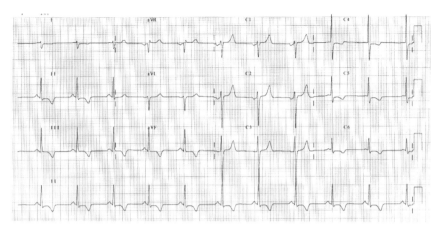

Fig. 43.1 12 lead ECG at first admission.

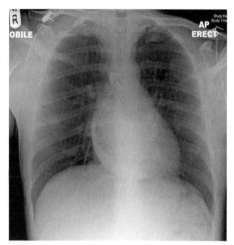

Fig. 43.2 Chest X-ray on re-referral.

Answers

1) **Report the ECG (Fig. 43.1).**

The ECG shows sinus rhythm at a rate of 65 bpm. The QRS axis is deviated to the right. There is mild inferolateral ST depression with asymmetrical T-wave inversion.

2) **What is the differential diagnosis for his initial clinical presentation and what is most likely?**

The differential diagnosis of precordial T-wave inversion poses a significant clinical challenge (Table 43.1). In view of the history of chest pain myocardial ischaemia, PE, pericarditis, and myocarditis (see Case 24) should be considered in the differential diagnoses. The localized sharp pain in the subscapular region would be atypical of a coronary syndrome. In this case pleurisy, pericarditis, myocarditis, or PE are more likely than MI as there is evidence of serosal inflammation (friction rub on auscultation).

The ECG changes in pericarditis vary with the duration and extent of inflammation. The first changes (stage 1) are ST elevation and PR segment depression due to abnormalities in the atrial repolarization (Tp) wave (see Case 24). These changes subsequently resolve and the T waves flatten and invert (stage 2). The T-wave inversion subsequently becomes generalized (stage 3) before returning to normal (stage 4). The absence of the typical concave upwards ST elevation (stage 1) on the ECG at presentation does not exclude a diagnosis of pericardits, but may represent a more subacute presentation. However, similar ECG findings can also be associated with PE.

A friction rub occurs in up to 80% of patients with pericarditis but fewer than 5% of patients with PE. The friction rub in this case is more suggestive of pericarditis. Although the pain increased with inspiration, the persistence of pain despite apnoea is more suggestive of pericarditis than pleurisy.

Serum cTn concentrations are elevated in around a third of patients with pericarditis, but abnormalities of serum CK are less common. In the majority of cases of pericarditis this represents epicardial inflammation rather than myocyte necrosis but an associated myocarditis may be present. Myopericarditis is more likely if the cTn concentration is raised above the threshold for diagnosis of MI in a patient with an ACS (cTnI > 1.5 ng/mL). Troponin concentrations usually normalize within 2 weeks of diagnosis in patients with pericarditis; however, prolonged elevation is suggestive of ongoing myocarditis and worse outcome. Patients with acute pericarditis usually have evidence of systemic inflammation, including leukocytosis, elevated erythrocyte sedimentation rate, and increased CRP. A low-grade fever is common, but purulent bacterial pericarditis should be considered if fevers are higher than 38°C.

Table 43.1 Differential diagnosis of ventricular repolarization abnormalities on ECG

Intrinsic cardiac causes of negative or flattened T waves	
Ischaemic heart disease	
Pericarditis	
LV hypertrophy	
LBBB	
Myocarditis and cardiomyopathies	
Cor pulmonale and pulmonary embolism	
Post-tachycardia	
Post-intermittent depolarization abnormalities ('electrical memory')	LBBB
	Pacemakers
	WPW syndrome
Extrinsic causes of negative or flattened T waves	
Normal variants: children, black race, women, athletes	
Hyperventilation	
Alcoholism	
Stroke	
Hypothyroidism	

3) **Report the chest X-ray (Fig. 43.2).**

The AP erect chest X-ray shows dense but localized pericardial calcification around the right-heart border. The lung fields are normal.

4) **Why is the patient breathless and what tests would confirm this?**

The patient was referred to the cardiology clinic with symptoms of heart failure. However, there is no evidence of pulmonary congestion or cardiomegaly on the chest X-ray (Fig. 43.2). The differential diagnosis of shortness of breath with signs of right-heart failure includes constrictive pericarditis, which should be considered in any patient with unexplained systemic venous congestion, restrictive cardiomyopathy (see Case 28), chronic PE, RV infarction, and chronic obstructive lung disease. Constrictive pericarditis is the most likely diagnosis in this case in view of the pericardial calcification and presentation with subacute pericarditis 2 years prior to this presentation. However, a definitive diagnosis requires exclusion of restrictive cardiomyopathy. Typically constriction results in prominent x and y descent of an elevated jugular venous pulse. This reflects the high filling pressure and rapid early ventricular filling but slowed late ventricular filling. An associated apical filling sound in mid or late diastole (muscle knock) is audible in 40% of patients presenting with constriction.

Doppler echocardiography has limited value in this condition. It commonly demonstrates restricted filling of both ventricles with a rapid deceleration of the early diastolic mitral inflow velocity (E wave) and small or absent A wave. The mitral inflow velocity also varies significantly (>25%) during normal respiration.

Traditionally, constriction and restriction are differentiated by haemodynamic criteria obtained at cardiac catheterization. In constriction, there is usually high and equal end-diastolic pressure in all four cardiac chambers, with low early diastolic pressures in both ventricles. With restriction, LV end-diastolic pressure exceeds RV pressure by at least a few mmHg and rises more gradually in diastole in contrast to the 'dip and plateau' pattern of constriction. Pulmonary hypertension is often associated with restriction but is not typically present with constriction. However, these classic haemodynamic criteria have a limited specificity for constriction (24–57%). Variations in RV pressure are more sensitive (>90%). Pericardial constriction causes RV systolic pressures to rise during inspiration (see Kussmaul's sign), while LV systolic pressure falls as ventricular pressures are interdependent.

5) **How would you have managed the patient at the initial presentation?**

The initial assessment and investigation of patients presenting with pericarditis should determine:

1. whether or not admission to hospital is indicated (risk of short-term, immediately threatening complications)

2. probable aetiology.

The significant potential short-term complications of pericarditis include cardiac tamponade and disability due to pain, fever, sepsis, or the precipitant of the pericarditis (e.g. malignancies, vasculitides, and sepsis). A policy of admitting all patients presenting with pericarditis could be considered 'safe'. However, in the vast majority of cases, pericarditis is benign and self-limiting. A policy of universal admission would be inconvenient, inefficient, and expensive, and would unnecessarily expose many patients to the not insignificant risks of admission to hospital.

Patients with high-risk features of pericarditis (Table 43.2) are at increased risk of short-term complications and have a higher probability of there being a specific (i.e. non-viral) cause of pericarditis. Admission and/or further investigation should be considered if patients present with or subsequently develop any high-risk features. Patients who are not admitted require outpatient follow-up to determine the risk of significant long-term complications (e.g. recurrence, chronic pericarditis, and pericardial constriction).

In this case, the patient was was febrile on admission and the initial episode of pericarditis was slow to resolve (subacute; >6 weeks). The patient received several courses of NSAIDs during this time with little benefit and subsequently developed chronic relapsing pericarditis.

Table 43.2 High-risk features at initial presentation with acute pericarditis

Fever (>38°C)

Subacute course (6 weeks to 6 months)[1]

An immunosuppressed state

Traumatic pericarditis

Use of oral anticoagulants

A large pericardial effusion at presentation (>20 mm)

Failure to respond to NSAIDs

The aim of the management of chronic relapsing pericarditis is the prevention of recurrence. The COlchicine for acute PEricarditis (COPE) trial found that the addition of colchicine to standard NSAID therapy significantly reduced the risk of recurrence in idiopathic pericarditis (number needed to treat = 5).

However, if a specific cause can be identified, specific interventions may be possible. For example, steroids should be considered for patients with connective tissue diseases and for autoreactive or uraemic pericarditis. Whilst steroid therapy may be considered for patients with recurrent or chronic pericarditis, use of steroids during the index attack may paradoxically increase the risk of recurrence.

In this case, constrictive pericarditis was confirmed on cardiac catheterization 2 years after the initial presentation. The patient had pericardiectomy. He recovered well after the operation, noticing almost immediate benefit, describing the feeling of 'being able to breathe normally again'. No specific cause of the pericarditis was identified despite thourough investigation. The patient returned to work at the steel mill with a normal exercise tolerance 2 years later.

The most common causes of pericardial constriction are mediastinal radiation, chronic idiopathic pericarditis, previous cardiac surgery, tuberculous pericarditis (see Case 23), and trauma. Scarred, thickened, and frequently calcified pericardial tissue can impair cardiac filling by limiting the total cardiac volume. In early diastole, initial ventricular filling occurs rapidly as blood moves under pressure from atria to ventricles without much change in the total cardiac volume; a prominent x and y descent on JVP ensues, giving the pulsating neck veins that were so prominent in the clinic. Once the pericardial constraining volume is reached, diastolic filling stops abruptly. This causes the diastolic knock and the characteristic dip and plateau seen on invasive ventricular pressures measurements, and equalizes the end-diastolic pressures in the four cardiac chambers. In the face of continuing venous return, systemic congestion is much more marked than pulmonary congestion. The stiff pericardium isolates the cardiac chambers from respiratory changes in intrathoracic pressures, resulting in Kussmaul's sign: a paradoxical rise in JVP in inspiration. Treatment with diuretics can provide symptomatic relief. However, persistent symptoms require excision of the pericardium and perioperative mortality is 4–12%. The major perioperative complications include cardiac failure, ventricular perforation, and excessive epicardial bleeding.

Further reading

Little WC, Freeman GL (2006). Pericardial disease. *Circulation*; **113**: 1622–1632.

Imazio M, Demichelis B, Parrini I, Giuggia M, Cecchi E, Gaschino G, Demarie D, Ghisio A, Trinchero R. (2004). Day-hospital treatment of acute pericarditis. *J Am Coll Cardiol*; **43**: 1042–1046.

Imazio, M Bobbio M, Cecchi E, Demarie D, Demichelis B, Pomari F, Moratti M, Gaschino G, Giammaria M, Ghisio A, Belli R, Trinchero R. (2005). Colchicine in Addition to Conventional Therapy for Acute Pericarditis: Results of the COlchicine for acute PEricarditis (COPE) Trial. *Circulation*; **112**: 2012–2016.

ESC. (2004). Clinical Practice Guidelines on the Diagnosis and Management of Pericardial Diseases. *Eur Heart J*; **25**: 587–610.

Maisch B, Seferović PM, Ristić AD *et al.* (2004). ESC Clinical Practice Guidelines on the Diagnosis and Management of Pericardial Diseases. *Eur Heart J*; **25**: 587–610.

Case 44

A 51-year-old man received a 240-V, 50-Hz alternating current electrical injury whilst trying to repair his household washing machine. He was unable to release the appliance until his wife switched off the electricity approximately 1 minute later. He then noticed a severe painful burn in his left elbow and fast irregular palpitations, but was otherwise asymptomatic. The only significant past history was of hypertension, treated with enalapril 5 mg daily. He denied any previous episodes of palpitations.

He presented to the ED 30 minutes later. He denied any previous episodes of palpitations. On examination, a 5-cm^2 third-degree burn was present in the left antecubital fossa, HR was 190 bpm and BP 130/70 mmHg. Physical examination was otherwise unremarkable. An ECG was obtained (Fig. 44.1).

Intravenous metoprolol 10 mg reduced the HR to 170 bpm. Thirty minutes later flecainide 50 mg was administered intravenously. This did not restore sinus rhythm or reduce the HR. Routine blood tests, including full blood count, serum potassium, serum magnesium and thyroid function, were normal. Plain chest radiography was unremarkable.

Six hours after the onset of AF the patient reported dull central chest pain, dizziness, and sweating. His HR was 180 bpm and BP was 80/40 mmHg. There were no clinical signs of heart failure. An ECG was performed and was similar to that shown in Fig. 44.1.

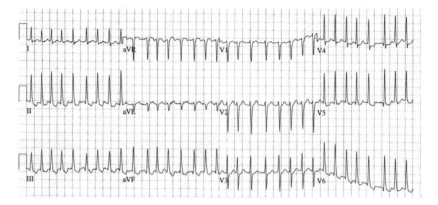

Fig. 44.1 ECG on admission.

Questions

1. What does the ECG (Fig. 44.1) show?
2. What is the most likely cause of this arrhythmia?
3. How is this arrhythmia classified clinically?
4. How would you manage this patient acutely?
5. 10 years later the patient was incidentally found to be in persistent AF at a preoperative assessment for a knee replacement. What is the most likely cause?
6. How can the risk of thromboembolism after elective DC cardioversion be reduced?
7. How would you assess the long-term risk of thromboembolism due to AF?
8. How would you assess the risk of haemorrhage with anticoagulation?

Answers

1) **What does the ECG (Fig. 44.1) show?**

   Figure 44.1 demonstrates an irregularly irregular narrow-complex tachycardia with a ventricular rate around 200 bpm. There are no P waves. The irregular baseline consists of rapid oscillations (fibrillatory waves) that vary in size, shape, and timing. The rhythm is AF.

   There is ST-segment depression and T-wave inversion in leads II, III, aVF, and V4–V6. In the absence of symptoms suggestive of ischaemia these widespread non-specific ST-segment and T-wave changes are most likely to be rate related. However, in this case myocardial ischaemia and CAD should be considered in view of the subsequent clinical deterioriation.

2) **What is the most likely cause of this arrhythmia?**

   Electrical injury to the heart is likely to have triggered the AF in the present case. Electrical injury to the heart often causes ECG changes and arrhythmias, the most serious of which are asystole and VF. The initiation of AF after electrical injury is rare. Table 44.1 lists some of the more common causes of AF.

Table 44.1 Cardiac and non-cardiac causes of AF

Cardiac causes of AF
Hypertension
Ischaemic heart disease
Valvular heart disease (particularly mitral stenosis)
Sick sinus syndrome
Pre-excitation syndromes (e.g. WPW syndrome; see Case 2)
Cardiomyopathy
Pericardial disease (including effusion and constrictive pericarditis)
Atrial septal defect
Cardiothoracic surgery
Atrial myxoma
Non-cardiac causes of AF
Electrolyte depletion (particularly K^+ and Mg^{2+})
Excessive alcohol or caffeine consumption
Sepsis, particularly respiratory tract
Pulmonary embolism
Intrathoracic pathology (eg lung cancer, pleural effusion)
Thyrotoxicosis

3) **How is this arrhythmia classified clinically?**

Classification of AF should link the presentation of AF to a suggested management strategy. The classification should therefore include symptoms, risks of thromboembolism and haemorrhage with anticoagulation as well as type of AF.

1. Patients may be asymptomatic, symptomatic, or both.

2. Risks of thromboembolism and haemorrhage may be simply estimated and be high or low.

3. The presentation may be the first detected episode or a recurrence (Table 44.2).

Recurrent AF may be paroxysmal, persistent, or permanent.

This case describes a first presentation with AF.

Table 44.2 Classification of AF

First presentation	Management strategy
Initial event (first detected episode) – may or may not recur	Rhythm control
Symptomatic	
Asymptomatic (first detected)	
Onset unknown (first detected)	
Recurrent AF (two or more episodes)	
Paroxysmal AF[1]	
Spontaneous termination within 7 days and usually within 48 hours	Rate or rhythm control
Persistent AF	
Not self-terminating	Rate or rhythm control
Lasting more than 7 days or required cardioversion	
Permanent AF	
Not terminated	Rate control
Terminated but relapsed	
No attempt at cardioversion	

[1] Use of pharmacological or DC cardioversion to reduce time to conversion does not change the classification of paroxysmal AF to persistent as AF would have terminated on its own.

4) **How would you manage this patient acutely?**

If acute AF causes haemodynamic instability, as in the present case, urgent electrical cardioversion is required, irrespective of the duration of the AF. If there is any delay in organizing electrical cardioversion, intravenous amiodarone should be administered via a central vein.

Patients with acute AF should be started on heparin (unfractionated or LMWH) at the initial presentation unless contraindicated (or already adequately anticoagulated). This should not delay emergency cardioversion. Heparin should be continued until a full assessment has been made and appropriate antithrombotic therapy has been started, based on risk stratification (see below).

In this case, LMWH was administered and sinus rhythm restored by a single 200-J biphasic shock under general anaesthesia. A 12 lead ECG performed after cardioversion was normal. Serum troponin I taken 12 hours after the onset of haemodynamic compromise was not raised and echocardiography was normal. The patient was monitored in the CCU for 24 hours. The AF did not recur and the patient was transferred to a burns unit for skin grafting.

On review 3 months later, the patient remained well and denied any recurrence of palpitations. ECG confirmed normal sinus rhythm and exercise tolerance testing was unremarkable.

Arrhythmia management

Atrial fibrillation is both the most common sustained arrhythmia and the most common cause of presentation to hospital due to arrhythmia. The prevalence of AF increases with age from 0.5% at 50–59 years to almost 9% at 80–89 years. It causes substantial mortality and morbidity due to stroke, thromboembolism, heart failure, reduced quality of life, and impaired cognitive function.

Rapid atrial stretch shortens the refractory period and can cause acute AF. This is often associated with ACS or LV failure. Management includes volume unloading and rate slowing. This may increase the atrial refractory period, improving the chance of cardioversion.

AF can be managed by either restoring and maintaining sinus rhythm (rhythm control) or ventricular rate control (rate control). There are no significant differences between these management strategies in relief of symptoms or mortality. Aggressive rhythm control is most appropriate for first presentations of AF or if symptoms persist despite control of the ventricular rate. Rhythm control increases admission to hospital and treatment-related side effects so rate control is recommended for the elderly and the minimally symptomatic.

Pharmacological therapy for rate control

AF is considered rate controlled if the resting ventricular response is 60–80 bpm and 90–115 bpm on moderate exertion. In the elderly, conduction disease is common so medication may not be required for rate control.

Beta blockade directly prolongs the refractory period of the AVN and antagonises sympathetic activity. Although beta-blockers are the first-line therapy, caution is required in patients with asthma, COPD, or heart failure.

The Calcium channel blockers CCBs verapamil and diltiazem prolong the refractory period of the AV node. These are commonly used for rate control, reducing heart rate at rest and during exercise. However, CCBs are negatively inotropic, so caution is required in patients with acute heart failure.

Digoxin is commonly used for rate control in patients with heart failure or limited activity. It blocks parasympathetic effects on the AV node but has little effect in terminating AF. It is less effective if AF is driven by sympathetic stimulation (e.g. sepsis, exercise, and hyperthyroidism). However, the combination of digoxin and beta-blockers is more effective than the combination of digoxin and diltiazem.

Amiodarone is sympatholytic and antagonises calcium, which therefore depresses AV conduction. Amiodarone is used in acute AF when conventional drugs have failed to control the ventricular rate. Rhythm control can be achieved in a significant number of cases.

Pharmacological therapy for rhythm control

The duration and type of AF should guide drug therapy for pharmacological cardioversion. Acute AF is associated with normal atrial refractory periods and relatively short excitable gaps. Slowing of conduction by drugs such as flecainide (class IC) is effective. Prolonged AF and strongly remodelled dilated atria rarely respond to classical antiarrhythmics. However, rhythm control may still be possible with class III drugs (e.g. amiodarone) or prolonged drug administration. Newer agents such as dronaderone, structurally related to amiodarone, may offer efficacy with less risk of side effects compared to amiodarone.

A consequence of AF-induced electrical remodelling is that the efficacy of secondary prophylaxis after cardioversion may depend on the type of recurrence. To prevent immediate recurrence of AF, class IC drugs and amiodarone are most effective. Amiodarone reduces all types of postcardioversion recurrence.

Electrophysiological and surgical techniques

Reducing atrial size or confining atrial electrical activity may eliminate re-entrant AF by reducing the volume of muscle in which re-entry can occur and thus reducing the number of circulating wavelets below a critical number. This is the principle of the Maze operation and of linear catheter ablation (left-atrial circumferential ablation).

Curative treatment of AF, such as ablation and surgery, requires understanding of the underlying mechanism. In patients with AF and atrial flutter or other supraventricular arrhythmias, including WPW syndrome, radiofrequency ablation or cryoablation aimed at these arrhythmias may also cure the AF. Furthermore, if focal AF is proven, ablation of the foci may be curative.

5) **10 years later the patient was incidentally found to be in persistent AF at a preoperative assessment for a knee replacement. What is the most likely cause?**

   Hypertension is the most common cause of AF. Structural change to the left atrium often develops long before AF. The 5-year risk of chronic AF in hypertensive subjects is highest in those with the greatest LV mass and largest LA diameter. Management of hypertension is important to reduce the incidence of AF. Medical treatment of hypertension is important in the primary prevention of AF.

6) **How can the risk of thromboembolism after elective DC cardioversion be reduced?**

   The risk of thromboembolism is increased after cardioversion. The cause is complex. Pre-existing thrombus may embolize from the endocardial wall.

Furthermore, thrombus may form after sinus rhythm is restored because the mechanical function of the atria is impaired.

If AF has been present for over 48 hours full anticoagulation is usually required for at least 4 weeks before and after elective cardioversion. Thromboembolism occurs in up to 2% of cardioversions despite these precautions.

TOE-guided cardioversion

The need for adequate anticoagulation prior to urgent cardioversion can be avoided if TOE excludes LA thrombus. TOE can reveal thrombus within the left atrium and appendage and identify indicators for thrombus formation. If thrombus is seen the patient is at high risk of postcardioversion thromboembolism. The safety and applicability of TOE-guided cardioversion is reasonably established. After exclusion of thrombus, LMWH anticoagulation should start. Anticoagulation is still required for a minimum of 4 weeks after cardioversion so warfarin is generally started at the same time. After that time risk persists in patients with typical stroke risk factors so anticoagulation should be continued even if sinus rhythm is maintained and particularly if the risk of recurrence is high (Table 44.3).

A TOE-guided cardioversion may also be used to minimize precardioversion anticoagulation to reduce bleeding risk or reduce delays to other treatments, for example surgery.

Table 44.3 Factors indicating a high risk of AF recurrence

Previous failed cardioversion
Structural heart disease (mitral valve disease, LV dysfunction or large LA)
Long duration of AF (>12 months)
Previous recurrence

7) **How would you assess the long-term risk of thromboembolism due to AF?**

The relative risk of thromboembolism is increased around five-fold by non-rheumatic AF. Non-rheumatic AF impairs atrial mechanical function by electrical and mechanical remodelling, which can occur within days. Subsequent structural remodelling further impairs atrial function, promoting blood stagnation and increasing the risk of thrombus formation. Long-term thromboprophylaxis is therefore required in persistent AF. The risk of thromboembolism is affected by age and coexisting disease. The CHADS2 score (Table 44.4) is a validated clinical prediction score for estimating the risk of stroke in non-rheumatic AF (Table 44.5).

Anticoagulation with warfarin reduces the relative risk of stroke by 66%. However, the risk of haemorrhagic stroke and significant extracranial bleeding is increased, therefore in the lower risk groups aspirin, which provides a 33% relative risk reduction, is more appropriate. Recommended strategies for anticoagulation are listed in Table 44.6.

Other independent risk factors for stroke in AF include structural heart disease and previous MI. The relative risk of thromboembolism is increased 17 times if AF is associated with rheumatic mitral valve disease so warfarin is strongly recommended.

In the present case, the patient was anticoagulated with warfarin for 4 weeks before and after elective DC cardioversion. Thereafter he was treated with aspirin 75 mg daily as the CHADS2 score was 1. The knee replacement was performed 3 weeks later without complication.

Table 44.4 CHADS2 score

	Condition	Points
C	Congestive heart failure	1
H	Hypertension (or treated hypertension)	1
A	Age >75 years	1
D	Diabetes	1
S2	Prior stroke or TIA	2

Table 44.5 The association between CHADS2 score and risk of stroke in non-rheumatic AF

CHADS2 Score	Stroke risk (%)	95% CI
0	1.9	1.2–3.0
1	2.8	2.0–3.8
2	4.0	3.1–5.1
3	5.9	4.6–7.3
4	8.5	6.3–11.1
5	12.5	8.2–17.5
6	18.2	10.5–27.4

Table 44.6 Strategies for anticoagulation based on the CHADS2 score

CHADS2 score	Risk	Anticoagulation therapy	Considerations
0	Low	Aspirin	75 mg/day lower doses may be equally efficacious
1	Moderate	Aspirin or warfarin	Aspirin daily or raise INR to 2.0–3.0, depending on factors such as patient preference
≥2	Moderate or high	Warfarin	Target INR range 2.0–3.0, unless contraindicated (e.g. history of falls, clinically significant gastrointestinal bleeding, inability to monitor INR regularly)

8) **How would you assess the risk of haemorrhage with anticoagulation?**

Anticoagulation is associated with an increased risk of spontaneous and traumatic haemorrhage. Assessment of bleeding risk is an important part of the clinical assessment and must be discussed with the patient before starting anticoagulation therapy.

The annual rate of major haemorrhage (defined as intracranial haemorrhage, requiring transfusion of at least two units of blood, or requiring hospital admission) was 1% in controls and 1.3% in warfarin-treated patients. The annual risk of intracranial haemorrhage increases from 0.1% in control to 0.3% in warfarin-treated groups (excess of two intracranial bleeds per annum per 1000 patients treated). Factors that increase the risk of haemorrhage in patients on warfarin therapy are listed in Table 44.7

To provide adequate thromboprophylaxis and minimize the risk of bleeding, aim for INR 2.5 (acceptable range 2.0–3.0). INR >3.0 is associated with increased bleeding and INR <2.0 with increased stroke risk.

Table 44.7 Factors that increase risk of haemorrhage with anticoagulation therapy

Age over 75 years
Polypharmacy
Antiplatelet drugs (e.g. aspirin or clopidogrel) or NSAIDs
History of poorly controlled anticoagulation therapy
Uncontrolled hypertension
History of bleeding (e.g. peptic ulcer or cerebral haemorrhage)

Low-dose aspirin also increases the risk of major haemorrhage, especially if hypertension is not well controlled. The addition of aspirin to oral anticoagulation therapy does not further reduce the risk of thromboembolism but increases bleeding risk. Warfarin should not be prescribed with aspirin or clopidogrel to reduce the risk of strokes in patients with AF.

Further reading

National Collaborating Centre for Chronic Conditions (2006). Atrial fibrillation: national clinical guideline for management in primary and secondary care. London: Royal College of Physicians.

Androulakis A, Aznaouridis KA, Aggeli CJ, Roussakis GN, Michaelides AP, Kartalis AN, Stougiannos PN, Dilaveris PE, Misovoulous PI, Stefanadis CI, Kallikazaros IE. (2007). Transient ST-segment depression during paroxysms of atrial fibrillation in otherwise normal individuals: relation with underlying coronary artery disease. *J Am Coll Cardiol*; **50**: 1909–1911.

Case 45

An 80-year-old man with an asymptomatic 6.5-cm abdominal aortic aneurysm (AAA) was referred to the cardiology outpatient clinic for assessment prior to elective AAA repair. The referral letter from the consultant anaesthetist who reviewed him in the preanaesthesia assessment clinic is given below.

Dear consultant cardiologist,

Thank you for reviewing this 80-year-old man with an asymptomatic 6.5-cm AAA, who is scheduled for elective AAA repair. He has hypertension, hypercholesterolaemia, renal impairment (creatinine 180 µmol/L), and smokes 20 cigarettes per day. He was diagnosed with mild exertional angina by his GP 10 years prior to this referral but never had an exercise test or angiogram. He has not suffered from angina or used sublingual GTN for several years. He lives in a ground-floor flat and so does not need to climb stairs. However, he is unable to walk more than 100 m on the flat because of arthritis in his knees. His regular medication includes aspirin 75 mg daily, simvastatin 20 mg daily, and ramipril 2.5 mg daily.

His 12 lead ECG and chest X-ray were normal. I am organizing cardiopulmonary exercise (CPEX) testing for risk stratification.

I would be grateful for your opinion on the need for further investigation and treatment to optimize this gentleman's cardiovascular status prior to elective AAA repair.

Thank you.

Questions

1. What factors affect the perioperative risk of morbidity and mortality associated with non-cardiac surgery? How does this affect the need for specialist cardiorespiratory preoperative assessment?
2. What is the prognosis of the medical management of AAA?
3. What is the pathophysiological cause of perioperative cardiac morbidity and mortality?
4. What is the risk of perioperative mortality for elective AAA repair?
5. When should an AAA be operated on electively?
6. What medical therapy may influence perioperative cardiac risk?
7. What are the indications for preoperative coronary revascularization in patients with stable cardiovascular disease awaiting non-cardiac surgery?
8. Does this patient require pre-operative stress testing?
9. Cardiopulmonary exercise testing was performed and revealed an anaerobic threshold (AT) of 10 mL/kg/min. What is a CPEX test? What is the significance of the AT?

Ten days later the patient presented to the ED with severe diffuse chest and abdominal pain. The ECG demonstrated sinus tachycardia. An ACS was suspected. He was treated with aspirin 300 mg and clopidogrel 300 mg. He subsequently became hypotensive and developed abdominal distension.

10. What is the most likely diagnosis on the patient's admission to the ED? What is the mortality associated with this?
11. How would you manage this patient?

Answers

1) **What factors affect the perioperative risk of morbidity and mortality associated with non-cardiac surgery? How does this affect the need for specialist cardiorespiratory preoperative assessment?**

Surgery results in dehydration, blood loss, and an inflammatory and endocrine stress response. The factors that affect the stress response and the perioperative risk of morbidity and mortality are listed in Table 45.1. Operations are classed as low, intermediate, or high risk of morbidity and mortality (Table 45.2).

Patients with pre-existing cardiac disease are at increased risk of perioperative morbidity and mortality after non-cardiac surgery. The American College of Cardiology/American Heart Association (ACC/AHA) guidelines recommend a stepwise approach to perioperative cardiac risk assessment and optimization of patients before non-cardiac surgery(see below).

Table 45.1 Factors which determine the perioperative cardiac risk associated with operations

Preoperative haemodynamic state
Surgery-specific factors which determine stress response (e.g. site, fluid shifts, duration, blood loss)
Comorbidity (incidence of cardiac and respiratory associated with the disease requiring surgery)
Time available for preoperative optimization (emergency, urgent or elective surgery)

Table 45.2 Risk of perioperative cardiovascular morbidity and mortality after non-cardiac surgery

1. High risk (>5%)
Aortic surgery
Major vascular surgery (supra-inguinal)
Peripheral vascular surgery
2. Intermediate risk (1–5%)
Abdominal and thoracic surgery
Endovascular aortic aneurysm surgery
Infrainguinal vascular surgery carotid endarterectomy
Head and neck surgery
Orthopaedic surgery
3. Low risk (<1%)
Endoscopy
Superficial procedures
Cataract surgery
Breast surgery

2) **What is the prognosis of the medical management of AAA?**

The normal diameter of the aorta is 2 cm. The aorta is aneurysmal if the outer diameter is over 3 cm. AAAs enlarge up to 0.8 cm/year and eventually rupture. The annual risk of rupture of an asymptomatic AAA is related to its size. In the present case, the annual risk of rupture is 10–20%. To reduce the rate of expansion and risk of rupture advise the patient to stop smoking, control hypertension, and consider beta blockade to reduce arterial wall tension.

Abdominal aortic aneurysms require elective surgical intervention because the inevitable outcome of medical management is death from rupture. Other complications include peripheral embolization (stroke or limb ischaemia), acute aortic occlusion, and aortocaval or aortoduodenal fistulae. However, in the elderly or those with limited life expectancy, repair may be inappropriate.

3) **What is the pathophysiological cause of perioperative cardiac morbidity and mortality?**

Perioperative cardiac complications are caused by either myocardial ischaemia or acute coronary thrombosis. The physiological demand of major surgery is similar to walking briskly for a few days. Oxygen consumption increases by 40%. Myocardial ischaemia occurs when myocardial oxygen demand exceeds supply. Tachycardia, hypertension, and pain increase oxygen demand, whilst hypotension, vasospasm, tachycardia, hypoxia, and anaemia reduce oxygen supply. The sympathetic stimulation, hypercoagulable state, leucocyte activation, and inflammation caused by the stress response may precipitate coronary artery occlusion or rupture of a pre-existing atherosclerotic plaque.

4) **What is the risk of perioperative mortality from elective AAA repair?**

Elective AAA repair is high-risk surgery with reported perioperative mortality rates of 2% for endovascular and up to 4% for open approaches. The perioperative cardiovascular risk in this case therefore depends on whether open or endovascular aortic aneurysm repair is performed.

Cardiovascular mortality mainly results from perioperative MI (up to 40% postoperative deaths). Non-fatal perioperative MI increases late mortality and morbidity, worsening long-term outcomes. Major open vascular surgery has the highest risk. Preoperative cardiorespiratory assessment and intervention may be beneficial in this population. Unlike open vascular procedures, endovascular aortic aneurysm repair is intermediate risk.

The precise morbidity and mortality associated with operations classed as intermediate risk, depending on the site of surgery and nature of the procedure. Some are short, with minimal fluid shifts, whereas others are longer, with large fluid shifts and higher risk of complications. Clinical judgement is required to correctly stratify perioperative risks and the need for further assessment on a case-by-case basis.

5) **When should an AAA be operated on electively?**

The timing of elective AAA repair is based on perioperative risk, risk of rupture, and the estimated life expectancy of the patient. The factors which determine the perioperative risk from elective AAA repair include comorbidities (age, gender, renal function, and cardiorespiratory disease) and hospital factors (e.g. the number of procedures performed annually).

Elective repair should be performed when the risk of rupture exceeds the risk associated with the operation.

The vast majority of AAAs are asymptomatic. However, AAA may cause pain in the abdomen, chest, back, or scrotum. The risk of rupture of a symptomatic AAA is high. This is therefore an indication for elective surgery.

Small (<4 cm) asymptomatic AAA should be measured with ultrasound every 6 months and managed medically initially. Offer elective surgical intervention if the aneurysm expands or causes symptoms. Four to five centimetre AAAs warrant consideration of elective repair if patients have low perioperative risk and good life expectancy.

Current guidelines recommend consideration of elective repair of asymptomatic AAA when the diameter of the aorta is 5.5 cm. Patients with 5–6-cm AAAs often benefit from repair, especially if other factors increase risk of rupture (e.g. hypertension, continued smoking, or COPD). At this size, the annual risk of rupture is approximately 10%. The mortality associated with aortic rupture is over 50%. In the UK, mortality after elective AAA repair is around 6–8%.

However, for high-risk patients, the threshold for repair may be 6–7 cm, depending on the perioperative risk. Correct timing of AAA repair is difficult and must involve the patient in the decision-making process.

6) **What medical therapy may influence perioperative cardiac risk?**

Optimization of medical therapy may improve perioperative outcome. Beta-blockers, statins, and aspirin have the strongest evidence base.

The patient in this case was started on bisoprolol and advised to continue all other medications in the perioperative period.

Beta-blockers

Several studies have reported improved outcome from perioperative beta blockade. However, the safety of this has been questioned since the Perioperative Ischemic Evaluation (POISE) trial. High-dose controlled-release metoprolol reduced risk of perioperative MI. However, risk of stroke and overall mortality were increased. The timing and titration of beta-blockers to control heart rate may affect perioperative outcome.

Continue beta-blockers if patients are already beta-blocked. Unless contraindicated beta-block high-risk patients prior to vascular surgery if coronary heart disease is found on preoperative testing. Beta-blockers are probably also of benefit to high-risk patients (more than one clinical risk factor) undergoing intermediate-risk or high-risk surgery.

The benefit of beta-blockers is less clear for lower risk patients awaiting intermediate or high-risk surgery and in high-risk surgery patients. Beta-blockers should not be given to patients with absolute contraindications to such therapy.

Statins

Besides lipid lowering, statins may have other beneficial effects on atherosclerotic vascular disease. These effects include plaque stabilization and reduction of oxidative stress and vascular inflammation. Statins reduce postoperative cardiovascular morbidity and mortality from major non-cardiac surgery.

Statins should be continued in the perioperative period if a patient is already taking statins. Consider starting statins in all patients awaiting vascular surgery and patients awaiting intermediate risk surgery with at least one clinical risk factor.

Aspirin

Aspirin is important in the secondary prevention of cardiovascular disease but the potential benefit in the perioperative period of non-cardiac surgery is less well established. Concerns about perioperative bleeding are often cited to justify stopping aspirin.

However, increasing evidence supports the view that aspirin does not greatly increase the severity of perioperative bleeding complications or mortality for most non-cardiac surgery. Furthermore, withdrawal of aspirin precedes 10% of perioperative acute coronary events.

Aspirin should only be stopped if the associated bleeding risks could increase morbidity and mortality more than the expected cardiovascular risks of aspirin withdrawal. It therefore seems sensible to continue aspirin use in most cases. The only absolute contraindications to the perioperative administration of aspirin are some neurosurgical procedures.

7) **What are the indications for preoperative coronary revascularization in patients with stable cardiovascular disease awaiting non-cardiac surgery?**

Randomized trial data suggest that if cardiac symptoms are stable routine 'prophylactic' preoperative coronary revascularization does not improve long- or short-term risk of death or MI after elective vascular surgery. Preoperative PCI does not prevent perioperative cardiac events after non-cardiac surgery, unless independently indicated for high-risk coronary anatomy, unstable angina, MI, or haemodynamically or arrhythmogenic unstable active coronary disease.

Similarly, PCI performed months to years before non-cardiac surgery has not been shown to reduce perioperative MI or death. However, coronary restenosis is unlikely more than 8–12 months after PCI. So it is probably reasonable to consider asymptomatic, active individuals 8–12 months after PCI to be at low risk of perioperative ischaemic complications.

8) **Does this patient require preoperative stress testing?**

In this case, the patient is scheduled for high-risk vascular surgery and has a reduced exercise tolerance. He has three risk factors from the revised cardiac risk index (RCRI; Table 45.3) so is classed at high risk (Table 45.4). He was unable to perform an exercise ECG so stress echocardiography was requested.

Preoperative non-invasive stress testing for high-risk patients (RCRI >3) increases survival at 1 year and reduces length of stay in hospital. However, stress testing is

Table 45.3 Revised Cardiac Risk Index

High-risk surgical procedure
Ischaemic heart disease
Congestive heart failure
Cerebrovascular accident
Preoperative treatment with insulin
Serum creatinine >170 μmol/L

Table 45.4 Estimated risk of major cardiac complications based on revised cardiac risk index

Risk factors	Cardiac risk
0	0.5%
1	1.0%
2	2.5%
≥3	5%

of limited benefit to intermediate-risk patients (RCRI 1–2) and may harm those at low risk.

The ACC/AHA guidelines propose a stepwise approach for the preoperative cardiac assessment and management of cardiac patients before non-cardiac surgery. This approach is based on:

- the urgency of surgery
- the presence of active cardiac conditions (Table 45.5) and/or risk factors (Table 45.3)
- the risk associated with the operation to be performed (Table 45.2)
- the patient's functional capacity
- the risk:benefit ratio of delaying surgery for preoperative optimization.
    1. Determine the urgency of the operation. Preoperative cardiac assessment may not be possible before emergency surgery.
    2. If preoperative assessment is possible, screen for active major cardiac disease (Table 45.5). Further assessment and treatment may be required if

Table 45.5 Major risk factors for perioperative cardiac morbidity and mortality

1. Unstable coronary syndromes (unstable angina or recent MI – within 30 days)
2. Decompensated heart failure
3. Significant arrhythmias
4. Severe valvular disease (severe aortic stenosis, symptomatic mitral stenosis)

any of these are present. However, the potential benefits of preoperative optimization must be greater than the risk of delaying the operation.

3. If no major risk factors are present, assess the risk of surgery (Table 45.2). Low-risk operations do not require specialist preoperative assessment even if patients are high risk.

4. Assess the patient's functional capacity prior to intermediate or high-risk surgery. If greater than four metabolic equivalents of task (METs) without symptoms, proceed to surgery. However, further assessment is needed if the patient is symptomatic or the functional capacity cannot be determined.

5. If the patient's functional capacity is less than four METs, screen for clinical risk factors from the revised Cardiac Risk Index (Table 45.3).

If there are no clinical risk factors, proceed to surgery. If the patient has one or two risk factors, consider proceeding to planned surgery with adequate heart rate control or consider further non-invasive testing if it will change management. If high-risk surgery is planned for a patient with three or more risk factors, consider further non-invasive testing if it will change management.

The best strategy for patients awaiting intermediate-risk surgery remains unclear. Consider either further testing or proceeding to surgery with heart rate control on a case-by-case basis.

9) **Cardiopulmonary exercise testing was performed and revealed an AT of 10 mL/kg/min. What is a CPEX test? What is the significance of the AT?**

Cardiopulmonary exercise testing is an objective test to determine preoperative fitness and examine the ability of the cardiovascular system to deliver oxygen to tissues under stress. If a patient is unable to increase oxygen delivery sufficiently a worse outcome is more likely. The results of CPEX testing correlate with perioperative mortality and morbidity. This allows identification of patients in whom the perioperative risk is so high that surgery may not be appropriate. Patients who are identified as 'fit' may be managed in high dependency or post-anaesthesia care areas rather than an ITU. This is particularly useful because nearly 20% of elective AAA repairs are cancelled because ITU beds are not available.

Cardiopulmonary exercise testing involves measurement of exhaled gas during graded exercise (usually on a bicycle or hand cycle). Exercise ECG testing is performed simultaneously. This provides information on the cardiorespiratory and metabolic function of the whole body and has a low complication rate.

The AT is the oxygen consumption in mL/kg/min when the rise in CO_2 production becomes disproportionate to the rise in O_2 consumption. This indicates that the body has reached maximal aerobic capacity and the higher the AT the better. Patients with AT <11 mL/kg/min may not be able to increase O_2 delivery to the level demanded by major surgery and are a high-risk group. Perioperative invasive monitoring and optimization of cardiac function may improve the outcome of these patients.

10) **What is the most likely diagnosis on the patient's admission to the ED? What is the mortality associated with this?**

A ruptured AAA is a clinical diagnosis based on the presence of abdominal pain, shock, and a pulsatile abdominal mass. In the present case, this is the most likely diagnosis given that the patient is known to have a 6.5-cm AAA. This may be confirmed by FAST or aortic ultrasound scan in the ED. No further diagnostic investigations or cardiac assessments are needed before surgery. The perioperative mortality for a ruptured AAA has gradually improved but remains over 50%. Cardiovascular risk stratification could be considered in the postoperative period.

11) **How would you manage this patient?**

Ruptured AAA is a life-threatening emergency associated with very high mortality. Although palliation should be considered in view of the significant cardiovascular comorbidities in this case.

Surgery should not be delayed if active management is appropriate. In addition to the standard preoperative management of ruptured AAA the effects of aspirin and clopidogrel should be reversed.

The evidence base to guide reversal of antiplatelet therapy prior to urgent operations is poor. Transfusion of platelets is the only way to reverse antiplatelet therapy quickly. However, this will need to be repeated if, as in this case, active drug is still present in the blood. Clopidogrel, a prodrug, acts irreversibly on the platelet ADP receptor and remains active throughout the life of the platelet (up to 5 days). Meticulous surgical technique and several transfusions of platelets are often required. Platelet transfusions should therefore be guided by assessment of platelet function if possible.

In this case, the management was discussed with a consultant haematologist. Two units of pooled platelets were transfused immediately. In all, 16 units of blood, 8 units of FFP and 4 more units of platelets were required in theatre during emergency repair of the ruptured AAA. The patient made a good postoperative recovery, TTE was normal, and he was discharged home 10 days later. Stress echocardiography performed 2 months later was normal.

Further reading

Wijeysundera DN, Beattie WS, Austin PC, Hux JE, Laupacis A. (2010). Non-invasive cardiac stress testing before elective major non-cardiac surgery: population based cohort study. *BMJ*; **340**: 252.

POISE Study Group, Devereaux PJ, Yang H, Yusuf S, Guyatt G, Leslie K, Villar JC, Xavier D, Chrolavicius S, Greenspan L, Pogue J, Pais P, Liu L, Xu S, Málaga G, Avezum A, Chan M, Montori VM, Jacka M, Choi P. (2008). Effects of extended-release metoprolol succinate in patients undergoing non-cardiac surgery (POISE trial): a randomised controlled trial. *Lancet*; **371**: 1839–1847.

Fleisher LA, Beckman JA, Brown KA, Calkins H, Chaikof EL, Fleischmann KE, Freeman WK, Froehlich JB, Kasper EK, Kersten JR, Riegel B, Robb JF. (2009). 2009 ACCF/AHA focused update on perioperative beta blockade incorporated into the ACC/AHA 2007 guidelines on perioperative cardiovascular evaluation and care for noncardiac surgery: a report of the American college of cardiology foundation/American heart association task force on practice guidelines. *Circulation*; 120:e169–276.

Case 46

A 70-year-old man with hypertension treated only with amlodipine 5 mg a day was brought to hospital by ambulance 1 hour after the onset of severe central crushing chest pain and breathlessness at rest. The paramedics had performed an ECG at the scene (Fig. 46.1) and transmitted this to the CCU. On admission to the CCU the patient was alert, orientated, and haemodynamically stable. Cardiovascular examination was unremarkable. Aspirin and high-flow oxygen had already been administered by the paramedics. Clopidogrel, intravenous morphine, and sublingual GTN were given in CCU before the patient was transferred to the cardiac catheter laboratory.

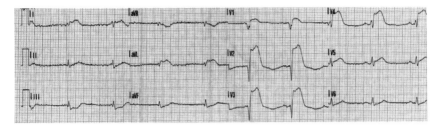

Fig. 46.1 ECG transmitted to the CCU.

Angiography was performed (Fig. 46.2). However, shortly after completion of the angiogram the patient developed further chest pain and then became drowsy and less responsive. He was peripherally cool and diaphoretic. His BP was 85/30 mmHg and HR was 110 bpm (sinus rhythm). A central venous catheter and a urinary catheter were inserted. Infusions of dobutamine and noradrenaline were started but failed to improve organ perfusion. An 8 French gauge IABP was placed percutaneously through the right femoral artery. Balloon counterpulsation was initiated at a 1:1 ratio with 100% augmentation. The BP improved to 98/47, the heart rate fell to 90 pbm, and the patient's level of consciousness improved.

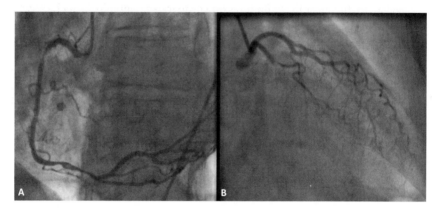

Fig. 46.2 Coronary angiogram. A, RCA angiogram in LAO view; B, LCA angiogram in PA view.

Questions

1. What does the ECG (Fig. 46.1) show?

2. Define cardiogenic shock.

3. What is the most likely cause of cardiogenic shock in this case?

4. What is an IABP? What is its main limitation?

5. What are the contraindications to the use of an IABP?

6. What are the complications associated with the use of an IABP?

7. What are the most likely findings on coronary angiography in such cases? Report the angiogram (Fig. 46.2).

8. Could this patient benefit from thrombolysis?

9. What is the definitive treatment of choice?

10. When should weaning from the IABP begin?

11. How should the patient be weaned from the IABP?

Answers

1) **What does the ECG (Fig. 46.1) show?**

The HR is 60 bpm in sinus rhythm. There is marked ST elevation in leads I, aVL, and V1–V5. There is ST depression in III and aVF. In conjuction with the history of typical cardiac chest pain this fulfils the diagnostic criteria for ST-elevation MI.

2) **Define cardiogenic shock.**

Cardiogenic shock occurs when inadequate tissue perfusion results from cardiac dysfunction. It is characterized by both systolic and diastolic dysfunction. Management requires a rapid, well-organized response.

Cardiogenic shock may be defined as decreased cardiac output and evidence of tissue hypoxia in the presence of adequate intravascular volume.

Diagnostic criteria for cardiogenic shock are sustained hypotension (systolic BP <90 mmHg for over 30 minutes) with a reduced cardiac index (<2.2 L/min/m^2) but raised pulmonary capillary wedge pressure (>15 mmHg).

Cardiogenic shock may be diagnosed clinically by observing hypotension and clinical signs of poor tissue perfusion, which include oliguria, cyanosis, cool peripheries, prolonged capillary refill time, and confusion. These signs usually persist despite correction of hypoxia, hypovolemia, acidosis, and arrhythmias.

3) **What is the most likely cause of cardiogenic shock in this case?**

Postmortem studies demonstrate that cardiogenic shock is usually associated with the loss of over 40% of the LV muscle mass. Causes of cardiogenic shock are listed in Table 46.1. The most common cause is a large MI. This is most likely in this case in view of the acute onset of chest pain and anterior ECG changes diagnostic of ST-elevation MI. A mechanical complication of acute MI, which could cause cardiogenic shock, should be excluded. Acute MR, large RV infarction, or rupture of the interventricular septum or left ventricular free wall, for example, could be revealed by echocardiography.

A small MI in a previously compromised left ventricle also may precipitate shock. After MI, stunned (non-functional but viable) myocardium may contribute to cardiogenic shock. Cardiogenic shock is the most common cause of death after acute MI. Although recent studies report in-hospital mortality rates of 55–65%, this may decline with improved treatment of MI and heart failure.

Coronary angiography is urgently indicated in patients with myocardial ischaemia or MI who also develop cardiogenic shock. Angiography is required to assess the anatomy of the coronary arteries and the need for urgent revascularization.

Table 46.1 Causes of cardiogenic shock

Cardiogenic shock	
Left ventricular failure	**Right ventricular failure**
Systolic dysfunction (decreased contractility)	
Ischaemia/MI	
Global hypoxemia	
Valvular disease	
Drugs—myocardial depressants (e.g. beta-blockers, calcium channel blockers, antiarrhythmics)	
Myocardial contusion	
Respiratory acidosis	
Metabolic (e.g. acidosis, hypophosphataemia, hypocalcaemia)	
Diastolic dysfunction/increased myocardial diastolic stiffness	
Ischaemia	
Ventricular hypertrophy	
Restrictive cardiomyopathy	
Prolonged hypovolemic or septic shock	
Ventricular interdependence	
Pericardial tamponade	
Greatly increased afterload	**Greatly increased afterload**
Aortic stenosis	Pulmonary embolism
Hypertrophic cardiomyopathy	Pulmonary vascular disease (e.g. pulmonary arterial hypertension, veno-occlusive disease)
Dynamic aortic outflow tract obstruction	
Coarctation of the aorta	Hypoxic pulmonary vasoconstriction
Malignant hypertension	Peak end-expiratory pressure
	High alveolar pressure
	Acute respiratory distress syndrome
	Pulmonary fibrosis
	Sleep disordered breathing
	Chronic obstructive pulmonary disease
Valvular or structural abnormality	
Mitral stenosis	
Endocarditis	
Mitral or aortic regurgitation	
Papillary muscle dysfunction or rupture	
Ruptured septum or free wall	
Obstruction (atrial myxoma or thrombus)	

(Continued)

Table 46.1 (continued) Causes of cardiogenic shock

Decreased contractility
RV infarction
Ischaemia
Hypoxia
Acidosis

Arrhythmias
Atrial and ventricular arrhythmias (tachycardia-induced cardiomyopathy)
Conduction abnormalities (e.g. atrioventricular blocks, sinus bradycardia)

4) **What is an IABP? What is its main limitation?**

If cardiogenic shock fails to improve with medical therapy, mechanical circulatory support or cardiac transplantation are the only therapeutic options.

The IABP is the most widely used device for circulatory support. Balloon counter-pulsation involves balloon inflation in diastole and deflation in systole. Intra-aortic balloon inflation at the onset of diastole increases diastolic pressure, displacing blood in the aorta proximally and distally. This improves coronary blood flow and systemic perfusion. The balloon deflates just before systole, reducing LV afterload. The magnitude of these effects depends on the following:

   (i) Balloon volume: volume of blood displaced is proportional to the volume of the balloon.

  (ii) Heart rate: LV and aortic diastolic filling times are inversely proportional to heart rate. Shorter diastolic time (tachycardia) reduces balloon augmentation per unit time. Left ventricular perfusion occurs mainly during diastole and so tachycardia also reduces myocardial perfusion.

 (iii) Aortic compliance: as aortic compliance increases (SVR decreases), the magnitude of diastolic augmentation decreases.

Left ventricular function improves as myocardial oxygen supply increases and oxygen demand is reduced. Right ventricular function may also improve as offloading the LV reduces left atrial and pulmonary vascular pressures (RV afterload). Right ventricular myocardial perfusion is also increased.

The indications for using an IABP are listed in Table 46.2. The contraindications are listed in Table 46.3.

The main limitation of using an IABP is that cardiac support is passive so some level of intrinsic LV function is required. The IABP must also be synchronized with the cardiac cycle. If cardiac function is severely depressed or in the presence of persistent arrhythmias, haemodynamic support from the IABP may not be sufficient to treat cardiogenic shock.

Table 46.2 Indications for using an IABP

Indications for use of an IABP
Treatable primary cardiac causes of haemodynamic compromise
Acute MI ± complications
Refractory unstable angina
Refractory LV failure
Cardiogenic shock
Acute MR and VSD
Refractory ventricular arrhythmias
Cardiomyopathy
Perioperative haemodynamic compromise (expected to recover)
Cardiac catheterization and angioplasty
Cardiac surgery
Weaning from cardiopulmonary bypass
Bridge to other ventricular assist devices

Table 46.3 Contraindications to the use of IABP therapy

Absolute	Relative
Technical	**Technical**
Aortic regurgitation	Abdominal aortic aneurysm
Aortic dissection	Major arterial reconstruction surgery
Aortic stents	Severe peripheral vascular disease
	Tachyarrhythmias
Futility	**Risk of infection**
Irreversible brain damage	Uncontrolled sepsis
Chronic end-stage cardiac disease	

Left ventricular assist devices (LVADs) can provide short-term haemodynamic support. Percutaneous LVADs that actively support the circulation may benefit patients in cardiogenic shock who do not respond to standard treatment.

Use of an LVAD during reperfusion after acute MI can improve cardiac function by reducing LV preload and increasing regional myocardial blood flow. The LVAD maintains coronary blood flow by maintaining cardiac output and aortic pressure, and reducing LV wall tension.

A recent meta-analysis compared the potential benefits of percutaneous LVAD with the IABP on haemodynamics and 30-day survival. Patients who received percutaneous LVAD had better haemodynamic profiles (higher cardiac index and mean BP) than patients who received IABP treatment. However, there was no difference in 30-day mortality or leg ischaemia.

Thus although percutaneous LVADs provide better haemodynamic support than an IABP, the use of an LVAD currently does not improve 30-day mortality. The indications for insertion of a LVAD are therefore uncertain but should be considered if medical therapy and an IABP fail to support the circulation and the cause of cardiogenic shock is potentially reversible.

5) **What are the contraindications to the use of an IABP?**

There are relatively few absolute contraindications to the use of an IABP. Severe aortic-iliac atherosclerosis may prevent IABP placement

6) **What are the complications associated with the use of an IABP?**

The incidence of complications has reduced as experience with IABPs has increased. However, as the patients are vasculopathic the most common complication is limb ischemia, which occurs in up to 45% of patients. Patients must be monitored for symptoms and signs of limb ischaemia if an IABP is in situ. If signs of ischaemia appear the IABP should be removed. Complications are listed in Table 46.4.

Table 46.4 Complications associated with IABPs

Vascular injury
Local injury—bleeding, haematoma, pseudoaneurysm
Transient loss of peripheral pulse
Limb ischaemia
Aortic dissection
Cardiac tamponade
Compartment syndrome
Mechanical
Thromboembolism
Balloon rupture (can cause gas embolus)
Balloon entrapment
Incorrect positioning (compromise organ circulation)
Haematological changes, e.g. thrombocytopenia, haemolysis
Infection

7) **What are the most likely findings on coronary angiography in such cases? Report the angiogram (Fig. 46.2).**

In patients with myocardial ischaemia who develop cardiogenic shock coronary angiography often demonstrates multivessel CAD. Compensatory hyperkinesis cannot occur in the non-infarct territory in the presence of severe coronary artery atherosclerosis.

In the present case, the angiogram (Figs 46.2 and 46.3) demonstrates severe steno-sis in the proximal dominant RCA with further severe distal stenosis. The left main stem was short, with an occlusion in the LAD at the first diagonal origin. The circumflex was small, with minor atheroma only.

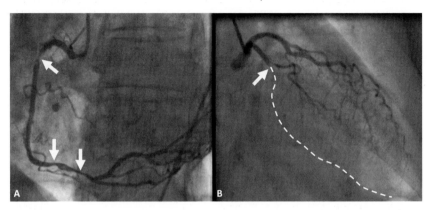

Fig. 46.3 Labelled coronary angiogram. A, RCA angiogram in LAO view: severe proximal and distal stenoses in a large dominant vessel. B, LCA angiogram in PA view: occluded proximal LAD involving ostium of small first diagonal. Circumflex has minor proximal plaque. left main stem is short and unobstructed.

8) **Could this patient benefit from thrombolysis?**

Used early in the course of MI, thrombolysis reduces mortality and the risk of subsequently developing cardiogenic shock. Once cardiogenic shock has developed the results are disappointing.

A prospective study used the SHould we emergently revascularize Occluded Coronaries for cardiogenic shock (SHOCK) trial registry to investigate the poten-tial benefit of thrombolysis and IABP use on in-hospital mortality from cardio-genic shock due to MI. Patients in cardiogenic shock who were thrombolysed had lower in-hospital mortality than those who were not (54% vs 64%). Patients who received IABP treatment had lower in-hospital mortality than those who did not (50% vs 72%). The in-hospital mortality of the group that received thrombolysis and IABP counterpulsation (47%) was the lowest of the four study groups. However, revascularization resulted in the greatest reduction in-hospital mortality (39% with revascularization vs 78% without revascularization).

The benefit of thrombolysis in this case would be slight. Only patients who cannot receive invasive therapy should be considered for thrombolysis.

9) **What is the definitive treatment of choice?**

Revascularization is the treatment of choice for patients with cardiogenic shock due to MI. The SHOCK trial demonstrated this. Patients were assigned to receive either optimal medical management, including use of an IABP and thrombolysis, or coronary angiography and revascularization (angioplasty or CABG).

At 6 months the mortality was significantly lower in the early intervention group (50% vs 63%) and at 1-year the survival rate of the early revascularisation group was 46.7% and of the medically managed group was 33.6%. However, only patients under 75 years benefitted from revascularization.

In this case, the angiographic findings shown in Fig. 46.2 did not preclude PCI as a possible mode of full revascularization. It seemed possible to reopen the acutely blocked LAD artery and dilate and stent the dominant RCA lesions.

However, reperfusion injury may occur during PCI and exacerbate the cardiogenic shock. As the patient's condition was critical, the cardiothoracic surgical team were asked to consider the place of emergency CABG. In this setting emergency CABG is associated with a high morbidity and mortality. The surgeons agreed that PCI should be the attempted as the initial revascularization strategy, with surgery if PCI was unsuccessful.

The cardiothoracic anaesthetist was asked to attend and induced anaesthesia and mechanical ventilation prior to angioplasty. Under these conditions, the LAD was successfully wired and TIMI grade 3 flow restored after thrombus aspiration (Table 46.5). A 3.5 × 15 mm bare-metal stent was placed in the proximal vessel. The three lesions in the RCA were stented with 3.5 × 15 mm and 3.0 × 24 mm bare-metal stents. The patient remained haemodynamically stable throughout and was recovered and extubated in the cardiac catheter laboratory before being transferred back to the CCU with the IABP in situ.

Table 46.5 TIMI flow grading system

Grade	Description of flow
Grade 0	No perfusion. No antegrade flow beyond point of occlusion
Grade 1	Penetration without perfusion. Contrast passes beyond the area of obstruction but fails to opacify the entire coronary bed distal to the obstruction for the duration of the cineangiographic filming sequence.
Grade 2	Partial perfusion. Contrast passes across the obstruction and opacifies the coronary bed distal to the obstruction. However, the rate of entry of contrast material into the vessel distal to the obstruction or its rate of clearance from the distal bed (or both) is perceptibly slower than its entry into or clearance from comparable areas not perfused by the previously occluded vessel (e.g. the opposite coronary artery or the coronary bed proximal to the obstruction).
Grade 3	Complete perfusion. Antegrade flow into the bed distal to the obstruction occurs as promptly as antegrade flow into the bed from the involved bed and is as rapid as clearance from an uninvolved bed in the same vessel or the opposite artery.

10) **When should weaning from the IABP begin?**

Weaning from the IABP should be considered when the inotropic requirements are minimal, which allows increased inotropic support if necessary.

In this case the IABP was kept *in situ* for 48 hours after the PCI whilst the dobutamine and noradrenaline were weaned. Recovery of myocardial function after successful revascularization may take several days and reperfusion injuries may initially cause deterioration in cardiac function.

11) How should the patient be weaned from the IABP?

Weaning is achieved by gradually (over 6–12 hours) decreasing the ratio of augmented to non-augmented beats from 1:1 to 1:2 to 1:3 and less frequent inflations. The balloon volume can also be reduced. The balloon should never be turned off whilst in situ because thrombus may form.

In this case, the IABP support was gradually weaned and stopped 24 hours after the inotropes were stopped. The patient remained haemodynamically stable and the next day was transferred from the CCU to the cardiology ward. Echocardiography demonstrated hypokinesia of the apex and lateral wall of the LV with an estimated ejection fraction of 40%.

The patient did not experience any further chest pain but he was short of breath on exertion (NYHA class III). He was started on bisoprolol and ramipril. These were both slowly titrated to 5 mg daily over the next 10 days.

On discharge his HR and BP were 60 bpm and 105/55 mmHg, respectively. His ECG showed sinus rhythm with poor R-wave progression and T-wave inversion in leads I, aVL, and V1–V5.

On review in clinic 6 months later the patient reported that his breathlessness had improved (NYHA class II) and there were no clinical signs of cardiac failure. On echocardiography the apex and lateral wall of the LV remained mildly hypokinetic but the LV function appeared to have improved (EF 55%). The ECG findings were similar to those on discharge from hospital.

Further reading

Hochman JS, Sleeper LA, Webb JG, Dzavik V, Buller CE, Aylward P, Col J, White HD (1999). Early revascularisation in acute myocardial infarction complicated by cardiogenic shock. SHOCK Investigators. Should We Emergently Revascularize Occluded Coronaries for Cardiogenic Shock. *New Engl J Med*; **341**: 625–634.

Hochman JS, Sleeper LA, White HD, Dzavik V, Wong SC, Menon V, Webb JG, Steingart R, Picard MH, Menegus MA, Boland J, Sanborn T, Buller CE, Modur S, Forman R, Desvigne-Nickens P, Jacobs AK, Slater JN, Le Jemtel TH (2001). One-year survival following early revascularisation for cardiogenic shock. *JAMA*; **285**: 190–192.

Sanborn TA, Sleeper LA, Bates ER, Jacobs AK, Boland J, French JK, Dens J, Dzavik V, Palmeri ST, Webb JG, Goldberger M, Hochman JS (2000). Impact of thrombolysis, intra-aortic balloon pump counterpulsation, and their combination in cardiogenic shock complicating acute myocardial infarction: a report from the SHOCK Trial Registry. SHould we emergently revascularize Occluded Coronaries for cardiogenic shocK? *J Am Coll Cardiol*; **36**: 1123–1129.

Cheng JM, den Uil CA, Hoeks SE, vander Ent M, Jewbali LS, van Domburg RT, Serruys PW, (2009). Percutaneous left ventricular assist devices vs. intra-aortic balloon pump counterpulsation for treatment of cardiogenic shock: a meta-analysis of controlled trials. *Eur Heart J*; **30**: 2102–2108.

Case 47

A 16-year-old girl who had had a total cavopulmonary connection (TCPC) procedure for tricuspid atresia completed 10 years previously was admitted with a 2-month history of worsening breathlessness, reduced appetite, abdominal distension, and swelling of the ankles.

The patient initially had a right-modified Blalock–Taussig shunt (systemic-to-pulmonary artery shunt) formed on the third day of life. At 6 months of age she had a bidirectional Glenn procedure (superior cavopulmonary anastamosis) and the right-modified Blalock–Taussig shunt was closed. At 6 years of age, a Fontan-type circulation (TCPC) was completed with the formation of an extracardiac cavopulmonary shunt (Fig. 47.1).

Since then her development, exercise tolerance, and quality of life had been good. However, at her annual review with a paediatric cardiologist 1 month prior to this presentation she reported mild breathlessness on exertion and pedal oedema.

At that time ECG demonstrated sinus rhythm. Transthoracic echocardiography findings were no different from those of the routine TTE performed at the previous annual clinic review. The systolic and diastolic function of the systemic ventricle was good, with no evidence of atrioventricular valve regurgitation, shunts, obstruction in the TCPC, or spontaneous echo contrast within the atrium. A bubble contrast study did not identify pulmonary arteriovenous malformations.

Her GP was asked to perform routine blood tests and outpatient cardiac catherization was planned. She was started on furosemide 40 mg daily. Her only other regular medication was aspirin 75 mg daily. However, 1 month later she presented to hospital because her symptoms had progressed to the point that she was unable to walk more than 50 m and she 'looked pregnant'.

On admission her observations were HR 70 bpm (sinus rhythm), BP 95/45 mmHg, temperature 36.7°C, and O_2 saturations 95% on air. Examination revealed a median sternotomy scar, a raised JVP, a distended abdomen with palpable liver edge, and shifting dullness. There was pitting oedema up to the abdominal wall. Examination of the chest was normal.

On admission to hospital laboratory investigations were Hb 17 g/dL, WBC 8.7 × 10^9 cells/L, platelets 276 × 10^{12} cells/L, INR 0.9, serum sodium 135 mmol/L, potassium 4.5 mmol/L, creatinine 53 μmol/L, urea 5 mmol/L, bilirubin 23 μmol/L, albumin 23 g/L, total protein 43 g/L, alanine transaminase 62 iu/L, alkaline phosphatase 53 iu/L, gamma-glutamyltransferase 52 u/L, calcium 1.72 mmol/L, and CRP <5 mg/L. Urine dipstick and pregnancy test were negative. ECG confirmed sinus rhythm and there were no significant abnormalities on the chest X-ray. Abdominal ultrasound demonstrated an enlarged liver with moderate ascites.

The symptoms and peripheral oedema did not improve despite treatment with intravenous furosemide (80 mg twice daily). Cardiac catheterization and angiography were performed (Table 47.1).

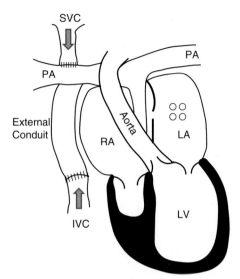

Fig. 47.1 TCPC (Fontan-type) with an extracardiac conduit. This figure illustrates the Fontan circulation with an extracardiac conduit for total cavopulmonary connection. The systemic and pulmonary circulations are connected in series. The right atrium (RA) or systemic veins are connected to the pulmonary artery (PA) via an extracardac conduit. The single ventricle pumps blood into the systemic circulation. Blood flow through the pulmonary circulation is passive. In the absence of fenestration, mixing of systemic and pulmonary venous blood does not occur. However, systemic venous pressure is raised and drives pulmonary blood flow.

Table 47.1 Cardiac catheterization report

	Pressure (mmHg)	Oxygen saturation
Superior vena cava	14 (mean)	64%
Inferior vena cava	14 (mean)	68%
External venous conduit	14 (mean)	
Right pulmonary artery	14 (mean)	66%
Left pulmonary artery	14 (mean)	66%
Systemic ventricle	100/8	
Aorta	100/60	94%

Angiography report

No areas of obstruction within the external conduit for systemic venous blood or the pulmonary arteries. Satisfactory shortening of the systemic left ventricle. No atrioventricular valve regurgitation.

Questions

1. Describe the stages that are likely to have preceded completion of the TCPC in this case.
2. What are the indications for formation of a TCPC?
3. How does a TCPC differ from the normal circulation and congenital heart disease with a single functional ventricle?
4. Why is the TCPC circulation not formed at birth?
5. What is the likely cause of the diuretic resistant oedema and ascites in this case?
6. What investigations are required?
7. What are the options for medical therapy in this case?
8. If medical management fails, what other options are available for treatment?
9. What is the prognosis in this case?
10. What difficulties are associated with cardiac transplantation in these patients?

Answers

1) **Describe the stages that are likely to have preceded completion of the TCPC in this case.**

   Creation of the TCPC for surgical palliation of patients with a single ventricle is usually a staged procedure involving

   (1) systemic–pulmonary shunt (within first few days of life)

   (2) superior cavopulmonary connection (2–6 months of age)

   (3) completion of the Fontan circulation (TCPC; 1–5 years).

Systemic–pulmonary shunt

The first stage of the palliation is lesion specific but results in common physiology regardless of the initial pathology:

- unobstructed venous return to the single ventricle from the pulmonary circulation
- unobstructed ventricular outflow to the systemic circulation
- mixing of systemic and pulmonary venous return
- limited pulmonary blood flow (enough for tissue O_2 delivery and growth of pulmonary arteries).

This palliative procedure involves placement of a synthetic or subclavian atrial conduit (3–4 mm internal diameter) between a major systemic central vessel and a proximal pulmonary artery. Optimizing pulmonary blood flow keeps PVR and the ventricular volume load low.

Superior cavopulmonary connection

The second stage of the procedure involves formation of a bidirectional Glenn shunt procedure. The first shunt is usually ligated at this stage. Cardiopulmonary bypass is usually required to anastomose the SVC to the proximal right pulmonary artery. Blood drains directly from the SVC to the pulmonary arteries.

This is operation is usually performed at 2–6 months of age, when the pulmonary arteries have grown sufficiently to reduce PVR.

This allows low-pressure pulmonary blood flow and reduces the ventricular volume load. However, the patient remains cyanosed (peripheral O_2 saturations of 80–85%). The single ventricle still receives mixed oxygenated and deoxygenated blood from the functionally single atrium: deoxygenated blood from the IVC and oxygenated blood via the pulmonary veins. After surgery, intrapulmonary arteriovenous shunts may develop and exacerbate the shunting of deoxygenated blood.

Completion of the Fontan-type circulation

The final stage of Fontan palliation (completion) is usually performed at 1–5 years of age, when restriction of activity affects the child's lifestyle and pulmonary vasculature is grown and has a low PVR.

Blood in the IVC is directed into the pulmonary circuit to complete the TCPC. There are numerous variations in the surgical approach but the most commonly encountered Fontan circulations are:

(1) direct RA–PA connection

(2) intra-atrial tunnel (SVC to PA and IVC to PA through an intra-atrial tunnel)

(3) extracardiac conduit (SVC to PA and IVC to PA through an external conduit; Fig. 47.1).

If PVR is suboptimal (10–25%) a small fenestration between the conduit and the atrium is required to allow a residual right-to-left shunt. The shunt reduces pulmonary blood flow, caval pressure, and congestion, and increases preload and cardiac output, at the expense of slight desaturation.

2) **What are the indications for formation of a TCPC?**

Conversion to a TCPC is considered if a biventricular repair is not possible for complex congenital heart disease. In 1971, Fontan and Baudet first described the technique for palliation of tricuspid atresia using the right atrium to complete the cavopulmonary connection. Other indications include pulmonary atresia with an intact ventricular septum, double inlet left ventricle, hypoplastic left heart, double outlet right ventricle, and complete atrioventricular septal defects.

3) **How does the TCPC differ from the normal circulation and congenital heart disease with a single functional ventricle?**

In the normal postnatal circulation, the pulmonary circulation is connected to the systemic circulation in series and each is powered by a separate pump (the right and left ventricles, respectively).

Some patients with complex congenital heart disease are born with only one functional ventricle. The single functional ventricle must maintain both the systemic and pulmonary circulations, which are connected in parallel. This has two major disadvantages:

(1) hypoxia and cyanosis at rest, increasing during exercise

(2) chronic volume overload of the single functional ventricle.

The chronic volume overload will gradually impair ventricular function. Life expectancy is reduced, with mortality mainly due to congestive heart failure.

With TCPC, systemic venous return is diverted directly to the pulmonary arteries, bypassing the right heart. The single functional ventricle must still maintain both the systemic and pulmonary circulations but these are now connected in series. This reduces the volume load on the single ventricle and reduces or abolishes mixing of oxygenated and deoxygenated blood. Systemic venous hypertension (mean pressure >10 mmHg) and pulmonary arterial hypotension (mean pressure <15 mmHg) develop because blood flow through the lungs is passive. However, obstruction to blood flow can reduce cardiac output and precipitate circulatory failure.

The pathophysiology of the failing TCPC differs from both biventricular heart failure and the failure of the untreated univentricular heart. In TCPC a change in systemic vascular resistance has a direct effect on the PVR and vice versa.

4) **Why is the TCPC circulation not formed at birth?**

With TCPC, blood flow into the lungs is passive. Blood is not pumped into the lungs by a right ventricle. In the neonatal period the physiologically high PVR would restrict passive flow of blood. A staged formation of the circulation allows adaptation of the heart and lungs. This reduces perioperative morbidity and mortality.

5) **What is the most likely cause of the diuretic resistant oedema and ascites in this case?**

In the present case, the patient is hypoalbuminaemic and hypocalcaemic (corrected calcium 2.06 mmol/L). Hypoalbuminaemia can result from:

◆ decreased production
◆ increased loss
◆ haemodilution
◆ inflammation.

However, in the present case, serum biochemistry demonstrates normal renal function. The normal CRP excludes an acute phase response. Although the bilirubin, alanine tranaminase, and gamma-glutamyltransferase are raised, the INR is normal. Liver disease is unlikely to explain the degree of hypoproteinaemia in the present case. Mildly deranged liver function tests are a common finding in patients with a TCPC (discussed below). The ECG excluded an arrhythmia. Cardiac catheterization data (Table 47.1), angiography, and TTE demonstrate 'normal' TCPC anatomy and haemodynamics.

Protein loss via the gastrointestinal (GI) tract (protein-losing enteropathy; PLE) is the most likely diagnosis. Up to 13% of patients with a TCPC develop PLE, which usually presents with complications of hypoproteinaemia, including oedema and ascites. Other complications include immunodeficiency from loss of immunoglobulins, thrombophilia, fat malabsorption, hypocalcaemia, and hypomagnesaemia.

The diagnosis of PLE should only be considered after exclusion of other causes of fluid retention, hypoproteinaemia, and protein loss, such as malnutrition or cardiac, hepatic, or renal disease. The symptoms of reduced cardiac output and systemic venous congestion may be due to obstruction of the TCPC. This must be excluded before the diagnosis of PLE is made.

Cardiac catheterization should be performed by an adult congenital heart disease specialist. Transoesophageal echocardiography and MRI are often helpful. However, pulmonary artery pressure or resistance cannot be measured directly by MRI.

In congested low-output TCPCs, small pressure gradients across venous connections are often missed by non-invasive investigation. Angiography can detect obstructions at suture lines or within the pulmonary arteries, which may cause resistance to flow. These obstructions can be dilated or stented. Alternatively, an atrial shunt (Fontan fenestration) may be formed in the cardiac catheter laboratory or surgically, perhaps as a bridge to transplantation. This increases cardiac output and oxygen delivery at the cost of some cyanosis. If collaterals between the aorta and pulmonary artery are found, coil embolization may prevent a competitive high-pressure circuit.

Some protein is normally lost from the GI tract in secretions and sloughed enterocytes. However, PLE is characterized by the severe loss of protein into the intestine. Mechanisms include lymphatic obstruction and mucosal disease (erosion, ulceration, or increased mucosal permeability to proteins). Proteins are digested into amino acids by enzymes and reabsorbed in the GI tract. Hypoproteinaemia develops when the rate of protein loss exceeds the rate of protein synthesis. The aetiology of PLE in patients with a TCPC is unclear. The true prevalence is unknown as GI protein loss begins before patients present with symptoms of oedema.

The high systemic venous pressure of the TCPC is transmitted to the splanchnic venous and lymphatic circulation. This may affect the intestinal mucosal cell function and induce apoptosis with subsequent loss of integrity and protein leakage. Systemic venous hypertension (>15 mmHg) increases the risk of PLE but is not the only cause. As the present case demonstrates, satisfactory haemodynamics (systemic venous pressures of 10–15 mmHg) may be found on cardiac catheterization. However, these pressure measurements may be affected by the hypovolaemia and reduced cardiac output caused by severe PLE and exacerbated by diuretic therapy. Regardless, venous pressure in the TCPC is higher than with normal biventricular circulation.

6) **What investigations are required?**

Investigation for PLE requires measurement of the GI clearance of α1-antitrypsin, a non-specific marker of protein loss. Scintigraphy with intravenous administration of technetium labelled (Tc-99m) dextran or human serum albumin is more accurate. Endoscopy or barium studies can also be used to further localize the GI protein loss.

In the present case, faecal α1-antitrypsin was markedly elevated (448 mg/g stool normal range <2 mg/g stool). Further investigation was not considered necessary in view of the associated hypoalbuminaemia and hypocalcaemia.

7) **What are the options for medical therapy in this case?**

Cardiac catheterization and angiography are required to assess the haemodynamics and anatomy of the circulation. If there are no treatable problems, medical management of PLE should be considered.

The options for the medical management of PLE are limited, but include:

♦ improving Fontan-type circulatory haemodynamics medically (ACE inhibitors)

♦ symptomatic relief by using diuretics, albumin infusions, and dietary changes (low in salt but high in calories, protein, and medium-chain triglycerides, supplementation with fat-soluble vitamins)

♦ reduction of intestinal protein loss (steroids, octreotide, or heparin).

Medical management of PLE

Treatment should be tailored to the severity of the disease. Initial management should include ACE inhibitors. These may improve haemodynamics by improving blood flow through the TCPC and increasing cardiac output.

Palliation of symptoms should then be considered. Diuretics may reduce oedema. Increasing dietary protein and medium-chain triglycerides can be helpful. Medium-chain triglycerides are rapidly absorbed and reduce the amount of protein in the intestinal lymph, reducing protein loss. These simple measures can increase serum proteins and relieve oedema in patients with mild PLE. However, serum protein concentrations rarely normalize and regular monitoring of nutritional status is required. Supplementation of fat-soluble vitamins may be helpful.

Pleural or pericardial effusions may develop if PLE is severe, with very low serum protein concentrations. Intravenous 20% human albumin solution can rapidly increase serum protein levels. However, the effect is temporary as the administered albumin is eventually lost into the GI tract. However, in combination with the use of diuretics, increasing serum protein concentrations with albumin infusion can significantly improve symptoms, buying time for other treatments to take effect.

Protein loss from the GI tract may be reduced by high-dose steroids. However, the doses required can cause severe side effects. Furthermore, as the primary problem persists, weaning steroids may be difficult. The risk-to-benefit ratio should be discussed with the patient prior to treatment. Continuous heparin infusions also improve serum protein concentrations and relieve symptoms, but the mechanism is unclear. Octreotide, a somatostatin analogue, may be useful. It inhibits several GI hormones and reduces GI blood flow. However, further research is required to define the roles of octreotide and heparin infusions in the management of PLE.

In the present case, oral diuretics were continued (frusemide 80 mg twice daily), dietary advice was given, and enalapril and oral prednisolone were started (2 mg/kg/day). In view of the increased risk of thromboembolism warfarin was started and the aspirin was stopped. The oedema improved, but did not resolve completely and the serum protein concentrations stabilized but did not improve significantly. However, attempts to wean the dose steroid resulted in falls in serum albumin and total protein, accompanied by worsening oedema.

8) **If medical management fails, what other options are available for treatment?**

If medical therapy fails to improve symptoms or steroid therapy cannot be weaned, the remaining surgical options are:

◆ resection of enteropathic bowel.

◆ improving Fontan-type circulatory haemodynamics (conversion or fenestration, ventricular assist device).

◆ cardiac transplantation.

In the present case surgical fenestration of the TCPC conduit to the left atrium was performed using cardiopulmonary bypass. The post-operative course was remarkable. Within 1 week of the operation, the oedema resolved completely.

Steroid therapy was weaned. One month after fenestration serum albumin concentration was 32 g/L, total protein was 62 g/L, and calcium was 2.10 mmol/L. Although O_2 saturation by pulse oximetry was 89% on air, exercise tolerance was not affected.

9) **What is the prognosis in this case?**

In the present case, the development of protein-losing enteropathy suggests a poor prognosis with a 5-year survival rate of 45–60% without cardiac transplantation.

In a registry of 261 patients who underwent Fontan surgery before 1985 30% died, 2% received heart transplants, 2% required Fontan revision, and 8.0% had Fontan conversion. Perioperative deaths were responsible for 70% of mortality but decreased steadily over time. The crude perioperative mortality rate for initial Fontan surgery was 17%. In the last three decades, surgical mortality has substantially improved.

Of those who survived surgery, survival rate (without transplant) was good (90% at 10 years, 83% at 20 years, 70% at 25 years). Mortality was mainly due to thromboembolism, heart failure, or sudden death (0.15% per year, probably due to arrhythmias). As increasing numbers of patients survive into adulthood it is important to be aware of the potential complications of the TCPC.

Complications of the Fontan-type circulation

Most patients with a Fontan circulation have a good quality of life for many years. However, several potential complications may develop.

Reduced exercise tolerance and Fontan failure

The cardiac response to exercise is abnormal. The heart rate response is blunted. The increase in stroke volume with exercise is limited by impaired ventricular function and difficulty increasing ventricular preload. The ventricle hypertrophies, dilates, and contractility are impaired. Both systolic and diastolic function decline. The main determinant of ventricular function is preload, so inotropes, vasodilators, and beta-blockers have limited effect. Myocardial dysfunction and grade II heart failure develop in about 70% of patients by 10 years post Fontan.

Tachyarrhythmias and bradyarrhythmias

Atrial arrhythmias are the most common of the late complications of the TCPC. These occur in 45% of patients within 10 years of surgery. The aetiology is multifactorial and includes the multiple suture lines near the sinus node, atrial hypertension, and dilation. Arrhythmias may be poorly tolerated and DC cardioversion may be required. Treatment is difficult because sinus node dysfunction often coexists. Apart from amiodarone, medical therapy is rarely successful. Ablation of atrial re-entry circuits is challenging. Bradycardia or junctional rhythms require medical therapy or a pacemaker to maintain AV synchrony. Anticoagulation is required as the risk of thromboembolism is high.

Shunts

Patients with a TCPC, particularly those with a fenestration and right-to-left shunt, have slightly low resting O_2 saturation and desaturate on exertion. Drainage of deoxygenated blood from the coronary sinus into the systemic circulation contributes to this. As PVR increases, left-to-right shunt may develop through aorta–pulmonary collaterals or incomplete occlusion of previous artificial shunts. These shunt volumes overload the ventricle and may induce an irreversible increase in PVR secondary to high regional pulmonary blood flow.

If cyanosis develops, careful angiographic assessment of the circulation is required. Right-to-left shunts through venous collaterals may be embolized or intracardiac shunts closed. However, sealing the 'release valve' from the high-resistance pulmonary circulation may reduce cardiac output and cause systemic venous congestion.

Thromboembolism

About 30% of patients have thromboembolic events within 10 years. Arrhythmias, atrial scars, the low-flow circulation, hypovolaemia, and hypercoagulability all increase the risk. However there is no robust long-term data or clear guidance on prophylaxis. Whilst some retrospective studies recommend antiplatelet therapy, others suggest anticoagulants are more effective. However, some experts discourage routine anticoagulation. A recent retrospective case series found that the absence of aspirin or warfarin therapy was a powerful independent predictor of mortality from thromboembolism. Antiplatelet therapy should probably be prescribed for patients with a Fontan circulation with no other risk factors for thromboembolism.

Plastic bronchitis

This rare complication of Fontan failure presents with chronic respiratory symptoms, including cough with expectoration of bronchial casts, breathlessness, and wheeze. It is associated with systemic venous hypertension and increased PVR. The aetiology is unclear but the pathogenesis may be similar to PLE.

Liver disease

The elevated systemic venous pressure of the TCPC is transmitted to the subdiaphragmatic veins. The splanchnic and the hepatic portal veins are affected. Elevated transaminases, raised bilirubin, and abnormal clotting are common findings suggestive of liver dysfunction. Studies using computed tomography, liver biopsy, and postmortem assessment of patients with this physiology have demonstrated various stages of hepatic disease from chronic passive congestion to hepatocellular carcinoma.

10) **What difficulties are associated with cardiac transplantation in these patients?**

Replacement of Fontan physiology with cardiac transplantation is the definitive surgical palliation for the patient with a TCPC. However, the transplant operation is very challenging and donors limited. The systemic venous connections and the pulmonary arterial pathways must be reconstructed. The multiple previous cardiac surgeries cause scarring and adhesions. Chronic hypoxia results in polycythemia and coagulopathy. The coagulopathy is exacerbated by liver dysfunction.

The risk of perioperative bleeding is further increased in the presence of acquired systemic-to-pulmonary artery and systemic venous collaterals.

Despite these problems transplantation is generally well tolerated and has good outcomes. The 5-year survival after cardiac transplantation for 'failing Fontan' is approximately 70%. Although similar to other congenital heart disease, the post-transplant mortality remains higher than in patients without acquired heart disease.

The potential long-term complications are similar to those of any other cardiac transplant patient. However, unlike the patients transplanted for cardiomyopathy there are initially no perioperative complications related to pulmonary hypertension. However, the improved cardiac output post transplant may increase PVR and cause hypertension in the abnormal pulmonary vasculature of the previous Fontan circulation.

Further reading

The Task Force on the Management of Grown Up Congenital Heart Disease of the European Society of Cardiology (2003). Guidelines on the Management of Grown Up Congenital Heart Disease. *Eur Heart J*; 24: 1035–1084.

Sørensen TS, Therkildsen SV, Hansen OK, Sørensen K, Pedersen EM. (2002). Total cavo-pulmonary connection. a virtual 3-dimensional fly-through. *Circulation*; **105**: e176.

Khairy P, Fernandes SM, Mayer JE Jr, Triedman JK, Walsh EP, Lock JE, Landzberg MJ. (2008). Long-term survival, modes of death, and predictors of mortality in patients with Fontan surgery. *Circulation*; **117**: 85–92.

Case 48

A 19-year-old man with a history of repair of tetralogy of Fallot (TOF) was brought into the ED by ambulance. He had lost consciousness whilst walking to catch a bus with his father. He fell but was caught by his father, who lowered him to the ground. His father reported that the patient initially appeared pale but regained consciousness over about 2 minutes. There was no convulsion, urinary incontinence, or tongue biting. On waking he was mildly disorientated for a few minutes.

On arrival in the ED 30 minutes after the collapse he was alert, orientated, and could clearly recall events before the collapse and after regaining consciousness. He denied any previous episodes of palpitations, dizziness, or syncope. He did not take any regular medication and denied preceding ingestion of caffeine, alcohol, and illicit drugs.

Repair of TOF was performed at 8 months of age with a right ventriculotomy, closure of a subaortic VSD with a Dacron patch and a subannular pericardial patch to relieve the RVOT obstruction.

On admission his observations were HR 80 bpm (sinus rhythm), BP 115/65 mmHg, temperature 36.5°C, and O_2 saturations 98% on air. A median sternotomy scar was present. Examination was otherwise unremarkable.

Routine laboratory blood tests were normal. The 12 lead ECG showed sinus rhythm, axis +100 and RBBB (QRS duration 190 ms).

The patient was admitted to a monitored bed for overnight observation. There were no further clinical events, and atrial and ventricular ectopics were shown on telemetry.

Transthoracic echocardiography findings were similar those of the routine TTE performed at the previous annual clinic review. The gradient across the RVOT was 14 mmHg. There was mild pulmonary regurgitation (PR), mild tricuspid regurgitation, and mild RV dilation. There was no residual VSD. Left and right ventricular function appeared normal.

Questions

1. What are the features of TOF?
2. What is the most likely cause of syncope in the present case?
3. What risk factors suggest increased risk of SCD after repair of TOF?
4. What investigations would you consider for the present case?
5. Further investigation suggests increased risk of SCD. How would you manage the patient?
6. What is the prognosis after repair of TOF? What are the common late cardiac complications after repair of TOF?

Answers

1) **What are the features of TOF?**

   Tetralogy of Fallot includes the following major features:

   1. RVOT obstruction, which may be subvalvar (muscular), valvar and/or supravalvular
   2. concentric RV hypertrophy
   3. subaortic perimembraneous VSD
   4. over-riding aorta (deviation of the origin of the aorta to the right so that it overrides the VSD).

   Tetralogy of Fallot results from the deviation and hypertrophy of the infundibular septum, which causes muscular outflow tract obstruction.

2) **What is the most likely cause of syncope in the present case?**

   The most likely cause of syncope in the present case is a transient tachyarrhythmia.

   The patient was haemodynamically stable prior to loss of consciousness and shortly after regaining consciousness. The TTE excluded significant structural abnormalities and demonstrated normal left and right ventricular function.

   Both atrial and ventricular arrhythmias are common after repair of TOF. Repair of TOF usually causes RBBB as a result of injury to myocardium and the conducting system. However, prolongation of the QRS duration >180 ms is associated with RV dilation, VT, and SCD after repair of TOF. There was no evidence of heart block on the 12 lead ECG so bradycardia is less likely to have caused syncope. The atrial and ventricular ectopics are not clinically significant.

3) **What risk factors suggest increased risk of SCD after repair of TOF?**

   Several risk factors for the occurrence of VT or SCD after repair of TOF have been identified (Tables 48.1 and 48.2). The risk factors in this case include male sex, ventriculotomy, and QRS duration 190 ms.

Table 48.1 Risk factors for VT or SCD after repair of TOF

Clinical risk factors
Older age at repair
Male
Heart failure
Right ventriculotomy for repair of TOF
Electrocardiographic risk factors
QRS duration ≥180 ms
Echocardiographic risk factors
RV dilatation
Chronic RV pressure overload
Higher residual RVOT gradient
Moderate to severe pulmonary regurgitation
Electrophysiologic testing
Inducible sustained monomorphic or polymorphic VT

4) **What investigations would you consider for the present case?**

Patients who present with pre-syncope, syncope, or non-sustained VT require comprehensive investigation, including electrophysiological assessment with programmed atrial and ventricular stimulation. Cardiac magnetic resonance imaging and on occasions cardiac catheterization and angiography may be necessary where anatomical and haemodynamic information is in doubt. In the present case, this was not necessary as there were no significant abnormalities on TTE.

Programmed ventricular stimulation was performed during electrophysiological studies. No atrial tachyarrhythmia was inducible. However, sustained monomorphic VT (180 bpm) developed after two ventricular extrastimuli from the RV apex. The QRS complexes had LBBB morphology consistent with a focus in the RVOT. Blood pressure fell 50% but there were no overt symptoms. The arrhythmia was terminated without acceleration by programmed ventricular stimulation.

Inducible sustained monomorphic or polymorphic VT on electrophysiological testing is associated with increased risk of spontaneous VT and SCD during long-term follow-up. The prognosis is better if sustained VT is not inducible. Electrophysiological studies may allow assessment of other potential triggers, including atrial tachyarrhythmias.

Patients with negative electrophysiological studies, minimal symptoms, and good haemodynamics do not require further treatment. Beta-blockers can be used to suppress symptomatic ectopics.

5) **Further investigation suggests increased risk of SCD. How would you manage the patient?**

In the present case, an ICD was implanted to reduce the risk of SCD. The device was programmed to provide antitachycardia pacing as well as defibrillation. There were no procedural complications. Amiodarone and bisprolol were then started.

Sudden cardiac death due to presumed arrhythmia is the most common cause of death in adults after repair of TOF. Implantable cardioverter defibrillator placement and antiarrhythmic drug treatment may prevent life-threatening arrhythmias and should be considered for patients with inducible VT or severe symptoms.

However, transvenous implantation of ICD is challenging. The cardiac anatomy is complex and there may be associated intracardiac shunts, difficult vascular access, and extracardiac malformations. Furthermore, inappropriate ICD shocks and lead-related complications are common in this patient group. The challenge is therefore to identify the patients at highest risk of SCD within a population already at increased risk. See Cases 10 and 33 for further discussion of SCD and ICD.

There are no prospective RCTs specific to congenital heart disease to guide practice in the present case. A retrospective, multicentre cohort study found a high rate of appropriate shocks in patients who had received an ICD for primary prevention after repair of TOF (Khairy et al., 2008). Factors associated with appropriate ICD shocks were identified (Table 48.2). These were used to produce a scoring system to determine the probability of receiving an appropriate shock after ICD implantation for primary prevention after repair of TOF (Khairy et al., 2008). Although the study had several limitations, patients with these characteristics may be more likely to benefit from ICD than those without.

Table 48.2 Risk factors associated with appropriate ICD discharge

Risk factor	Points
Surgical	
Prior palliative shunt	2
Ventriculotomy incision	2
Electrophysiological	
Inducible sustained VT2	2
Nonsustained VT	2
QRS duration ≥180 ms	1
Haemodynamic	
LV end diastolic pressure ≥12 mmHg	3

Total score 0–12. Low risk (0–1), annual risk of appropriate ICD discharge 0%; intermediate risk (3–5), annual risk of appropriate ICD discharge 3.8%; high risk (3–5), annual risk of appropriate ICD discharge 17.5%. Data and scoring system from Khairy et al. (2008).

In the 2 years since implantation of the ICD for the patient in this case the device has not delivered a shock or antitachycardia pacing. The device has, however, captured several episodes of asymptomatic non-sustained VT.

6) **What is the prognosis after repair of TOF? What are the common late cardiac complications after repair of TOF?**

Of the various causes of cyanotic congenital heart disease TOF is the most likely to reach adulthood without surgical repair. However, without surgical intervention the mortality is 25% within 1 year, 40% within 3 years, 90% within 25 years, and 95% within 40 years. The mortality depends on the precise nature of the cardiac defects. Progressive RVOT obstruction gradually increases right-to-left shunting, cyanosis, and hypoxia.

The majority of patients with TOF in developed countries are now repaired before adulthood. A single-centre study reported the outcomes of patients of over 1000 patients born before 1984. Overall survival was 85% at 10 years, 82% at 20 years, 80% at 30 years, and 77% at 40 years. However, the early mortality has declined as surgical techniques have improved. The survival of patients repaired in 1965 was 72% at 1 year and 63% at 40 years. The survival of patients repaired after 1985 was significantly better (survival was 97% at 1 year and 94% at 20 years). Early surgical mortality is the main determinant of the numbers of patients reaching adulthood.

Long-term survival after repair is good. However, unlike early mortality, the late risks of death and reintervention have not improved with improvements in surgical techniques. The specific anatomy of the TOF subtype and any other associated cardiovascular lesions are important determinants of late outcome. Late risk of mortality is low (0.5% per year 30 years after correction) but increases with age. The most common cause of death is SCD.

Quality of life is generally good after repair of TOF. Most patients have few symptoms, if any, and do not require treatment. The most common cardiac complications after repair of TOF in adults are cardiac failure and arrhythmias (atrial 20% and ventricular 14%). Pulmonary regurgitation is increasingly recognized as an important late contributer to symptoms and RV dysfunction and may be suitable for percutaneous valve replacement provided the pulmonary annulus is not too large. As the surgical technique for repair has improved, the incidence of bradyarrhythmias has reduced significantly.

Other late cardiac complications of surgical repair of TOF include tricuspid regurgitation, pulmonary artery branch stenosis, RV aneurysms, residual or recurrent RVOT obstruction, residual or recurrent ventricular septal defects, aortic root dilation, and infective endocarditis.

The morbidity and mortality of children currently undergoing repair is likely to be even lower. The 40-year survival of a cohort who had TOF repaired after 1985 is predicted to be 87%. Repair of TOF in infancy and improved surgical techniques should improve long-term survival and quality of life.

Reference

Khairy P *et al.* (2008). Implantable cardioverter-defibrillators in tetralogy of Fallot. *Circulation*; 117: 363.

Further reading

Apitz C, Webb GD, Redington AN. (2009). Tetralogy of Fallot. *Lancet*; 374: 1462–1471.

Engelfriet P, Boersma E, Oechslin E, Tijssen J, Gatzoulis MA, Thilén U, Kaemmerer H, Moons P, Meijboom F, Popelová J, Laforest V, Hirsch R, Daliento L, Thaulow E, Mulder B. (2005). The spectrum of adult congenital heart disease in Europe: morbidity and mortality in a 5 year follow-up period. The Euro Heart Survey on adult congenital heart disease. *Eur Heart J*; 26: 2325–2333.

Gatzoulis MA, Balaji S, Webber SA, Siu SC, Hokanson JS, Poile C, Rosenthal M, Nakazawa M, Moller JH, Gillette PC, Webb GD, Redington AN. (2000). Risk factors for arrhythmia and sudden cardiac death late after repair of tetralogy of Fallot: a multicentre study. *Lancet*; 356: 975.

Hickey EJ, Veldtman G, Bradley TJ, Gengsakul A, Manlhiot C, Williams WG, Webb GD, McCrindle BW. (2009). Late risk of outcomes for adults with repaired tetralogy of Fallot from an inception cohort spanning four decades. *Eur J Cardiothorac Surg*; 35: 156–164.

Khairy P, Harris L, Landzberg MJ, Viswanathan S, Barlow A, Gatzoulis MA, Fernandes SM, Beauchesne L, Therrien J, Chetaille P, Gordon E, Vonder Muhll I, Cecchin F. (2008). Implantable cardioverter-defibrillators in tetralogy of Fallot. *Circulation*; 117: 363.

Case 49

A 54-year-old obese man with severe rheumatic mitral stenosis and paroxysmal AF had a mechanical mitral valve replacement (MVR) with an Omniscience disc valve. There were no complications reported during the perioperative period. His only regular medications were bisoprolol, perindopril, and warfarin.

One year after the operation the patient presented to his GP complaining that his voice had become hoarse. On direct questioning the patient then reported that his breathlessness on effort had deteriorated despite the MVR. The GP noted jaundice, severe peripheral oedema, and a pansystolic murmur, and so referred the patient to the on-call medical registrar.

On admission to the medical assessment unit observations were O_2 saturations 89% on air, BP 175/80 mmHg, HR 78 bpm (AF), and temperature 36.3°C. Examination revealed a median sternotomy scar, jaundice, pallor, pitting oedema to the thighs, and elevation of the jugular venous pulsation to the angle of the jaw sitting upright. On auscultation of the heart the first heart sound was prosthetic. Although the second heart sound was normal, a loud pansystolic murmur was audible all over the praecordium. Breath sounds were vesicular but fine inspiratory crepitations were audible to the midzones. The abdomen was soft, with a palpable liver edge two fingerbreadths below the costal margin. There was no other palpable organomegaly and the rectum contained only soft brown stool.

High-flow oxygen and intravenous frusemide were administered and a GTN infusion was started.

Laboratory investigations revealed Hb 7 g/dL, mean cell volume 104 fl, WBC 7.5 × 10^9 cells/L, platelets 300 × 10^{12} cells/L, INR 3.0, serum sodium 140 mmol/L, potassium 4.8 mmol/L, creatinine 90 μmol/L, urea 7 mmol/L, bilirubin 70 μmol/L, albumin 35 g/L, alanine transaminase 34 iu/L, alkaline phosphatase 63 iu/L, gamma-glutamyltransferase 35 u/L, and CRP <5 mg/L. Urine dipstick showed positive urobilinogen only. A 12 lead ECG demonstrated rate-controlled AF (80 bpm).

Chest X-ray confirmed the presence of the mechanical MVR and showed interstitial pulmonary oedema. Trans-thoracic echocardiography was attempted but due to body habitus and the presence of the mechanical MVR adequate views could not be obtained. Transoesophageal echocardiography was performed (Fig. 49.1). Coronary angiography had been performed prior to the MVR was reported to be normal.

The ear, nose, and throat (ENT) surgeon on call performed oropharyngeal examination with flexible nasendoscopy. The left cord was partially abducted and did not move, suggesting a left vocal cord palsy. The rest of the ENT examination was normal.

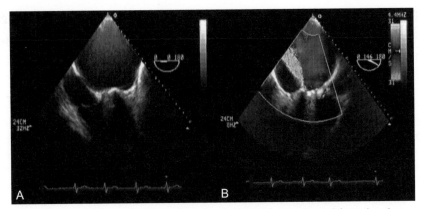

Fig. 49.1 Transoesophageal echocardiogram. A, The mid-oesophageal four-chamber view. B, The mid-oesophageal long-axis view with colour Doppler overlay. (See colour plate 22)

Questions

1. What types of heart valve prosthesis are available?
2. What does the TOE (Fig. 49.1) show?
3. What is the most likely cause of the anaemia in the present case? What further investigations would confirm this?
4. What is the definitive management for the present case?
5. What intervention should be considered if the 'gold standard' is not appropriate?
6. What caused the hoarse voice in the present case?

Answers

1) **What types of heart valve prosthesis are available?**

   Prosthetic heart valves can be:

   1. mechanical (only synthetic material)
      - lateral flow – ball and cage (Starr–Edwards; highest thrombogenic risk)
      - central flow – tilting disc (Medtronic-Hall, Omniscience)
      - bileaflet (St Jude Medical, ATS medical).
   2. bioprosthetic (synthetic and biological material)
      - xenografts, (donor species different to recipient)
      - homografts (donor same species as recipient; rarely used in mitral position).

   Mechanical valves can last more than 30 years but are thrombogenic. Lifelong anticoagulation is required. Aortic bioprosetheses are more durable than those in the mitral position (smaller diameter and lower closing pressure); 60% of mitral bioprosthesis fail within 15 years. However, most bioprosthetic valve replacements do not per se require anticoagulation.

2) **What does the TOE (Fig. 49.1) show?**

   The mid oesophageal four-chamber view (Fig. 49.1A) demonstrates a giant left atrium (12 × 14 cm; Fig. 49.2A). The colour Doppler overlay on the mid-oesophageal long-axis view (Fig. 49.1B) demonstrates severe mitral regurgitation due to a paraprosthetic valve leak (PVL; Fig. 49.2B). There was no evidence of endocarditis.

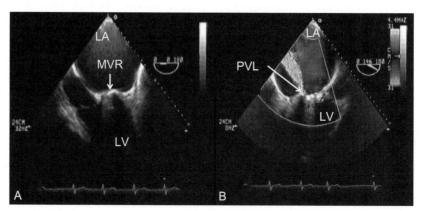

Fig. 49.2 Transoesophageal echocardiogram demonstrating PVL. A, The mid-oesophageal four-chamber view demonstrates a giant left atrium (LA; 12 × 14 cm). B, The colour Doppler overlay on the mid-oesophageal long-axis view demonstrates severe mitral regurgitation due to PVL. (See colour plate 23)

3) **What is the most likely cause of the anaemia in the present case? What further investigations would confirm this?**

The macrocytic anaemia in the present case which was associated with jaundice, a mechanical MVR, and PVL was most likely due to mechanical intravascular haemolysis. Bleeding should always be considered in anticoagulated patients. In the present case, there was no evidence of acute haemorrhage. Chronic bleeding is usually associated with iron deficiency and a hypochromic, microcytic picture.

Raised serum LDH, reduced or absent haptoglobulins, and reticulocytosis are markers of intravascular haemolysis. Other causes of anaemia can limit the bone marrow capacity to compensate for increased red cell destruction. Measurement of haematinics (iron, vitamin B12, and folate) and thyroid function is therefore important. A blood film is useful to confirm intravascular haemolysis. A negative Coombs test differentiates mechanical haemolysis from autoimmune haemolytic anaemia.

These laboratory findings are common in patients with mechanical valve prostheses. Mechanical haemolysis is common but is usually mild and subclinical. Patients with valve prostheses who develop severe haemolysis require investigation for PVL and infection.

In this case, the reticulocyte count was raised (10%), serum LDH was raised (3500 iu/L) and serum haptoglobulins were reduced (<6 mg/dL). The blood film revealed normochromic, macrocytic anaemia with red cell fragments, schistocytes, and polychromasia. Mild macrocytosis may be associated with reticulocytosis because the immature red cells (reticulocytes) are slightly larger than mature red cells. Coombs test was negative. Blood cultures were taken and subsequently demonstrated no growth despite prolonged culture for atypical causes of endocarditis.

In this case, three units of blood were transfused and folate and iron supplements were started. Severe haemolysis requiring blood transfusion is an indication to consider surgical revision of the valve. If intervention is not appropriate, treatment with erythropoietin may reduce the need for blood products.

Causes of paraprosthetic valve leaks

Leak around the circumference of the sewing ring of a valve prosthesis (paravalvular leak; PVL) is a well-recognized complication of valve replacement. A leak develops if the seal between the sewing ring and valve annulus is incomplete.

Small haemodynamically insignificant PVLs are commonly seen on intraoperative TOE or postoperative TTE. The incidence of PVL reported after a mitral or aortic valve replacement in various studies ranges from 20% to nearly 50%. The majority are trivial and do not progress over follow-up.

There are several causes of early dehiscence of a prosthetic valve. The retention sutures may loosen, break, or cut through the surrounding tissue. Technical factors that affect tissue–suture integrity include the preparation of the bed prior implantation of the valve, size of valve prosthesis, type of suture (fine monofilament polypropylene) and technique of suturing (continuous or interrupted), type of sewing ring, and method of myocardial preservation used. Surgery for revision of valve replacement is also associated with increased risk of PVL.

Patient-related factors that compromise tissue integrity include calcification, friability, and infective endocarditis. Annular calcification increases the risk of PVL because the bed created after removal of the calcified tissue during surgery is not always circular or robust. Endocarditis is the most significant risk factor for PVL as infected tissue is friable.

As surgical techniques have improved, the incidence of severe PVL has fallen to less than 1.5% per patient-year for both mechanical and bioprosthetic valves. The majority (60%) of PVL develop within 1 year of valve replacement and may increase over time. Mitral valve PVL is more common than aortic, and pulmonary and tricuspid valve prostheses rarely develop PVL.

The late development of a new PVL may be due to structural failure but endocarditis must be excluded.

4) **What is the definitive management for the present case?**

Surgical revision of MVR is currently the definitive treatment for patients with PVL who are symptomatic or transfusion dependent. The prosthesis can either be resutured or replaced.

However, the mortality and morbidity associated with revision valve surgery is significant. In one study, 96 patients with mitral PVL were observed over 5 years. Of these 50 underwent revision valve surgery and the rest were managed medically. The 30-day mortality after revision valve surgery was 6%. At 3 years the mortality in the surgical group (12%) was still high but significantly lower than the group managed medically (26%). The symptoms and mean Hb of the group who underwent revision valve surgery also improved significantly. This supports the role of early surgery in patients with mitral PVL.

In the present case, revision MVR (29 mm ATS Medical) was performed. On review 2 months later the patient's functional state was NYHA II. On examination there was only mild pitting oedema of the ankles and scattered bibasal crepitations on auscultation of the lungs. Clinical tricuspid regurgitation was reduced. The MVR was functioning well with no paraprosthetic regurgitation visible on TOE. There was no clinical or laboratory evidence of haemolysis.

5) **What intervention could be considered if the 'gold standard' is not appropriate?**

Surgical resuture or replacement of the implanted prosthesis is the current 'gold standard' treatment for severe PVL. However, the risks of revision surgery may preclude surgery in those with multiple comorbidities. In this situation percutaneous closure of the PVL should be considered as a possible alternative to surgery.

A few case series have reported the outcomes of percutaneous device closure of PVL. At the time of writing there are no transcatheter devices available that are specifically designed for the PVL closure, so various devices have been used to attempt closure. However, percutaneous device closure of PVL is less invasive and may be associated with fewer risks.

Procedural complications include bleeding, embolization (thrombus, air, atheroma, valve material, or the device), and mechanical disruption of the prosthetic valve, resulting in severe PVL and infection. Long-term complications include haemolysis, infection, and late device dislodgement.

Contraindications to percutaneous PVL closure include active local or systemic infection, mechanical instability of the prosthetic valve, and intracardiac thrombus.

6) **What caused the hoarse voice in the present case?**

In the present case, the hoarse voice was due to Ortner's cardiovocal syndrome, and the cardiothoracic anaesthetic and surgical teams requested that vocal cord palsy was confirmed by nasendoscopy prior to surgery.

Left recurrent laryngeal nerve RLN palsy secondary to mitral valve disease is rare. Ortner thought that RLN palsy resulted from compression by the enlarged left atrium. However, observation at operation has demonstrated that the nerve is compressed between an enlarged tense pulmonary artery and the aorta at the ligamentum arteriosum. Left RLN palsy has also been described in other conditions that cause pulmonary hypertension.

In the present case, the hoarse voice and vocal cord function recovered several months after revision of the MVR. Doppler echocardiography confirmed postoperative reduction of RV systolic pressure.

Further reading

Bhindi R, Bull S, Schrale RG, Wilson N, Ormerod OJ. (2008). Surgery Insight: percutaneous treatment of prosthetic paravalvular leaks. *Nat Clin Pract Cardiovasc Med*; **5**: 140–147.

Genoni M, Franzen D, Vogt P, Seifert B, Jenni R, Künzli A, Niederhäuser U, Turina M. (2000). Paravalvular leakage after mitral valve replacement: Improved long-term survival with aggressive surgery? *Eur J Cardiothorac Surg*; **17**: 14.

Bonow RO, Carabello BA, Chatterjee K, de Leon AC Jr, Faxon DP, Freed MD, Gaasch WH, Lytle BW, Nishimura RA, O'Gara PT, O'Rourke RA, Otto CM, Shah PM, Shanewise JS; American College of Cardiology/American Heart Association Task Force on Practice Guidelines. (2008). ACC/AHA VHD Guidelines: 2008 Focused Update Incorporated Into the ACC/AHA 2006 Guidelines for the Management of Patients With Valvular Heart Disease. A Report of the American College of Cardiology/American Heart Association Task Force on Practice Guidelines (Writing Committee to Revise the 1998 Guidelines for the Management of Patients With Valvular Heart Disease). *JACC*; **52**: e1–e142.

Case 50

A 75-year-old man who had had a mechanical MVR (Bjork-Shiley) performed for mitral stenosis 20 years previously presented with worsening breathlessness and reduced exercise tolerance. He had NYHA class IV heart failure, rate-controlled chronic AF and a pansystolic murmur.

Laboratory investigations revealed haemolytic anaemia (Hb 7.9 g/dL) but were otherwise unremarkable. Symptoms persisted despite transfusion to a haemoglobin of 11 g/dL.

Transoesophageal echocardiography demonstrated severe paravalvular regurgitation with impaired LV function (LVEF 45%) and raised pulmonary artery pressure (estimated at least 50 mmHg).

Coronary angiography demonstrated a right dominant coronary system with a distal left main severe stenosis involving the ostia of the LAD and small circumflex artery. The distal LAD territory was extensively collateralized via septal perforators and around the apex from a large unobstructed RCS. There was a good distal target on the LAD for surgical revascularization with an arterial graft.

Elective revision of the MVR (29 mm model, ATS Medical) with coronary artery bypass grafting was performed. Although this was complicated by *Pseudomonas pneumonia*, 6 weeks after the operation, the patient's functional state was NYHA II–III. Laboratory investigations were unremarkable; the INR was 2.5.

Limited views were obtained when TTE was attempted as the sternal wound was still healing and painful. In order to visualize the MVR clearly TOE was performed. This confirmed that the MVR was functioning well with no paravalvular regurgitation. However, an unexpected finding was noted (Fig. 50.1).

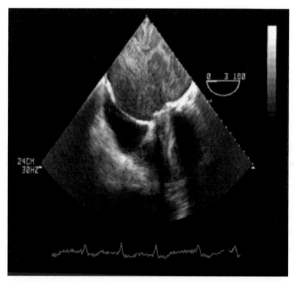

Fig. 50.1 Transoesophageal echocardiography. The mid-oesophageal four-chamber view is shown.

Questions

1. What are the principles of medical treatment of chronic mitral regurgitation?
2. How is the risk of complications from cardiac surgery assessed?
3. What specific difficulties are associated with revision cardiac sternotomy?
4. Is there a level of pulmonary hypertension that would prohibit MV surgery?
5. What is the prevalence of CAD in patients with valvular heart disease? What are the indications for preoperative cardiac catheterization prior to valve surgery?
6. When should simultaneous valve replacement and coronary artery bypass grafting be considered?
7. What proportion of patients have undiagnosed cardiac pathology at the time of operation?
8. What was found on TOE (Fig. 50.1)? What is the significance of this observation?

Answers

1) **What are the principles of medical treatment of chronic mitral regurgitation?**

   Congestive heart failure due to chronic mitral regurgitation is treated with diuretics and oral vasodilators. Vasodilators reduce peripheral vascular resistance. This reduces the regurgitant volume into the LA, increasing forward cardiac output. If the patient is in rapid AF, digoxin, beta-blockers, and occasionally calcium channel antagonists may help to slow down the ventricular rate. However, bradycardia may increase the regurgitant fraction and should be avoided.

2) **How is the risk of complications from cardiac surgery assessed?**

   Cardiac surgery is associated with a significant risk of morbidity and mortality. In an attempt to quantify these risks the Parsonnet score (Table 50.1) was developed in the 1980s. However, this scoring system now overestimates the complication rates of most modern cardiothoracic units. This reduces the utility of the Parsonnet score as a measure of risk or surgical performance.

   In the late 1990s, the European System for Cardiac Operative Risk Evaluation (EuroSCORE; Table 50.2) was developed and validated. The additive EuroSCORE correlates well with most cardiothoracic units but tends to overestimate risk at low scores and underestimate risk at high scores. The logistic EuroSCORE provides a more accurate risk assessment for high-risk patients. These scores are validated principally for first-time coronary artery surgery so have limited applicability to the present case.

   To use the standard EuroSCORE to estimate risk of death as described in Nashef *et al.* (1999), EuroSCORE values are simply added. If the logistic EuroSCORE is used the predicted mortality is calculated as described in Roques *et al.* (2003). Although developed to predict perioperative risk, the EuroSCORE has been used in an attempt to predict long-term mortality in patients with valvular heart disease after valve surgery.

   In the present case, the additive EuroSCORE was 10% (4 + 3 + 2 + 1) but the logistic score was 15.8%. The logistic score is probably more representative of the actual perioperative risk in this case. Combining CABG and valve replacement does not change the EuroSCORE but does increase the Parsonnet score.

Table 50.1 The Parsonnet stratification score for cardiac surgery

Factor	Points
Demographics	
70–74 years	7
74–79 years	12
>84 years	20
Female	1
Preoperative cardiovascular status	
LV function	
Good (LVEF >50%)	0
Moderate (LVEF 30–49%)	2
Poor (LVEF <30%)	4
Pulmonary artery pressure >60 mmHg	3
Preoperative intra-aortic balloon pump	2
'Catastrophic state'	10–50
LV aneurysm	5
Indication for surgery	
Catheter laboratory complication	10
'Rare conditions'	2–10
Redo procedure	
First	5
Second/subsequent	10
Mitral valve surgery	5
Aortic valve surgery	5
Aortic valve gradient >120 mmHg	2
Valve + CABG surgery	2
Comorbidities	
Diabetes mellitus	3
Hypertension	3
Morbid obesity	3

Table 50.2 The EuroSCORE additive risk stratification model (http://www.euroscore.org)

Factor	Points
Demographics	
Age per 5 years or part thereof over 60	1
Female sex	1
Comorbidities	
Chronic lung disease	
Long-term use of bronchodilators or steroids for lung disease	1
Non-cardiac vasculopathy	
Any one or more of: claudication, carotid occlusion or >50% stenosis, previous or planned intervention on the abdominal aorta, limb arteries or carotids	2
Neurological dysfunction severely affecting ambulation or day-to-day functioning	2
Previous cardiac surgery that opened the pericardium	3
Preoperative serum creatinine >200 mmol/L	2
Active endocarditis (still requiring treatment for endocarditis)	3
Preoperative cardiovascular status	
Critical preoperative state	
Any one or more of: VT or VF or aborted sudden death, preoperative cardiac massage, preoperative ventilation, preoperative inotropic support, IABP, or preoperative acute renal failure (anuria or oliguria <10 mL/h)	2
Unstable angina requiring intravenous nitrates Liver function	2
Moderate (LVEF 30–50%)	1
Poor (LVEF<30%)	3
Recent MI (<90 days)	2
Pulmonary hypertension: systolic pulmonary artery pressure >60 mmHg	2
Indication for surgery	
Emergency surgery performed before the next working day after a patient was referred	2
Other than isolated CABG: major cardiac procedure other than or in addition to CABG	2
Surgery on thoracic aorta (disorder of ascending or descending aortic arch)	3
Post MI septal rupture	4

3) **What specific difficulties are associated with revision cardiac sternotomy?**

Cardiac surgery can cause adhesions that fix the heart close to the sternum, requiring careful and often time-consuming dissection. So, if revision sternotomy is required, the right ventricle or brachiocephalic vein may be at risk of laceration from the sternal saw.

If CABG has previously been performed, the internal mammary artery or a saphenous graft may be at risk of damage. The potential complication of graft damage should be clear from the operation note and preoperative cardiac catheterization report. Operative damage to a functioning graft may cause severe myocardial ischaemia. If the grafts are occluded and not functional the risks are lower.

4) **Is there a level of pulmonary hypertension that would prohibit MV surgery?**

Although pulmonary artery hypertension substantially increases the risk of cardiac surgery (see Tables 50.1 and 50.2), there is no definitive answer to this question. Most teams would consider operating on patients with severe pulmonary hypertension. However, intensive postoperative respiratory support and diuresis are required to reduce the risk of RV failure and pulmonary oedema. After MV replacement for mitral stenosis, pulmonary artery pressure decreases. This effect usually occurs within hours but can be more gradual over weeks to months.

5) **What is the prevalence of CAD in patients with valvular heart disease? What are the indications for preoperative cardiac catheterization prior to valve surgery?**

The incidence and prevalence of ischaemic heart disease in the general population can be estimated on the basis of age, sex, and clinical risk factors. The prevalence of CAD in patients who have valvular heart disease is determined by the same risk factors. Patients with valvular disease and risk factors for IHD should be treated with the same strategies recommended for the general population.

Angina and equivalent symptoms are important predictors of IHD in the general population. However, in patients with valvular heart disease, angina is less specific. Other causes of angina in these patients include LV chamber enlargement, increased wall stress, or wall thickening with subendocardial ischaemia and RV hypertrophy.

Coronary artery disease is a common cause of MR. However, neither angina nor heart failure are reliable markers of CAD in patients with MR. In patients undergoing cardiac catheterization to assess the cause and severity of MR, CAD is present in a third. Around 20% of patients undergoing catheterization for acute coronary syndromes have associated MR.

However, CAD is uncommon in patients with degenerative MV disease undergoing surgery. In a large series, only 1% had CAD with single-vessel disease prominent. Thus, routine coronary angiography is not usually indicated in patients under 45 years of age undergoing MV surgery for degenerative MV disease in the absence of symptoms and risk factors.

Angina is common in young patients with severe congenital or rheumatic AS and normal coronary arteries. Coronary artery disease is, however, common in older men with symptomatic AS. In patients with AS and typical angina the prevalence of CAD is 40–50% and in those without chest pain around 20%. Some 25% of patients with AS and atypical chest pain have CAD. Even in patients under 40 years old without chest pain and no coronary risk factors, the prevalence of CAD is up to 5%. In patients over 70 years old, angina strongly suggests CAD (sensitivity 78%, specificity 82%). Calcification of the aortic valve is associated with a high prevalence of CAD (up to 90%).

As angina is an unreliable indicator of CAD in patients with AS, coronary angiography is recommended before AVR in symptomatic men over 35 years, premenopausal women over 35 years with coronary risk factors, asymptomatic men over 45 years, women over 55 years, and patients with two or more risk factors for CAD.

Coronary artery disease is less common in patients with AR, partly because of the younger age of such patients. The prevalence of CAD in patients with MS (around 20%) is also less than in patients with AS. However, as untreated CAD significantly impairs perioperative and long-term postoperative survival, preoperative identification of CAD is of importance in patients with AR or MS. Thus, preoperative coronary angiography is recommended in patients who are symptomatic and/or have LV dysfunction, men over 35 years, premenopausal women over 35 years with coronary risk factors and postmenopausal women.

6) **When should simultaneous valve replacement and coronary artery bypass grafting be considered?**

Simultaneous CABG should be considered with valve replacement for all patients with coexisting severe CAD. There are no RCTs comparing the outcomes of concomitant surgery with separate procedures. Concomitant CABG increases operative mortality, mainly because the duration of cardiopulmonary bypass is longer. The increased risk of a simultaneous procedure must be considered against the risks associated with a revision sternotomy and cardiac bypass at a later date in an older patient who may have greater comorbidity.

The decision is most difficult in patients with asymptomatic CAD. However, the final decision on whether to perform simultaneous CABG will depend on disease severity and the intraoperative haemodynamics.

Mitral regurgitation may result from CAD affecting the papillary muscle and the supporting LV wall. If so, CABG and valvuloplasty may be indicated. The decision to perform revascularization and MV repair is based on symptoms, severity of CAD, LV dysfunction, and evidence of inducible myocardial ischaemia.

If MV disease is not due to ischaemia but significant CAD is identified by preoperative cardiac catheterization, MV surgery and revascularization are generally performed together. There are no randomized data to guide this policy.

In the present case, simultaneous CABG was performed as the patient had significant proximal CAD and a good distal target vessel.

7) **What proportion of patients have undiagnosed cardiac pathology at the time of operation?**

Cardiac surgical patients are usually extensively investigated preoperatively. However, up to 5% of patients have additional previously undocumented pathology (e.g. valvular disease, patent foramen ovale) demonstrated by intraoperative TOE. Unexpected findings are more likely during emergency surgery.

Although in the present case there were no unexpected intraoperative findings, assiduous evaluation prior to surgery is essential.

8) **What was found on TOE (Fig. 50.1)? What is the significance of this observation?**

In the present case TOE (Fig. 50.1) unexpectedly revealed dense swirls within the giant LA (12 × 14 cm). This is spontaneous echo contrast (SEC). See Fig. 50.2.

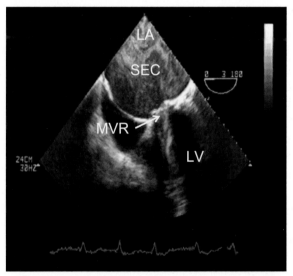

Fig. 50.2 Transoesophageal echocardiogram demonstrating spontaneous echo contrast (SEC) within a giant left atrium (LA; 12 × 12 cm).

The presence of SEC indicates increased risk of thromboembolism and may suggest prosthetic valve thrombosis (PVT). This must be excluded if SEC is observed in a symptomatic patient with a heart valve prosthesis in situ. Other indirect signs include the disappearance of 'physiological' prosthesis regurgitant flow, or the presence of central prosthesis regurgitation.

Direct echocardiographic evidence of PVT includes reduced leaflet mobility, leaflet immobility, and thrombus on either side of the prosthesis, with or without obstruction. Thrombus is more common on the atrial side of prosthetic MVs.

In the present case, there were no other clinical or echocardiographic features to suggest PVT. Even in the absence of PVT, AF and dense SEC increase the risk of thromboembolic events despite anticoagulation.

The pathogenesis of SEC is complex and remains unclear. Several factors of Virchow's triad are affected. Blood stasis promotes the development of SEC in areas of LA enlargement and impaired LV function. The velocity or shear rate of local blood flow is obviously affected by the presence of the valve prosthesis. Blood components are also affected. Rouleaux formation and increased serum fibrinogen or increased platelet aggregation may be involved.

In one case, a patient developed LV SEC despite treatment with heparin, and platelet aggregates were detected in the peripheral blood. Complete resolution occurred after antiplatelet treatment for 5 days.

There are no clear guidelines on the management of patients with SEC. Further studies are required to compare the effects of anticoagulation and antiplatelet drugs in patients with SEC.

In the present case, review of the anticoagulation record demonstrated that the INR had been below 2.5 on several occasions. The target INR was increased to 3.5. On review 6 months later the patient remained well with NYHA class II symptoms. Repeat TOE demonstrated resolution of the SEC and normal prosthetic valve function.

References

Nashef SA, Roques F, Michel P, Gauducheau E, Lemeshow S, Salamon R. (1999). European system for cardiac operative risk evaluation (EuroSCORE). *Eur J Cardiothorac Surg*; **16**: 9–13.

Roques F, Michel P, Goldstone AR, Nashef SA. (2003). The logistic EuroSCORE. *Eur Heart J*; **24**: 881–882.

Further reading

Toumpoulis IK, Anagnostopoulos CE, Toumpoulis SK, DeRose JJ Jr, Swistel DG. (2005). Euroscore predicts long-term mortality after heart valve surgery. *Ann Thor Surg*; **79**: 1905–1908.

Bonow RO, Carabello BA, Chatterjee K, de Leon AC Jr, Faxon DP, Freed MD, Gaasch WH, Lytle BW, Nishimura RA, O'Gara PT, O'Rourke RA, Otto CM, Shah PM, Shanewise JS; American College of Cardiology/American Heart Association Task Force on Practice Guidelines.Bonow et al. (2008). ACC/AHA VHD Guidelines: 2008 Focused Update Incorporated Into the ACC/AHA 2006 Guidelines for the Management of Patients With Valvular Heart Disease. A Report of the American College of Cardiology/American Heart Association Task Force on Practice Guidelines (Writing Committee to Revise the 1998 Guidelines for the Management of Patients With Valvular Heart Disease). *JACC*; **52**: e1–e142.

List of cases by diagnosis

Case 1: Atrial fibrillation in a patient with a DDDR pacemaker that did not mode switch
Case 2: Wolf-Parkinson White & atrial fibrillation
Case 3: Contrast induced nephropathy
Case 4: Posterior myocardial infarction and post-infarct angina
Case 5: Unstable angina due to severe triple vessel coronary artery disease
Case 6: Diabetic ketoacidosis
Case 7: Acute posterior myocardial infarction due to occlusion of the circumflex coronary artery
Case 8: Anterior ST elevation myocardial infarction due to critical stenosis of the left anterior descending artery
Case 9: Heterophile antibodies to troponin assay
Case 10: Alcohol-induced cardiomyopathy
Case 11: Post-partum cardiomyopathy
Case 12: Chronic aortic dissection
Case 13: Acute aortic dissection
Case 14: Candida endocarditis involving a mechanical mitral valve prosthesis
Case 15: Hypertrophic cardiomyopathy
Case 16: Aortic coarctation
Case 17: Malignant hypertension
Case 18: Secondary hypertension (idiopathic adrenal hypertrophy)
Case 19: Left Ventricular thrombus due to silent peri-operative antero-lateral myocardial
Case 20: Atrial myxoma
Case 21: Pulmonary embolism
Case 22: Iatrogenic pericardial effusion
Case 23: Tuberculous pericarditis
Case 24: Acute perimyocarditis
Case 25: Atrial septal defect
Case 26: Chronic thromboembolic pulmonary hypertension
Case 27: HIV induced pulmonary hypertension
Case 28: Restrictive cardiomyopathy secondary to amyloidosis
Case 29: Anomalous right coronary artery
Case 30: Ictal asystole
Case 31: Calcific aortic stenosis
Case 32: Mitral stenosis
Case 33: Ventricular tachycardia after silent inferior myocardial infarction caused by systemic lupus erythematosus
Case 34: Brugada syndrome
Case 35: Right ventricular outflow tract ventricular tachycardia
Case 36: Gastric volvulus
Case 37: Non-ST elevation myocardial infarction due to critical distal left main stem stenosis
Case 38: Ventricular tachycardia caused by drug-induced prolongation of QT interval
Case 39: Complete heart block due to anterior myocardial infarction
Case 40: Staphylococcal endocarditis of a native mitral valve
Case 41: Staphylococcal endocarditis involving a prosthetic aortic valve
Case 42: Patent foramen ovale
Case 43: Chronic pericarditis & pericardial constriction
Case 44: Acute onset atrial fibrillation
Case 45: Pre-operative cardiovascular assessment for abdominal aortic aneurysm repair
Case 46: Cardiogenic shock after anterior myocardial infarction
Case 47: Protein losing enteropathy in a patient with a total cavopulmonary circulation
Case 48: Ventricular tachycardia in a patient with Tetralogy of Fallot (corrected)
Case 49: Paravalvular leak after mechanical mitral valve prosthesis
Case 50: Spontaneous echo contrast after mechanical mitral valve replacement

List of cases by principal clinical features at diagnosis

Abnormalities on chest x-ray performed at pre-operative assessment: *12*
Abnormalities on ECG performed at pre-operative assessment: *39*
Abnormalities on ECG performed at pre-participation sports screening: *15*
Abnormalities on ECG performed for insurance medical: *34*
Acute chronic breathlessness: *26*
Acute respiratory distress post-partum: *11,*
Ascites: *10, 47*
Atypical chest pain: *4, 8, 9*
Back pain: *13,*
Blurred vision: *17*
Breathlessness: *1, 10, 23, 28, 32, 41, 47, 50*
Chest pain: *5, 6, 7, 13, 24, 33, 36, 37, 43, 46*
Confusion: *30*
Cough: *20, 41*
Dizziness: *17, 33, 35*
Exertional breathlessness: *25, 27, 31, 49*
Facial pallor and flushing: *35*
Fever: *20, 23*
General malaise: *24*
Growth of candida in blood cultures: *14,*
Haematuria after oesophagectomy for oesophageal cancer: *19*
Headache: *17,*
Hoarse voice: *49*
Hypertension: *16*
Hypertension in pregnancy: *18*
Increasing breathlessness: *43*
Left hemiparesis: *40*
Murmur detected on auscultation: *40, 41, 49, 50*
Non-productive cough: *23*
Oedema: *10, 47*
Oligoanuric renal failure: *3*
Palpitations: *2, 33, 44*
Peripheral oedema during pregnancy: *32*
Peripheral oedema: *27, 41*
Platypnoea-orthodeoxia: *42*
Pleuritic chest pain: *26*
Pre-operative assessment prior to AAA repair: *45*
Recurrent falls: *20*
Retrograde amnesia: *30*
Right loin pain: *19*
Seizures: *40*
Sudden onset breathlessness: *2*
Syncope: *6, 21, 29, 30, 40, 46, 48*
Syncope after percutaneous coronary intervention: *21*
Syncope post-partum: *38*

Index

Bold indicates the diagnosis of the case discussed within the page range.